AF126961

Application of Botulinum Neurotoxin in Lower Urinary Tract Dysfunctions: Where Are We Now?

Application of Botulinum Neurotoxin in Lower Urinary Tract Dysfunctions: Where Are We Now?

Editor

Hann-Chorng Kuo

MDPI • Basel • Beijing • Wuhan • Barcelona • Belgrade • Manchester • Tokyo • Cluj • Tianjin

Editor
Hann-Chorng Kuo
Buddhist Tzu Chi University
Taiwan

Editorial Office
MDPI
St. Alban-Anlage 66
4052 Basel, Switzerland

This is a reprint of articles from the Special Issue published online in the open access journal *Toxins* (ISSN 2072-6651) (available at: https://www.mdpi.com/journal/toxins/special_issues/botulinum_urinary).

For citation purposes, cite each article independently as indicated on the article page online and as indicated below:

LastName, A.A.; LastName, B.B.; LastName, C.C. Article Title. *Journal Name* **Year**, *Volume Number*, Page Range.

ISBN 978-3-0365-7938-2 (Hbk)
ISBN 978-3-0365-7939-9 (PDF)

© 2023 by the authors. Articles in this book are Open Access and distributed under the Creative Commons Attribution (CC BY) license, which allows users to download, copy and build upon published articles, as long as the author and publisher are properly credited, which ensures maximum dissemination and a wider impact of our publications.
The book as a whole is distributed by MDPI under the terms and conditions of the Creative Commons license CC BY-NC-ND.

Contents

About the Editor . . . . **vii**

Hann-Chorng Kuo
Botulinum Toxin Brings a Light to the Shadow of Functional Urology
Reprinted from: *Toxins* **2023**, *15*, 321, doi:10.3390/toxins15050321 . . . . **1**

Hann-Chorng Kuo
Clinical Application of Botulinum Neurotoxin in Lower-Urinary-Tract Diseases and Dysfunctions: Where Are We Now and What More Can We Do?
Reprinted from: *Toxins* **2022**, *14*, 498, doi:10.3390/toxins14070498 . . . . **5**

Ju-Chuan Hu, Lin-Nei Hsu, Wei-Chia Lee, Yao-Chi Chuang and Hung-Jen Wang
Role of Urological Botulinum Toxin-A Injection for Overactive Bladder and Voiding Dysfunction in Patients with Parkinson's Disease or Post-Stroke
Reprinted from: *Toxins* **2023**, *15*, 166, doi:10.3390/toxins15020166 . . . . **25**

Hsiang-Ying Lee and Hann-Chorng Kuo
Intravesical Injection of Botulinum Toxin Type A in Men without Bladder Outlet Obstruction and Post-Deobstructive Prostate Surgery
Reprinted from: *Toxins* **2023**, *15*, 221, doi:10.3390/toxins15030221 . . . . **39**

Po-Cheng Chen, Kau-Han Lee, Wei-Chia Lee, Ting-Chun Yeh, Yuh-Chen Kuo, Bing-Juin Chiang, et al.
Treating Neurogenic Lower Urinary Tract Dysfunction in Chronic Spinal Cord Injury Patients—When Intravesical Botox Injection or Urethral Botox Injection Are Indicated
Reprinted from: *Toxins* **2023**, *15*, 288, doi:10.3390/toxins15040288 . . . . **49**

Pedro Abreu-Mendes, António Ferrão-Mendes, Francisco Botelho, Francisco Cruz and Rui Pinto
Effect of Intratrigonal Botulinum Toxin in Patients with Bladder Pain Syndrome/Interstitial Cystitis: A Long-Term, Single-Center Study in Real-Life Conditions
Reprinted from: *Toxins* **2022**, *14*, 775, doi:10.3390/toxins14110775 . . . . **61**

Wan-Ru Yu, Yuan-Hong Jiang, Jia-Fong Jhang, Wei-Chuan Chang and Hann-Chorng Kuo
Treatment Outcomes of Intravesical Botulinum Toxin A Injections on Patients with Interstitial Cystitis/Bladder Pain Syndrome
Reprinted from: *Toxins* **2022**, *14*, 871, doi:10.3390/toxins14120871 . . . . **73**

Yao-Lin Kao, Yin-Chien Ou, Kuen-Jer Tsai and Hann-Chorng Kuo
Predictive Factors for a Successful Treatment Outcome in Patients with Different Voiding Dysfunction Subtypes Who Received Urethral Sphincter Botulinum Injection
Reprinted from: *Toxins* **2022**, *14*, 877, doi:10.3390/toxins14120877 . . . . **85**

Sheng-Fu Chen and Hann-Chorng Kuo
Urethral Sphincter Botulinum Toxin A Injection for Non-Spinal Cord Injured Patients with Voiding Dysfunction without Anatomical Obstructions: Which Patients Benefit Most?
Reprinted from: *Toxins* **2023**, *15*, 87, doi:10.3390/toxins15020087 . . . . **95**

Yin-Chien Ou, Yao-Lin Kao, Yi-Hui Ho, Kuan-Yu Wu and Hann-Chorng Kuo
Intravesical Injection of Botulinum Toxin Type A in Patients with Refractory Overactive Bladder—Results between Young and Elderly Populations, and Factors Associated with Unfavorable Outcomes
Reprinted from: *Toxins* **2023**, *15*, 95, doi:10.3390/toxins15020095 . . . . **105**

Po-Ming Chow and Hann-Chorng Kuo
Botulinum Toxin A Injection for Autonomic Dysreflexia—Detrusor Injection or Urethral Sphincter Injection?
Reprinted from: *Toxins* **2023**, *15*, 108, doi:10.3390/toxins15020108 . . . . **119**

Jia-Fong Jhang, Wan-Ru Yu and Hann-Chorng Kuo
Comparison of the Clinical Efficacy and Adverse Events between Intravesical Injections of Platelet-Rich Plasma and Botulinum Toxin A for the Treatment of Interstitial Cystitis Refractory to Conventional Treatment
Reprinted from: *Toxins* **2023**, *15*, 121, doi:10.3390/toxins15020121 . . . . **129**

Fan-Ching Hung and Hann-Chorng Kuo
Liposome-Encapsulated Botulinum Toxin A in Treatment of Functional Bladder Disorders
Reprinted from: *Toxins* **2022**, *14*, 838, doi:10.3390/toxins14120838 . . . . **141**

Wenshuang Li, Zhenming Zheng, Kaiqun Ma, Caixia Zhang, Kuiqing Li, Paierhati Tayier and Yousheng Yao
Preliminary Exploration of a New Therapy for Interstitial Cystitis/Bladder Pain Syndrome: Botulinum Toxin A Combined with Sapylin
Reprinted from: *Toxins* **2022**, *14*, 832, doi:10.3390/toxins14120832 . . . . **153**

About the Editor

Hann-Chorng Kuo

Dr. Hann-Chorng Kuo graduated from National Taiwan University (NTUH) in 1979. He underwent his residency training for four years after serving in the army. He was promoted to visiting staff in NTUH and became a lecturer at the National Taiwan University in 1985. Then he went to Hofuf, Saudi Arabia and served in Hofuf General Hospital for one year as a diplomatic supportive doctor. In 1988, Hann-Chorng moved to Tzu Chi General Hospital, Hualien, Taiwan and served as the chief of the department of Urology in Tzu Chi General Hospital (TCGH), where he remains to this day. During these years, Hann-Chorng devoted himself to clinical and research works in neurourology and urodynamics. He developed a videourodynamic laboratory and a wet lab for human bladder tissue and animal research in TCGH. Through detailed clinical observations and over 16,000 videourodynamic studies, Hann-Chorng has published more than 650 peer-reviewed papers and wrote more than 10 monographs in the fields of general urology, urodynamics, bladder outlet obstruction, neurogenic bladder, female urology, and overactive bladder. The interests of Hann-Chorng are numerous. Recently he has had interest in biomarkers for an overactive bladder, such as urinary nerve growth factor, serum CRP, cytokines, and bladder wall thickness; clinical application of botulinum toxin in lower urinary tract dysfunction; and pathophysiology of interstitial cystitis and painful bladder syndrome. He has also devoted a lot of time to continence promotion and the educational program of incontinence and voiding dysfunction as part of the Taiwanese Continence Society (TCS). Hann-Chorng gained his professor title from the Tzu Chi University School of Medicine in 2001, was the president of the TCS in 2006 through 2012, and was the president of the Taiwan Urological Association (TUA) from 2014 to 2016.

toxins

MDPI

Editorial

Botulinum Toxin Brings a Light to the Shadow of Functional Urology

Hann-Chorng Kuo

Department of Urology, Hualien Tzu Chi Hospital, Buddhist Tzu Chi Medical Foundation, Tzu Chi University, Hualien 970, Taiwan; hck@tzuchi.com.tw

Functional urology involves a large scale of lower urinary tract dysfunctions (LUTDs), including bladder dysfunctions and bladder outlet dysfunctions. The LUTDs can be neurogenic, inflammatory, or anatomical etiologies in male or female patients, and in elderly or pediatric patients. Currently, we can treat bladder overactivity by antimuscarinics and beta-3 adrenoceptor agonists and manage bladder outlet dysfunction by alpha-blocker, phosphodiesterase inhibitor, and 5-alpha-reductase inhibitors. However, there are still several LUTDs in the shadows of functional urology that are difficult to treat by currently available medications. Botulinum toxin A (BoNT-A) has been approved for treatment of neurogenic detrusor overactivity (NDO) and idiopathic overactive bladder (OAB) refractory to conventional medical therapy [1,2]. In addition to these indications, BoNT-A has been widely used in the treatment of several LUTDs which are not adequately treated by surgical or medical therapies. Currently, the applications of BoNT-A on LUTDs other than NDO and OAB include interstitial cystitis (IC) [3], neurogenic detrusor sphincter dyssynergia (DSD) in patients with spinal cord injury [4], autonomic dysreflexia in high-level spinal cord injury [5], adult non-neurogenic voiding dysfunction such as bladder neck dysfunction, dysfunctional voiding, or poor relaxation of the urethral sphincter [6,7], chronic prostatitis and pelvic pain [8], and pediatric detrusor overactivity and voiding dysfunction [9,10]. However, these indications have not been approved yet, most likely because of the uncertain treatment outcome and adverse events. Due to lack of phase 2 and phase 3 clinical trials, these clinical treatments in functional urology are off-labelled use and cannot be widely applied. Nevertheless, research is still ongoing because the treatment outcome of BoNT-A injections is beneficial for several LUTDs that are difficult to treat by conventional pharmacotherapies or surgical procedures.

In recent decades, clinical and basic research has shown that BoNT-A injections into the detrusor can improve urinary incontinence in elderly patients with OAB but intolerable to adverse events of antimuscarinics. BoNT-A injection into the bladder neck and urethral sphincter can effectively reduce the bladder outlet resistance and facilitate spontaneous voiding in patients with neurogenic or non-neurogenic voiding dysfunction. Repeated intravesical BoNT-A injections have been demonstrated to eliminate bladder inflammation and improve bladder irritative and painful symptoms in patients with IC or ketamine related cystitis. Moreover, clinical trials have shown that BoNT-A encapsulated by liposomes can facilitate BoNT-A protein to penetrate the cell membrane of the urothelium, therefore, the OAB or IC patients might be treated without intravesical injection [11]. Lower energy shock wave can also increase the permeability of urothelial cell membrane and help BoNT-A migrate into the suburothelium of the bladder. These preliminary results provide evidence that the large molecule BoNT-A might be efficiently managed to act on the suburothelial sensory nerves without traumatic injections [12]. In the future, with more clinical studies, we might have a chance to treat LUTDs in functional urology by the device of vehicles to carry BoNT-A into the bladder or urethral tissue without injections. In the shadow of functional urology where conventional medical treatment cannot reach, BoNT-A treatment may bring a light to treat LUTDs.

Citation: Kuo, H.-C. Botulinum Toxin Brings a Light to the Shadow of Functional Urology. *Toxins* **2023**, *15*, 321. https://doi.org/10.3390/toxins15050321

Received: 22 April 2023
Revised: 28 April 2023
Accepted: 1 May 2023
Published: 6 May 2023

Copyright: © 2023 by the author. Licensee MDPI, Basel, Switzerland. This article is an open access article distributed under the terms and conditions of the Creative Commons Attribution (CC BY) license (https://creativecommons.org/licenses/by/4.0/).

In this Special Issue, Ou et al. compared the clinical efficacy of BoNT-A injections between young and elderly patients with OAB and analyzed the factors associated with unfavorable outcome. They discovered that the therapeutic efficacy and safety profile of BoNT-A injection are comparable between young and elderly patients with OAB refractory to conventional medication. In the analysis of unfavorable treatment outcome in the elderly patients with OAB, they determined that female gender, presence of diabetes mellitus, and the baseline urodynamic parameters are potential factors. Therefore, before BoNT-A injection for the elderly patients with OAB, the possible treatment outcome should be informed. Hu, et al. reviewed the role of BoNT-A injections for OAB in patients with Parkinson's disease (PD) and stroke. They determined intravesical injection of 100U of BoNT-A is feasible for patents with PD and OAB to improve incontinence grade with acceptable adverse events of large post-void residual and urinary tract infection, while urethral sphincter BoNT-A injection can be used to treat voiding dysfunction in these patients with OAB due to central nervous lesions. Lee et al. reported the treatment outcome in male patients with OAB after surgery for bladder outlet obstruction. They determined that the therapeutic efficacy of BoNT-A to improve urgency and urinary incontinence is similar with that in female patients with OAB.

Chen et al. compared the therapeutic effects of urethral sphincter BoNT-A injections in patients with different non-neurogenic voiding dysfunction subtypes. Among the patients with detrusor underactivity, poor relaxation of urethral sphincter, and dysfunctional voiding, patients with dysfunctional voiding benefit most from BoNT-A treatment, both in subjective and objective parameters, and half of patients with detrusor underactivity and poor relaxation of urethral sphincter also had a fair response. A post-void residual volume of >250 mL was a negative predictor in patients with detrusor underactivity. Kao et al. also analyzed the predictive factors for the successful treatment outcome of BoNT-A urethral sphincter injections in patients with different subtypes of voiding dysfunctions. They determined that urethral sphincter BoNT-A injections provide comparative therapeutic efficacy in functional voiding dysfunction and non-neurogenic voiding dysfunction. Among the clinical characteristics of voiding dysfunction, detrusor underactivity and a low voiding efficiency could predict inferior therapeutic outcomes. For patients with NDO, Chen et al. compared the results of clinical treatment outcome between spinal cord injured patients receiving intravesical and urethral sphincter BoNT-A injections. Chow et al. analyzed the therapeutic efficacy of urethral or detrusor BoNT-A injections for patients with autonomic dysreflexia and determined detrusor BoNT-A injections superior to urethral sphincter BoNT-A injections in terms of symptomatic improvement of autonomic dysreflexia.

Five articles in this Special Issue reported the application of BoNT-A in the treatment of IC. Yu et al. reported the treatment outcomes of BoNT-A injections on patients with different subtypes of IC. Pedro Abreu-Mendes et al. reported the long-term real-life follow-up results of intratrigonal BoNT-A injections for patients with IC, and they discovered that intratrigonal BoNT-A injection is effective and durable for IC. Jhang et al. analyzed the therapeutic effects between BoNT-A and platelet-rich plasma (PRP) injections, and determined that BoNT-A injection is superior to PRP injection in reducing bladder pain score. Li et al. reported the results of a new therapy combining BoNT-A injection and Sapylin instillation and discovered significant superior outcome in the mixed group. Finally, Hung et al. reviewed the potential efficacy of intravesical instillation of liposomes and mixed liposomes and BoNT-A in treatment of functional bladder disorders. This treatment might improve LUTDs by BoNT-A without intravesical injection. These five articles provide excellent review and researches on the clinical application of BoNT-A treatment for IC refractory to conventional therapy. Based on previous basic studies of IC, the anti-inflammatory therapeutic effects of BoNT-A might have a chance to combat the inflammation in IC and improve the bladder pain symptoms.

This Special Issue collected original and review articles that focus on the novel applications of BoNT-A in LUTDs in functional urology. The collection of this Special Issue of

Toxins provides updated knowledge on the current and future position of BoNT-A in the shadows of functional urology and LUTDs.

Conflicts of Interest: The author declares no conflict of interest.

References

1. FDA. *FDA Approves Botox to Treat Specific Form of Incontinence*; The US Food and Drug Administration: Baltimore, MD, USA, 2011.
2. FDA. *Approves Botox to Treat Overactive Bladder*; The US Food and Drug Administration: Baltimore, MD, USA, 2013. Available online: https://www.fda.gov/NewsEvents/Newsroom/PressAnnouncements/ucm336101.htm (accessed on 22 April 2023).
3. Gao, Y.; Lai, F.; Liu, J.; Yang, D.; Huang, C. An indirect comparison meta-analysis of noninvasive intravesical instillation and intravesical injection of botulinum toxin-A in bladder disorders. *Int. Urol. Nephrol.* **2022**, *54*, 479–491.
4. Mehta, S.; Hill, D.; Foley, N.; Hsieh, J.; Ethans, K.; Potter, P.; Baverstock, R.; Teasell, R.W.; Wolfe, D. Spinal Cord Injury Rehabilitation Evidence Research Team. A meta-analysis of botulinum toxin sphincteric injections in the treatment of incomplete voiding after spinal cord injury. *Arch. Phys. Med. Rehabil.* **2012**, *93*, 597–603. [CrossRef]
5. Giannantoni, A.; Mearini, E.; Del Zingaro, M.; Porena, M. Six-year follow-up of botulinum toxin A intradetrusorial injections in patients with refractory neurogenic detrusor overactivity: Clinical and urodynamic results. *Eur. Urol.* **2009**, *55*, 705–711. [CrossRef]
6. Chen, G.; Liao, L.; Zhang, F. Efficacy and safety of botulinum toxin a injection into urethral sphincter for underactive bladder. *BMC Urol.* **2019**, *19*, 60. [CrossRef]
7. Kuo, H.C. Effectiveness of urethral injection of botulinum A toxin in the treatment of voiding dysfunction after radical hysterectomy. *Urol. Int.* **2005**, *75*, 247–251. [CrossRef] [PubMed]
8. Falahatkar, S.; Shahab, E.; Gholamjani Moghaddam, K.; Kazemnezhad, E. Transurethral intraprostatic injection of botulinum neurotoxin type A for the treatment of chronic prostatitis/chronic pelvic pain syndrome: Results of a prospective pilot double-blind and randomized placebo-controlled study. *BJU Int.* **2015**, *116*, 641–649. [CrossRef] [PubMed]
9. Kajbafzadeh, A.M.; Moosavi, S.; Tajik, P.; Arshadi, H.; Payabvash, S.; Salmasi, A.H.; Akbari, H.R.; Nejat, F. Intravesical injection of botulinum toxin type A: Management of neuropathic bladder and bowel dysfunction in children with myelomeningocele. *Urology* **2006**, *68*, 1091–1096. [CrossRef]
10. Horst, M.; Weber, D.M.; Bodmer, C.; Gobet, R. Repeated botulinum-A toxin injection in the treatment of neuropathic bladder dysfunction and poor bladder compliance in children with myelomeningocele. *Neurourol. Urodyn.* **2011**, *30*, 1546–1549. [CrossRef]
11. Janicki, J.J.; Chancellor, M.B.; Kaufman, J.; Gruber, M.A.; Chancellor, D.D. Potential Effect of Liposomes and Liposome-Encapsulated Botulinum Toxin and Tacrolimus in the Treatment of Bladder Dysfunction. *Toxins* **2016**, *8*, 81. [CrossRef] [PubMed]
12. Chuang, Y.C.; Huang, T.L.; Tyagi, P.; Huang, C.C. Urodynamic and immunohistochemical evaluation of intravesical botulinum toxin A delivery using low energy shock waves. *J. Urol.* **2016**, *196*, 599–608. [CrossRef] [PubMed]

Disclaimer/Publisher's Note: The statements, opinions and data contained in all publications are solely those of the individual author(s) and contributor(s) and not of MDPI and/or the editor(s). MDPI and/or the editor(s) disclaim responsibility for any injury to people or property resulting from any ideas, methods, instructions or products referred to in the content.

toxins MDPI

Review

Clinical Application of Botulinum Neurotoxin in Lower-Urinary-Tract Diseases and Dysfunctions: Where Are We Now and What More Can We Do?

Hann-Chorng Kuo

Department of Urology, Hualien Tzu Chi Hospital, Buddhist Tzu Chi Medical Foundation, Tzu Chi University, Hualien 97004, Taiwan; hck@tzuchi.com.tw; Tel.: +886-3-8561825 (ext. 2117); Fax: +886-3-8560794

Abstract: Botulinum toxin A (Botox) had been considered a promising drug that has an effect on functional disorders of the lower urinary tract. Because Botox exhibits anti-inflammatory and antispasmodic effects, Botox injection into the bladder can decrease detrusor contractility, reduce bladder hypersensitivity, and eliminate painful sensations. Injecting Botox into the bladder outlet can relax the hyperactivity of the bladder neck, and of the urethral smooth and striated muscles. Based on these therapeutic effects, Botox has been widely applied to treat lower-urinary-tract dysfunctions (LUTDs) such as overactive bladder and neurogenic detrusor overactivity. However, this treatment has not been licensed for use in other LUTDs such as interstitial cystitis, voiding dysfunction due to benign prostatic hyperplasia in men, and dysfunctional voiding in women. Botox has also not been approved for the treatment of children with overactive bladder and dysfunctional voiding; in patients with spinal cord injuries with detrusor sphincter dyssynergia and autonomic dysreflexia; or for poorly relaxed external sphincter in non-neurogenic patients. This article reviews the current knowledge regarding Botox treatment for LUTDs and discusses the potential clinical applications of Botox, as well as work that can be conducted in the future.

Keywords: adverse events; lower-urinary-tract dysfunction; therapeutic efficacy; urinary incontinence; voiding dysfunction

Key Contribution: Botulinum toxin A (Botox) treatment is effective in treating several lower-urinary-tract dysfunctions (LUTDs) in addition to overactive bladder and neurogenic detrusor overactivity. Although the clinical applications of Botox on these LUTDs are unlicensed, the careful selection of patients and diseases and the monitoring of adverse events can improve urinary incontinence or voiding dysfunction in patients whose LUTDs are refractory to conventional medical therapy.

Citation: Kuo, H.-C. Clinical Application of Botulinum Neurotoxin in Lower-Urinary-Tract Diseases and Dysfunctions: Where Are We Now and What More Can We Do?. *Toxins* **2022**, *14*, 498. https://doi.org/10.3390/toxins14070498

Received: 16 June 2022
Accepted: 14 July 2022
Published: 18 July 2022

Publisher's Note: MDPI stays neutral with regard to jurisdictional claims in published maps and institutional affiliations.

Copyright: © 2022 by the author. Licensee MDPI, Basel, Switzerland. This article is an open access article distributed under the terms and conditions of the Creative Commons Attribution (CC BY) license (https://creativecommons.org/licenses/by/4.0/).

1. Introduction

In recent decades, botulinum toxin A (Botox) has been widely used for the treatment of several different lower-urinary-tract dysfunctions (LUTDs), including overactive bladder (OAB), neurogenic detrusor overactivity (NDO), interstitial cystitis/bladder pain syndrome (IC/BPS), pediatric urinary incontinence and voiding dysfunction, voiding dysfunction due to benign prostatic hyperplasia (BPH) in men, dysfunctional voiding (DV) in women, detrusor sphincter dyssynergia (DSD) in patients with spinal-cord injury (SCI), and poorly relaxed external sphincter (PRES) in non-neurogenic patients. Despite the fact that Botox injection has only been licensed to treat OAB and NDO refractory to conventional treatment, the clinical applications of Botox on other LUTDs have been enthusiastically tried [1]. However, because some clinical experiences of adverse events have limited its widespread application, Botox injection treatment has not popularly used for LUTDs other than OAB and NDO. Nevertheless, evidence has shown that Botox has distinguished advantages related to functional alteration, chronic inflammation, and sensory disorders in some LUTDs that are difficult to treat with oral pharmacologic medications. Other than OAB and NDO, several other LUTDs can benefit from intravesical Botox injection, intravesical instillation, or urethral Botox injection. (Table 1) This article focuses on the off-label and novel applications of Botox on LUTDs. The content of this article may provide updated knowledge and information regarding the current situation and where Botox may be further applied in functional urology and LUTDs.

2. Clinical Application of Botox on OAB: Efficacy, Adherence, Adverse Events, and Novel Treatment without Injection

Botox treatment for OAB and NDO is becoming increasingly recognized as an effective therapeutic option for patients who are refractory to or cannot tolerate anticholinergic agents. The results from open-label studies have suggested that this therapy is effective in both neurogenic and idiopathic detrusor overactivity (DO) [2]. However, undesired adverse events and the need for repeat injections remain obstacles to the popularity of this treatment.

Botulinum toxin is a neurotoxin produced by *Clostridium botulinum* that inhibits signal transmission at the neuromuscular and neuroglandular junctions [3]. The most popular current clinical use of Botulinum toxin is onabotulinumtoxinA (Botox®, Allergan, Irvine, CA, USA). Botox has received regulatory approval for LUTDs, including OAB and NDO. The approved dose of Botox for NDO due to SCI or multiple sclerosis (MS) is 200 U by 1 mL for each injection into the detrusor at 30 sites on the bladder wall. For Botox treatment of OAB, the dose is 100 U by 0.5 mL for each injection into 20 sites on the bladder wall [4]. Botox has both a motor and sensory effect on the lower urinary tract; therefore, the therapeutic effects include not only a decrease in striated or smooth muscle contractility, but also effects on sensory dysfunction, including frequency urgency sensation and bladder pain [5,6].

Following the initial clinical trials of Botox injection for OAB, the recommended optimal dose was set at 100 U injected into 20 sites of the bladder wall [7,8]. Adverse events of this treatment include difficult urination, urinary-tract infection (UTI), and large postvoid residual (PVR) volume requiring clean intermittent catheterization [9]. For patients who are frail and old with a PVR > 100 mL, injecting at the bladder base and trigone is safer to avoid acute urinary retention and subsequent UTI [10]. Phase 3 clinical trials and pooled analysis have demonstrated that Botox injection is superior to placebo and that patients may have fewer episodes of urgency and urgency urinary incontinence (UUI) as well as experiencing an improvement in quality of life [11,12].

2.1. *Adherence of Botox Treatment in OAB and Causes of Discontinuation*

According to the guidelines of the American Urological Association and recommendations of the European Urological Association, Botox intravesical injection is the third-line treatment for OAB [13,14]. Repeated Botox injections have been reported to have a similar effect, and the interinjection interval has been reported to remain unchanged for up to five injections [15]. However, increasing age, a Botox dose of 200 U, higher body-mass index, and baseline UUI episodes were found to be associated with a shorter time to UUI recurrence after Botox injection [16]. In patients who have diminished Botox effect on OAB symptoms, adding mirabegron could increase the therapeutic effects, mainly on OAB symptoms and the Global Response Assessment scale [17].

A long-term follow-up study revealed a low rate of persistence of another brand of botulinum toxin A, abobotulinumtoxinA, as an injection for OAB. A total of 59.3% of patients were successfully treated with the first injection. The median number of injections per patient was only two, and the median reinjection interval was 10.7 months. The estimated 5-year discontinuation-free survival rate was 23.4%. The main cause of discontinuation was primary failure in 35.5% of patients, 23.7% of patients had persistent symptom improvement, and 20.3% stopped the injections because of tolerability issues [18]. In women with OAB, a significant reduction in the DO rate and an increase in the median maximum cystometric capacity were noted after Botox injection for idiopathic DO. The maximum flow rate (Qmax), detrusor pressure (Pdet), and PVR all showed no significant change, and no patient required catheterization after Botox injection [19].

2.2. Comparison of Repeat Botox Injections and Percutaneous Tibial Nerve Stimulation and Sacral-Nerve Neuromodulation

In addition to Botox injections, percutaneous tibial nerve stimulation (PTNS) and sacral-nerve neuromodulation (SNM) are two options for the treatment of refractory OAB. Because Botox injection requires local or general anesthesia, and repeated injections are necessary to maintain the therapeutic effect, patients might consider switching to another procedure for better convenience. A recent study revealed that PTNS and Botox resulted in a similar improvement in OAB symptom scores; however, Botox resulted in significantly greater improvement in urgency and UUI episodes than PTNS [20]. Overall, Botox, PTNS, and SNM were more efficacious than the placebo. However, the greatest reduction in UUI episodes and voiding frequency was observed with SNM. Botox resulted in a higher complication rate, including UTI and urine retention, as compared with PTNS [21].

Although SNM is an invasive procedure and requires a two-stage implantation, the therapeutic effectiveness is as high as 69%, and the battery lasts for up to 15 years [22]. SNM has become a well-accepted procedure for refractory OAB, especially in women. However, the high cost of SNM limits its wide application in treating UUI as compared with 200 U of Botox [23]. In patients who failed previous Botox treatment and in Botox-naïve patients, the therapeutic efficacy was shown to be similar between the Botox and SNM groups and similar between patients with a previously different volume of Botox injection [24]. Although the risks of UTI and urinary retention are higher in patients treated with Botox, the risk of revision or removal of the battery and implant also requires caution [25].

2.3. Potential Vehicle to Carry Botox across the Urothelium without Injection

Liposome-encapsulated Botox intravesical instillation had been demonstrated as effective in decreasing OAB symptoms without adverse events such as a PVR increase or the risk of UTI [26,27]. An immunohistochemistry study showed that Botox injection can effectively cleave the SNAP-25 protein, whereas liposome-encapsulated Botox can decrease urothelial P2 $\times$ 3 expression but does not cleave SNAP-25 [28]. The same formulation of liposome-encapsulated Botox had been applied in the treatment of patients with IC/BPS, and the results showed a positive effect on the decrease in IC symptoms, although the improvement was not superior to the placebo arm [29]. Nevertheless, these pilot studies demonstrated that, using liposomes encapsulation, the Botox protein can be delivered across the phospholipid layer of the cell membrane and act on the sensory receptors of the urothelial cells. However, the depth of Botox penetration might be too superficial to achieve a longer therapeutic effect. Thus, additional investigation of the treatment frequency and dosage of Botox are necessary [30].

LESW was shown to be effective for temporarily increasing tissue permeability and the intravesical delivery of Botox for the treatment of OAB in animal studies and in a human clinical trial [31]. Our preliminary study using LESW and intravesical BoNT-A instillation every week in OAB patients also demonstrated an improvement in the Global Response Assessment without any adverse events [32]. A prior immunohistochemistry study revealed the presence of cleaved SNAP-25 protein in the IC bladder suburothelium, suggesting that Botox molecules could be carried across the urothelial cell membrane with the assistance of LESW. These results provide evidence of the efficacy and safety of this novel treatment using LESW plus Botox instillation without anesthesia or bladder injection [32].

2.4. Perspectives of Researchers on Botox Injection Related to UTI, Difficult Urination, and Adverse Events after Treatment

The most common and frustrating adverse events after Botox injection for OAB are UTI and dysuria [33]. In patients with OAB, previous UTI is the strongest predictor of UTI after Botox injection. Men have 2.4 times higher odds of incomplete emptying than women, and 17% of men and 23.5% of women experience more than one episode of UTI in the first month following injection [34]. Although researchers have reported that aging is associated with a higher rate of large PVR and lower long-term success [35], the age-related outcomes of Botox for the treatment of OAB are significantly understudied [36]. Male gender, baseline large PVR (≥100 mL), comorbidity, and a Botox dose of >100 U are risk factors for increasing the incidence of adverse events after intravesical Botox injection for idiopathic detrusor overactivity [37]. Factors that can predict poor response and higher risk of UTI to Botox injection for OAB include female gender, retained prostate in men, and clean intermittent self-catheterization [38]. A recent meta-analysis also revealed a positive effect of Botox treatment on sexual function in patients with OAB. Significant improvement was observed in desire, arousal, lubrication, orgasm, and satisfaction after Botox injection; however, there was no improvement in pain [39].

Based on the results of previous studies, several topics of research remain to be investigated: (1) Can a small dose of Botox injection and combined medications (mirabegron or antimuscarinics) be used to treat patients with OAB to avoid undesired UTI and urinary retention? (2) Can the dose of Botox be flexibly adjusted to fit the needs of patients with different severities of OAB and neurologic lesions? (3) Can we use LESW on the bladder plus Botox instillation to treat patients with OAB or hypersensitive bladder without intravesical injection under anesthesia?

3. Clinical Application of Botox on NDO: Efficacy, Adherence, Adverse Events, and Conversion of Treatment

OnabotulinumtoxinA was first injected into the urethral sphincter to treat patients with SCI with DSD who did not desire surgery or were unable to perform self-catheterization [40]. Later clinical trials confirmed the therapeutic effectiveness of 200 U or 300 U of Botox detrusor injections on NDO due to SCI and MS [41,42]. In patients with Parkinson's disease and SCI, Botox detrusor injection can modulate bladder afferent activity, which explains why Botox can improve DO [43]. The therapeutic duration is about 6 to 9 months, and the significant reduction in detrusor pressure, increase in bladder capacity, improvement in hydronephrosis, and reduction in UTI episodes are remarkable after Botox injection [42,44]. After several repeated detrusor Botox injections, the therapeutic efficacy remains the same [45]. Currently, Botox detrusor injections are widely applied in the treatment of patients with chronic SCI or MS refractory to antimuscarinic therapy for NDO and UUI [46–48].

3.1. Therapeutic Efficacy, Adverse Events, and Tolerability of Botox Injection for NDO

In a post-market survey, intradetrusor Botox injections were reported to be safe and to be able to improve subjective measures related to NDO [49]. A meta-analysis also revealed that Botox can result in a significant reduction in UUI frequency and improvement in urodynamic parameters in patients with NDO at 6 weeks after treatment. No statistical or clinical difference in efficacy has been reported between 300 U and 200 U dosages of Botox [50]. Patients treated with 300 U of Botox had similar therapeutic efficacy after 200 U of Botox treatment. The number of episodes of urinary incontinence and daily pad use were similar between the two dosage phases [51]. However, quality-of-life measures were significantly improved, and an improvement in end-filling pressure and bladder compliance was also reported [52]. Although Botox detrusor injections are effective and tolerable for patients with NDO, adverse events related to Botox injection, including hematuria, UTI, urinary retention, urinary bladder hemorrhage, autonomic dysreflexia (AD), and epididymitis, warrant caution [53]. The results of a long-term follow-up study showed that only 50% of patients with SCI continuously received intradetrusor Botox injections for NDO after 10 years [54]. In patients with NDO, repeat Botox injections allow sustained improvements in UUI, with an acceptable rate of adverse events [55]. The efficacy of repeat detrusor Botox injections included significant improvement in urinary symptoms and bladder compliance in 52% of patients, and 31% of patients had an objective improvement in bladder compliance [56].

3.2. Switching from Botox to Augmentation Enterocystoplasty

After the initial Botox injections for NDO, some patients might not experience persistent improvement in symptoms, and some might prefer to have definite treatment without repeated injections. Augmentation enterocystoplasty (AE) is one option for patients with SCI and NDO and urinary incontinence [57]. Patients receiving AE had a statistically significant increase in bladder capacity and a decrease in detrusor pressure during voiding. Patients with SCI receiving Botox injections but who experience few improvements in their urodynamic parameters should consider switching from repeat Botox injections to AE to achieve better storage function and functional bladder capacity [58]. In patients who still have symptoms of NDO or AD after AE, the injection of Botox into the native bladder was effective in 58% of patients in increasing bladder capacity and decreasing detrusor pressure [59].

3.3. Causes of Discontinued Botox Injection in OAB and NDO

Although Botox injections are effective for treating urinary incontinence of OAB and NDO, more than half of patients with NDO discontinue Botox injections within the first 10 years after their first treatment [60]. Patients with spina bifida have a higher discontinuation rate. The most common cause of discontinuation is treatment failure (43.7%). In a long-term follow-up study of the satisfaction rate of patients with SCI and NDO who received detrusor Botox injections, only 48.4% of patients continued Botox injections over 7 years [61]. The presence of high detrusor pressure and higher-grade bladder outlet resistance are predictive of a decrease in incontinence. In total, 69.1% of patients expressed satisfaction with their current status.

4. Clinical Application of Botox on Interstitial Cystitis/Bladder Pain Syndrome: Efficacy, Adverse Events, and Perspectives

4.1. Current Strategy of Using Botox Injections on IC/BPS

IC/BPS has been classified into classic ulcer and non-ulcer types based on cystoscopic findings [30]. Although researchers have proposed many pathogeneses of IC/BPS, the actual etiology remains unclear. Possible etiologies include (1) the post-infection autoimmune process; (2) mast-cell activation induced by inflammation, toxins, or stress; (3) urothelial dysfunction and increased permeability of the urothelium; and (4) neurogenic inflammation resulting in increased urothelial permeability, mast-cell activation, the up-regulation of sensory fibers, the release of inflammatory neuropeptide, and bladder pain [62]. In addition, psychosomatic dysfunction has also been reported to be involved in the pathophysiology of IC/BPS, especially in the pain phenotype [63,64]. Conventional therapies include oral pentosan polysulfate [65], intravesical heparin instillation [66], intravesical hyaluronic acid instillation [67], and oral medications that target suburothelial inflammation. Although IC/BPS has not received regulatory approval for Botox use, current evidence supports that Botox injection can improve symptoms and bladder pain for IC/BPS as compared with a placebo [68].

Intravesical onabotulinumtoxinA injections might not only reduce bladder sensitivity in patients with IC/BPS but also induce desensitization in the central nervous system by affecting the overexpression of activated proteins in the dorsal horn ganglia [69]. The therapeutic effects of Botox on IC/BPS were confirmed by several clinical trials showing that Botox could effectively reduce bladder pain and urinary frequency and improve psychosocial functioning [70–72]. As compared with cystoscopic hydrodistention, intravesical Botox injection plus hydrodistention can improve IC symptom scores, reduce bladder pain, and increase functional bladder capacity [73]. In the first prospective, multicenter, randomized, double-blind, placebo-controlled clinical trial, we demonstrated a significantly greater reduction in pain in the Botox group compared with the normal saline group (-2.6 ± 2.8

vs. −0.9 ± 2.2, p = 0.021) at week 8. We also found that the cystometric bladder capacity was increased significantly in the Botox group. The overall success rates were 63% in the Botox group compared with 15% in the control group (p = 0.028), with a similar rate of adverse events between groups [74].

The injection of Botox into the pelvic floor muscles of women has also been shown to improve chronic pelvic pain syndrome; however, this treatment may worsen preexisting pelvic floor conditions such as constipation, stress urinary incontinence, and fecal incontinence [75,76].

4.2. Predictive Factors for a Successful or Failed Treatment Outcome

In patients with non-ulcer IC/BPS, intravesical Botox injections can effectively improve symptoms and reduce bladder pain, but these injections do not benefit patients with ulcer IC/BPS [77]. As compared with a single injection, repeat intravesical Botox injections were associated with a significantly higher success rate in a long-term follow-up. However, the incidence of adverse events did not increase with a higher number of Botox injections. A higher pretreatment interstitial cystitis symptom index and interstitial cystitis problem index score were predictive of a successful response to repeated intravesical Botox injections [78]. Injecting Botox into the bladder body and trigone did not result in a difference in treatment outcomes or rates of adverse events [79].

In a recently published analysis of factors predictive of successful Botox treatment outcomes for IC/BPS, patients with a maximal bladder capacity under hydrodistention of >760 mL had a satisfactory treatment outcome [80]. The improvement in bladder pain was remarkable in patients with a satisfactory treatment outcome. A maximal bladder capacity of ≥760 mL is a predictive factor for satisfactory treatment outcome, whereas glomerulation grade and urodynamic parameters do not have a predictive value for the IC/BPS treatment outcome. Only 10% of patients who were treated with Botox injection complained of difficulty in urination after treatment.

4.3. Comparison of Effects between Different Botox Injection Sites and between Botox and Sacral Neuromodulation in Treatment of IC/BPS

There has been debate regarding the effectiveness of Botox on IC/BPS between different sites of injection. The trigone has been considered to be rich in unmyelinated nociceptive C-fibers, and it may be a potential target for chemodenervation in patients with IC/BPS [81]. Giannantoni et al. injected Botox at the trigone and lateral bladder wall and reported symptomatic improvement in 86.6% of patients [70]. Pinto et al. injected 100 U of Botox into 10 trigonal sites and found an increase in bladder capacity and a transient reduction in urinary nerve growth factor and brain-derived neurotrophic factor [82]. However, in our study, after intravesical Botox injection in the bladder body or trigone, we did not find any significant difference in improvement in IC symptoms or urodynamic parameters [79]. Evans et al. compared the treatment outcomes between patients with IC/BPS who were randomly assigned to a trigone-including or trigone-sparing Botox injection template. They found no significant difference between groups or in the post-treatment complication profiles [83].

4.4. Perspectives of Future Research on Botox Treatment IC/BPS: Using Instillation with the Aid of LESW or Liposome but Not Injection

Although intravesical Botox injections of IC/BPS have been shown to be significantly superior to intravesical Botox instillation, the adverse event of difficult urination after Botox injection remains a problem to be solved [84]. The delivery of Botox via liposome encapsulation and gelation hydrogel intravesical instillation provided a potentially less invasive and more convenient form of application for patients with IC/BPS [85]. However, a pilot study showed only a short-term effect and limited improvement in IC symptoms in liposome-encapsulated Botox treatment [29]. Using LESW to increase urothelial permeability and facilitate the penetration of Botox intravesical instillation showed an early promising effect and the presence of cleaved SNAP-25 protein in the suburothelium [28].

These results provide evidence for the future treatment and safety of this novel treatment modality for patients with IC/BPS using LESW plus Botox instillation without bladder injection under anesthesia injection [32].

5. Clinical Applications of Botox on Pediatric OAB and DV: Efficacy, Adherence, and Adverse Events

5.1. Advantages of Botox Injection for Pediatric Refractory OAB

Although Botox is not licensed for use in children with neurogenic or non-neurogenic LUTD, this treatment has been widely applied to treat pediatric OAB and DV refractory to conventional therapy. At a dose of 5 U to 10 U/Kg detrusor injection in patients with myelomeningocele and NDO, an increase in bladder capacity, and a decrease in detrusor pressure were noted [86,87]. Vesicoureteral reflux resolved in 73% of patients after detrusor Botox injections [88]. An additional urethral sphincter Botox injection at a dose of 2 U/Kg could decrease PVR in children with DSD [89]. Pediatric patients with non-neurogenic OAB can also benefit from detrusor Botox injection for the reduction of urinary incontinence [90–92].

In children with urinary incontinence due to NDO or OAB, Botox detrusor injection results in a significant improvement and is well tolerated [93]. A high rate of urinary continence can be achieved, with improvements in urodynamic parameters, including a reduction in detrusor pressure to <40 cmH_2O and an increase in compliance to >20 mL/cmH_2O, without major adverse events. In children with NDO, a dose of 200 U of Botox was well tolerated and showed greater efficacy in bladder pressure reduction and bladder capacity increase [94]. Children with a high detrusor pressure and low bladder compliance had a significantly greater improvement in compliance after detrusor Botox injections [95]. It was reported that the therapeutic effects persisted in the first 6 months after Botox injection in children with severe OAB symptoms, urodynamic-confirmed DO, and reduced bladder volume [96]. When children are treated with Botox injections for OAB, mirabegron and anticholinergics may be used as an exit strategy for recurrent OAB symptoms after the Botox effect declines [97].

5.2. Do Children with OAB Need Continuous Repeated Botox Injections? Will OAB Resolve with Aging?

For children with neurogenic or non-neurogenic DO, repeat intravesical Botox injections are required to maintain therapeutic efficacy. In children with NDO, Botox may provide long-term urinary continence and upper urinary tract protection, and the results remain effective after up to 11 injections [98]. However, in children with DV or DSD, the response to Botox was less predictable, with <50% of patients experiencing symptom resolution [98]. In children with myelomeningocele, repeated Botox injections were found to be safe and effective for keeping the bladder and upper urinary tract in a stable condition [99]. A systematic review and meta-analysis also confirmed that repeated Botox injections provided sustainable improvement in children with NDO and an acceptable rate of adverse events [55]. Nevertheless, the failure rates were reported to be 12.6% after 3 years, 22.2% after 5 years, and 28.9% after 7 years of follow-up with a withdrawal rate of 11.3%. Patients with severe NDO at baseline might experience a less favorable treatment outcome [100]. For this reason, a prior study reported that, based on long-term follow-up, a bladder procedure was still required in 35.3% of children with NDO and a severely contracted bladder that could not be recovered to a stable condition after repeated Botox detrusor injections [101].

5.3. Therapeutic Efficacy of Urethral Sphincter Botox Injections for Children with Non-Neurogenic DV

DV is highly prevalent in pediatric patients with NDO or non-neurogenic OAB [102]. Urethral sphincter Botox injection at a dose of 50 to 100 U can normalize the voiding curve and decrease PVR in children with non-neurogenic DV [103,104]. In children with DV, a higher dose of Botox may increase the therapeutic efficacy without increasing morbidity.

Urethral sphincter Botox injection appears to be effective and safe in treating voiding dysfunction in children with DV or DSD [105].

6. Clinical Applications of Botox on Neurogenic and Non-Neurogenic Voiding Dysfunction: Efficacy and Perspectives

6.1. Current Treatment Outcome of Urethral Sphincter Botox Injection on DSD

Botox urethral-sphincter injection was first applied in patients with DSD due to SCI and MS [106]. Despite the lack of a phase 3 clinical trial and of licensed approval for clinical use, Botox has been widely applied for treating voiding dysfunction due to neurogenic or non-neurogenic voiding dysfunctions [107,108]. After the urethral sphincter Botox injection, patients with DSD or DV showed an improvement in voiding efficiency and a reduction in UTI episodes [109,110]. The dose of Botox for urethral-sphincter injections ranged from 100 U to 200 U for voiding dysfunction in patients with MS, cerebrovascular accident, or SCI [107,111]. After a urethral injection of 100 U of Botox, the indwelling catheter or clean intermittent catheterization can be discontinued in most patients [107,112]. In male patients with SCI with NDO and DSD who have received concomitant detrusor and urethral sphincter Botox injection, a significant reduction in detrusor pressure and maximal urethral closure pressure and an increase in maximal cystometric bladder capacity at 3 months after treatment were noted [113]. A better improvement rate was observed in patients with cervical SCI, the presence of NDO and DSD, partial hand function, and incomplete SCI. However, only 35.6% of patients continually received urethral sphincter Botox injections, and >60% of patients converted their treatment to another bladder outlet surgery to facilitate spontaneous voiding [57]. A meta-analysis showed that Botox was effective in 60–78% of patients with DSD for reducing PVR and lowering detrusor pressure and detrusor leak-point pressure after treatment. To maintain the therapeutic effect, reinjection is required after 4–9 months, without significant adverse events [114].

6.2. Current Treatment Outcome of Urethral Sphincter Botox Injection on Non-Neurogenic Voiding Dysfunction

In neurologically normal women, DV is characterized by an intermittent and/or fluctuating flow rate due to nonrelaxing or involuntary intermittent contractions of the periurethral striated or levator muscles during voiding [115]. Non-neurogenic DV may occur due to an enhanced guarding reflex against uninhibited detrusor contractions during the storage phase [116,117]. Treatment modalities for female DV include biofeedback pelvic-floor muscle training, medications such as alpha-blockers and skeletal muscle relaxants to decrease urethral resistance, antimuscarinic drugs for DO, and urethral Botox injection [118]. However, a urethral sphincter Botox injection can relieve voiding dysfunction in only about 67.9% of patients with DV. Patients with a tight bladder neck or with detrusor underactivity and low abdominal pressure to void might have a poor therapeutic result [119]. Multivariate analysis also revealed that narrowing of the bladder neck and history of catheterization were predictive factors for a negative outcome [120]. Another study reported a successful outcome in 59.4% of patients. There was no difference in treatment outcome between the different genders, voiding dysfunction subtype, bladder dysfunction, or sphincter dysfunction subtypes. In patients with DV, a significantly higher detrusor pressure might predict a successful treatment outcome of urethral sphincter Botox injection [121].

6.3. Perspectives of Urethral Sphincter Botox Injections for Patients with DSD or DV

Although urethral sphincter Botox injections comprise a safe and effective treatment for patients with urethral sphincter hyperactivity, the success rate has not been satisfactorily high. Currently, only 60% of patients with neurogenic DSD or non-neurogenic DV have benefited from this treatment [57,119]. No study has investigated whether an increase in Botox dose might result in a higher treatment success rate. In addition, because the pathophysiology of DV remains unclear, repeat urethral sphincter Botox injections could eliminate chronic inflammation in the central nervous system via the mechanism of afferent desensitization. Based on previous clinical trials of Botox injection at the trigone for eliminating bladder pain and sensory frequency in patients with IC/BPS [70,82], we might hypothesize that in patients with DV, injecting Botox into the trigone and bladder neck results in better therapeutic success than injecting into the urethral sphincter. Therefore, the following topics are of interest and could be investigated in the future: (1) whether the dose of Botox (100 U) and injection interval (once every 6 months) are enough to treat voiding dysfunction; (2) the adherence of urethral Botox injection for voiding dysfunction; and (3) whether voiding dysfunction improves with Botox injections into the trigone and bladder base, rather than into to the urethral sphincter.

7. Clinical Applications of Botox on Male LUTS and BPH: Efficacy and Perspectives

7.1. Current Evidence of Botox Injection in Treating Male LUTS/BPH

BPH is one of the main contributing diseases to LUTS in older men. However, not all men with LUTS are treated satisfactorily with BPH medication. Transurethral resection of the prostate is an established surgery for the rapid relief of LUTS in patients with BPH and bladder outlet obstruction (BOO). However, because of potential complications such as erectile dysfunction or urinary incontinence, patients might not accept this procedure. Therefore, minimally invasive procedures have been developed and tried in men with LUTS suggestive of BPH.

Several preliminary clinical trials have been reported. The injection of 200 U of Botox into the prostate has been shown to be effective with minimal side effects in patients with BPH and BOO who are poor surgical candidates [122]. Further clinical trials also revealed that Botox could relieve LUTS in patients with a small BPH of <30 mL [123]. Another study showed that an injection of 200 U of Botox into the prostate could improve LUTS and reduce the prostate volume by 50% in patients with large BPH, and the effect lasted for 12 months [15]. The transurethral injection method has been recommended as a preferable technique [124].

Several nonrandomized clinical studies have shown that Botox injection to the prostate can relieve LUTS in men with a small or large BPH. Intraprostatic Botox-A injection can reduce prostate volume, increase maximum flow rate and voided volume, and decrease PVR [125,126]. Patients with an International Prostate Symptom Score (IPSS) of $\leq$22, a Qmax $\leq$ 10 mL/min, and a prostate volume $\leq$ 56.5 mL had better treatment outcomes [127]. These results indicated that in patients with BPH, intraprostatic Botox injection is safe and effective for improving LUTS and quality of life. However, a randomized, double-blind, placebo-controlled clinical trial revealed an effect on LUTS/BPH symptoms, including IPSS, total prostate volume, transition zone volume, and Qmax, in both the Botox and placebo groups at week 12. Therefore, this study concluded that the therapeutic effects of Botox on BPH/LUTS are merely a placebo effect [128]. The results of a systematic review and meta-analysis of Botox injection for LUTS/BPH also showed no difference in the efficacy between Botox and a placebo. Thus, current evidence does not support the use of Botox injection for LUTS/BPH in real clinical practice [129].

7.2. Myth or Truth of Botox on BPH: Are We Treating Urethral Smooth Muscle or Prostatic Gland?

A previous study in patients with urethral sphincter pseudodyssynergia after cerebrovascular accidents or intracranial lesions reported that urethral sphincter Botox injection was effective and had no adverse effects [112], suggesting that Botox can relax the urethral smooth muscle or striated muscle and facilitate spontaneous voiding. Injecting Botox into the bladder neck and urethra has been shown to improve LUTS and increase Qmax in men with LUTS and a small prostate [130]. Botox prostatic injection has been demonstrated to be a promising treatment for patients with small prostates and symptomatic BPH. The mean prostate volume, symptom score, and quality-of-life index were significantly reduced after treatment. Because LUTS in men with a small BPH might relate more to urethral smooth muscle rather than to the prostate gland itself, the therapeutic effect of Botox on LUTS/BPH might relate to urethral dysfunction more than prostatic obstruction [131]. All of these pilot studies showed that LUTS does not result solely from BPH and obstruction. The functional inhibition of the voiding reflex or obstruction of the bladder outlet might play important roles in male LUTS, and Botox may eliminate these dysfunctions and improve LUTS. Despite the diverse results of clinical studies of Botox on LUTS/BPH, based on the current data, intraprostatic Botox still can be considered as a promising, safe, and minimally invasive procedure for patients with BPH who are not suitable for surgical intervention and who have an unsatisfactory response to standard drug therapy [132,133].

7.3. Perspectives of Botox Injections for Male LUTS/BPH

For men with symptomatic BPH, Botox injection into the prostate is a minimally invasive, safe, and effective procedure. The mechanisms of relief of LUTS might not depend completely on reducing prostate volume [123]. A previous study of Botox urethral-sphincter injection in patients with voiding dysfunction revealed that 61.1% of patients could benefit from this treatment [134]. In women with voiding dysfunction, Botox urethral injection can significantly improve LUTS without altering Qmax and voiding detrusor pressure [135]. These results indicate that the inhibitory effect on urethral smooth muscle or abnormal sensory function might play an important role in the therapeutic effects of Botox on voiding dysfunction and LUTS [123]. Furthermore, whether the dosage of Botox can affect therapeutic efficacy has not been well elucidated [136].

Based on the above evidence, there are several critical points that should be addressed in the future to clarify the therapeutic role of Botox on male LUTS/BPH: (1) the therapeutic effect of Botox injection to the bladder neck in the treatment of urodynamically proven bladder neck dysfunction in male LUTS; (2) the therapeutic effect of Botox prostatic injections between male patients with LUTS and different prostatic volumes and obstructive severity; (3) the therapeutic efficacy of Botox urethral injection in male patients with LUTS who have a small prostate volume and urodynamic BOO and non-BOO; and (4) the treatment outcomes of different doses of Botox (100 U or 200 U) and injecting sites (prostate gland or prostatic urethral smooth muscle) in male patients with LUTS who have a small prostatic volume.

8. Potential Clinical Applications of Botox on Recurrent UTI, Detrusor Underactivity, and AD

8.1. Will Botox Injection Reduce Episodes of UTI in Neurogenic LUTD?

Deficits and inflammation in the bladder urothelial barrier have been found to be increased in patients with chronic SCI, resulting in chronic inflammation and increased apoptosis and contributing to recurrent UTI in patients with NDO and DSD [137]. The expressions of the γEpithelial Na(+) channel and the acid-sensing ion channel 1 in the urothelium of patients with NDO have been found, which might have an impact on impaired mechanosensory function and low bladder compliance [138]. Because Botox can reduce detrusor pressure and episodes of involuntary detrusor contractions, intravesical Botox injections may decrease the incidence of symptomatic UTI in patients with NDO and low bladder compliance [139]. Women with recurrent UTI may have different voiding dysfunction due to DO or DV, resulting in damage to the integrity of the urothelial barrier and invasion by uropathogens [139]. Injecting Botox into the urethral sphincter may also decrease urethral resistance and voiding detrusor pressure, and patients with OAB and DV might experience fewer UTI episodes after Botox injections [140].

8.2. Risk of UTI after Botox Injection in Patients with OAB and IC/BPS

UTI is a major complication after intravesical Botox injections for NDO, OAB, and IC/BPS. Although UTI can be treated with antibiotics, the occurrence of this adverse event might prohibit patients from receiving this treatment after their first UTI experience following Botox injection. A recent study reported that the administration of a first Botox injection within 30 days of a UTI does not increase the risk of post-Botox UTI [141]. Patients with prior prolapse surgery or with recurrent UTI may have a higher risk of UTI after a Botox procedure [142]. Actually, Botox injection may improve bladder and bladder outlet functions, resulting in a reduction in UTI incidence [143]. In patients with NDO with 20 or 30 sites of Botox injections, the most common bacterium detected was *Escherichia coli*; however, the incidence of UTI was similar between groups [144].

8.3. What Are the Predictors for Successful Botox Treatment on DU?

Because Botox injection may decrease urethral resistance, it has been hypothesized that patients with DU or detrusor acontractility might benefit from urethral Botox injections. Chinese botulinum toxin A, Prosigne®, had been shown to be effective for treating an underactive bladder. After Botox injection, the Qmax increased, maximum urethral pressure decreased, and PVR decreased; however, the therapeutic effect seemed to last for only 3 months [145]. In a recently published article, female patients with DU showed improvement in voiding efficiency after urethral Botox injections, but patients with very low detrusor contractility, an absence of bladder sensation, and a tight bladder neck in a videourodynamic study showed less-favorable treatment outcomes [146].

Urethral sphincter Botox injections for voiding dysfunction were found to be effective in 60% of patients with DU, including 74.1% of patients with non-neurogenic DU and 48.5% of patients with neurogenic DU, yet the duration of the therapeutic effect was similar between patients with non-neurogenic and neurogenic DU [147]. The good treatment outcome was not related to age, gender, or videourodynamic subtypes. An open bladder neck during straining to voiding was the key factor in a successful result [147].

8.4. Perspectives of Botox Injections for Autonomic Dysreflexia (AD) in Patients with SCI and Neurogenic LUTD

Several issues are difficult to treat using medication or surgery. Because Botox has an anti-inflammatory mechanism of action, LUTDs related to chronic inflammation might be treated with Botox injection at the target organ or afferent nerves to achieve a satisfactory result [148]. In patients with chronic SCI, AD is a challenge for urological management, and Botox injection might reduce AD severity and improve the quality of life of these patients. There are some important questions to be resolved in future research: (1) Is AD an indication for Botox injection in patients with spinal cord lesion? (2) What is the optimal dose of Botox, and how frequently should patients be injected? (3) What is the therapeutic efficacy of the treatment of AD between injecting Botox into the detrusor and urethral sphincter? (4) Can Botox injection reduce the severity of AD after AE for patients with SCI who have a severely contracted bladder and AD?

Table 1 lists the clinical applications of Botox on lower urinary tract diseases or dysfunctions, and the dose, route, indications, adverse events after Botox injection or instillations. Although Botox has been launched for treatment of urological diseases for more than three decades, there should have more we can learn from the past researches and clinical trials. Through modification of dose adjustment, injection techniques, and the help of vehicles to carry Botox protein into the tissue, there should have more applications in the future to solve some urological diseases and dysfunctions that are not appropriately treated by the conventional medications.

Table 1. Current application of botulinum toxin A on lower-urinary-tract diseases or dysfunctions.

LUTD	Dose and Route	Indications	Adverse Events	References
Overactive bladder	100 U detrusor	Urinary incontinence Frequency urgency	Difficult urination Urine retention, UTI	[2,4,7–12,15,16,18,19,33,35–38]
Overactive bladder	200 U liposome encapsulated	Urinary incontinence Frequency urgency		[26,27]
Neurogenic DO	200 U–300 U	SCI, MS with UUI	Need CIC, UTI	[41–51,54–56,61,99]
IC/BPS	100 U detrusor	IC/BPS, ketamine cystitis	Difficult urination Urine retention, UTI	[70–72,74,76–84]
IC/BPS	100 U liposome encapsulated	IC/BPS	UTI	[29,85]
	200 U LESW	IC/BPS		[32]
Pediatric NDO and OAB	5 U/Kg detrusor	Non-neurogenic OAB, Urinary incontinence	UTI	[52,86–98,101]
Neurogenic DSD	100 U urethral sphincter	Dysuria, urine retention	Urinary incontinence, UTI, AD	[40,57,103–106,109–115]
Neurogenic AD	100 U bladder neck 200 U detrusor	Dysuria, AD	UTI	[148]
Male LUTS/BPH	200 U prostate	Dysuria, urine retention	UTI	[122–129,131–133,136]
Bladder neck dysfunction	100 U bladder neck	Dysuria,	Urinary incontinence	[130]
Non-neurogenic voiding dysfunction	100 U bladder neck, urethral sphincter	DV, DU, PRES	Urinary incontinence, UTI	[107,108,111,116–121,134,135,145–147]

9. Conclusions

Botox has been used in functional urology for more than 20 years. The licensed applications are limited to the treatment of OAB and NDO. However, because the pharmacologic mechanisms include inhibiting the release of neuropeptides, neuromodulation, anti-inflammatory effects, and antisense actions, Botox can be used in various LUTDs that are difficult to treat using conventional medications or surgical procedures. Advancing the clinical applications of Botox in LUTD necessitates further clinical and basic research to broaden the scope of its therapeutic effects.

Funding: This research received no external funding.

Institutional Review Board Statement: Not applicable.

Informed Consent Statement: Not applicable.

Conflicts of Interest: The authors declare no conflict of interest.

Abbreviations

AD	autonomic dysreflexia
AE	augmentation enterocystoplasty
BOO	bladder outlet obstruction
Botox	botulinum toxin A
BPH	benign prostatic hyperplasia
DO	detrusor overactivity
DSD	detrusor–sphincter dyssynergia
DV	dysfunctional voiding
IC/BPS	interstitial cystitis/bladder pain syndrome
IPSS	International Prostate Symptom Score
LESW	lower-energy shock wave
LUTD	lower-urinary-tract dysfunction
LUTS	lower-urinary-tract symptoms

MS	multiple sclerosis
NDO	neurogenic detrusor overactivity
OAB	overactive bladder
Pdet	detrusor pressure
PRES	poorly relaxed external sphincter
PTNS	percutaneous tibial nerve stimulation
PVR	post-void residual
Qmax	maximum flow rate
SCI	spinal-cord injury
SNM	sacral-nerve neuromodulation
UTI	urinary-tract infection
UUI	urgency urinary incontinence

References

1. Jhang, J.F.; Kuo, H.C. Botulinum toxin A and lower urinary tract dysfunction: Pathophysiology and mechanisms of action. *Toxins* **2016**, *8*, 120. [CrossRef] [PubMed]
2. Sahai, A.; Khan, M.S.; Gregson, N.; Smith, K.; Dasgupta, P.; GKT Botulinum Study Group. Botulinum toxin for detrusor overactivity and symptoms of overactive bladder: Where we are now and where we are going. *Nat. Clin. Pract. Urol.* **2007**, *4*, 379–386. [CrossRef]
3. Dolly, J.O.; O'Connell, M.A. Neurotherapeutics to inhibit exocytosis from sensory neurons for the control of chronic pain. *Curr. Opin. Pharmacol.* **2012**, *12*, 100–108. [CrossRef]
4. Mangera, A.; Apostolidis, A.; Andersson, K.E.; Dasgupta, P.; Giannantoni, A.; Roehrborn, C.; Novara, G.; Chapple, C. An updated systematic review and statistical comparison of standardised mean outcomes for the use of botulinum toxin in the management of lower urinary tract disorders. *Eur. Urol.* **2014**, *65*, 981–990. [CrossRef] [PubMed]
5. Chancellor, M.B.; Fowler, C.J.; Apostolidis, A.; de Groat, W.C.; Smith, C.P.; Somogyi, G.T.; Aoki, K.R. Drug insight: Biological effects of botulinum toxin A in the lower urinary tract. *Nat. Clin. Pract. Urol.* **2008**, *5*, 319–328. [CrossRef] [PubMed]
6. Apostolidis, A.; Popat, R.; Yiangou, Y.; Cockayne, D.; Ford, A.P.D.W.; Davis, J.B.; Dasgupta, P.; Fowler, C.J.; Anand, P. Decreased sensory receptors P2X3 and TRPV1 in suburothelial nerve fibers following intradetrusor injections of botulinum toxin for human detrusor overactivity. *J. Urol.* **2005**, *174*, 977–983. [CrossRef] [PubMed]
7. Nitti, V.W.; Dmochowski, R.; Herschorn, S.; Sand, P.; Thompson, C.; Nardo, C.; Yan, X.; Haag-Molkenteller, C.; EMBARK Study Group. OnabotulinumtoxinA for the treatment of patients with overactive bladder and urinary incontinence: Results of a phase 3, randomized, placebo controlled trial. *J. Urol.* **2013**, *189*, 2186–2193. [CrossRef]
8. Chapple, C.; Sievert, K.D.; MacDiarmid, S.; Khullar, V.; Radziszewski, P.; Nardo, C.; Thompson, C.; Zhou, J.; Haag-Molkenteller, C. OnabotulinumtoxinA 100 U significantly improves all idiopathic overactive bladder symptoms and quality of life in patients with overactive bladder and urinary incontinence: A randomised, double-blind, placebo-controlled trial. *Eur. Urol.* **2013**, *64*, 249–256. [CrossRef]
9. Kuo, H.C. Clinical effects of suburothelial injection of botulinum A toxin on patients with nonneurogenic detrusor overactivity refractory to anticholinergics. *Urology* **2005**, *66*, 94–98. [CrossRef]
10. Kuo, H.C. Bladder base/trigone injection is safe and as effective as bladder body injection of onabotulinumtoxinA for idiopathic detrusor overactivity refractory to antimuscarinics. *Neurourol. Urodyn.* **2011**, *30*, 1242–1248. [CrossRef]
11. Makovey, I.; Davis, T.; Guralnick, M.L.; O'Connor, R.C. Botulinum toxin outcomes for idiopathic overactive bladder stratified by indication: Lack of anticholinergic efficacy versus intolerability. *Neurourol. Urodyn.* **2011**, *30*, 1538–1540. [CrossRef] [PubMed]
12. Sievert, K.D.; Chapple, C.; Herschorn, S.; Joshi, M.; Zhou, J.; Nardo, C.; Nitti, V.W. OnabotulinumtoxinA 100 U provides significant improvements in overactive bladder symptoms in patients with urinary incontinence regardless of the number of anticholinergic therapies used or reason for inadequate management of overactive bladder. *Int. J. Clin. Pract.* **2014**, *68*, 1246–1256. [CrossRef] [PubMed]
13. Gormley, E.A.; Lightner, D.J.; Faraday, M.; Vasavada, S.P. Diagnosis and treatment of overactive bladder (Non-Neurogenic) in adults: AUA/SUFU guideline amendment. *J. Urol.* **2015**, *193*, 1572–1580. [CrossRef] [PubMed]
14. Apostolidis, A.; Dasgupta, P.; Denys, P.; Elneil, S.; Fowler, C.J.; Giannantoni, A.; Karsenty, G.; Schulte-Baukloh, H.; Schurch, B.; Wyndaele, J.J.; et al. Recommendations on the use of botulinum toxin in the treatment of lower urinary tract disorders and pelvic floor dysfunctions: A European consensus report. *Eur. Urol.* **2009**, *55*, 100–119. [CrossRef]
15. Veeratterapillay, R.; Harding, C.; Teo, L.; Vasdev, N.; Abroaf, A.; Dorkin, T.J.; Pickard, R.S.; Hasan, T.; Thorpe, A.C.; Veeratterapillay, R.; et al. Discontinuation rates and inter-injection interval for repeated intravesical botulinum toxin type A injections for detrusor overactivity. *Int. J. Urol.* **2014**, *21*, 175–178. [CrossRef]
16. Hendrickson, W.K.; Xie, G.; Rahn, D.D.; Amundsen, C.L.; Hokanson, J.A.; Bradley, M.; Smith, A.L.; Sung, V.W.; Visco, A.G.; Luo, S.; et al. Predicting outcomes after intradetrusor onabotulinumtoxina for non-neurogenic urgency incontinence in women. *Neurourol. Urodyn.* **2022**, *41*, 432–447. [CrossRef]
17. Wang, C.C.; Lee, C.L.; Hwang, Y.T.; Kuo, H.C. Adding mirabegron after intravesical onabotulinumtoxinA injection improves therapeutic effects in patients with refractory overactive bladder. Low. *Urin. Tract Symptoms* **2021**, *13*, 440–447. [CrossRef]

18. Baron, M.; Aublé, A.; Paret, F.; Pfister, C.; Cornu, J.N. Long-term follow-up reveals a low persistence rate of abobotulinumtoxinA injections for idiopathic overactive bladder. *Prog. Urol.* **2020**, *30*, 684–691. [CrossRef]
19. De Rienzo, G.; Minafra, P.; Iliano, E.; Agrò, E.F.; Serati, M.; Giammò, A.; Bianchi, F.P.; Costantini, E.; Ditonno, P.; Italian Society of Urodynamics (SIUD). Evaluation of the effect of 100 U of Onabotulinum toxin A on detrusor contractility in women with idiopathic OAB: A multicentre prospective study. *Neurourol. Urodyn.* **2022**, *41*, 306–312. [CrossRef]
20. Kopcsay, K.S.; Marczak, T.D.; Jeppson, P.C.; Cameron, A.P.; Khavari, R.; Tefera, E.; Gutman, R.E. Treatment of refractory overactive bladder with onabotulinumtoxinA vs. PTNS: TROOP trial. *Int. Urogynecol. J.* **2022**, *33*, 851–860. [CrossRef]
21. Lo, C.W.; Wu, M.Y.; Yang, S.S.; Jaw, F.S.; Chang, S.J. Comparing the efficacy of onabotulinumtoxinA, sacral neuromodulation, and peripheral tibial nerve stimulation as third line treatment for the management of overactive bladder symptoms in adults: Systematic review and network meta-analysis. *Toxins* **2020**, *12*, 128. [CrossRef] [PubMed]
22. High, R.A.; Winkelman, W.; Panza, J.; Sanderson, D.J.; Yuen, H.; Halder, G.; Shaver, C.; Bird, E.T.; Rogers, R.G.; Danford, J.M. Sacral neuromodulation for overactive bladder in women: Do age and comorbidities make a difference? *Int. Urogynecol. J.* **2021**, *32*, 149–157. [CrossRef] [PubMed]
23. Harvie, H.S.; Amundsen, C.L.; Neuwahl, S.J.; Honeycutt, A.A.; Lukacz, E.S.; Sung, V.W.; Rogers, R.G.; Ellington, D.; Ferrando, C.A.; Chermansky, C.J.; et al. Cost-effectiveness of sacral neuromodulation versus onabotulinumtoxinA for refractory urgency urinary incontinence: Results of the ROSETTA randomized trial. *J. Urol.* **2020**, *203*, 969–977. [CrossRef] [PubMed]
24. Reekmans, M.; Janssen, J.M.W.; Vrijens, D.M.J.; Smits, M.A.C.; van Koeveringe, G.A.; Van Kerrebroeck, P.E.V.A. Sacral neuromodulation in patients with refractory overactive bladder symptoms after failed botulinum toxin herapy: Results in a large cohort of patients. *Neurourol. Urodyn.* **2021**, *40*, 1120–1125. [CrossRef]
25. Amundsen, C.L.; Komesu, Y.M.; Chermansky, C.; Gregory, W.T.; Myers, D.L.; Honeycutt, E.F.; Vasavada, S.P.; Nguyen, J.N.; Wilson, T.S.; Harvie, H.S.; et al. Two-year outcomes of sacral neuromodulation versus onabotulinumtoxinA for refractory urgency urinary incontinence: A randomized trial. *Eur. Urol.* **2018**, *74*, 66–73. [CrossRef]
26. Kuo, H.C.; Liu, H.T.; Chuang, Y.C.; Birder, L.A.; Chancellor, M.B. Pilot study of liposome-encapsulated onabotulinumtoxina for patients with overactive bladder: A single-center study. *Eur. Urol.* **2014**, *65*, 1117–1124. [CrossRef]
27. Chuang, Y.C.; Kaufmann, J.H.; Chancellor, D.D.; Chancellor, M.B.; Kuo, H.C. Bladder instillation of liposome encapsulated onabotulinumtoxina improves overactive bladder symptoms: A prospective, multicenter, double-blind, randomized trial. *J. Urol.* **2014**, *192*, 1743–1749. [CrossRef]
28. Liu, H.T.; Chen, S.H.; Chancellor, M.B.; Kuo, H.C. Presence of cleaved synaptosomal-associated protein-25 and decrease of purinergic receptors P2X3 in the bladder urothelium influence efficacy of botulinum toxin treatment for overactive bladder syndrome. *PLoS ONE* **2015**, *10*, e0134803. [CrossRef]
29. Chuang, Y.C.; Kuo, H.C. A prospective, multicenter, double-blind, randomized trial of bladder instillation of liposome formulation onabotulinumtoxinA for interstitial cystitis/bladder pain syndrome. *J. Urol.* **2017**, *198*, 376–382. [CrossRef]
30. Jiang, Y.H.; Yu, W.R.; Kuo, H.C. Therapeutic effect of botulinum toxin A on sensory bladder disorders-fom bench to bedside. *Toxins* **2020**, *12*, 166. [CrossRef]
31. Chen, P.Y.; Cheng, J.H.; Wu, Z.S.; Chuang, Y.C. New frontiers of extracorporeal shock wave medicine in urology from bench to clinical studies. *Biomedicines* **2022**, *10*, 675. [CrossRef] [PubMed]
32. Jiang, Y.H.; Jhang, J.F.; Lee, Y.K.; Kuo, H.C. Low-energy shock wave plus intravesical instillation of botulinum toxin A for interstitial cystitis/bladder pain syndrome: Pathophysiology and preliminary result of a novel minimally invasive treatment. *Biomedicines* **2022**, *10*, 396. [CrossRef] [PubMed]
33. Truzzi, J.C.; Lapitan, M.C.; Truzzi, N.C.; Iacovelli, V.; Averbeck, M.A. Botulinum toxin for treating overactive bladder in men: A systematic review. *Neurourol. Urodyn.* **2022**, *41*, 710–723. [CrossRef] [PubMed]
34. Reynolds, W.S.; Suskind, A.M.; Anger, J.T.; Brucker, B.M.; Cameron, A.P.; Chung, D.E.; Daignault-Newton, S.; Lane, G.I.; Lucioni, A.; Mourtzinos, A.P.; et al. Incomplete bladder emptying and urinary tract infections after botulinum toxin injection for overactive bladder: Multi-institutional collaboration from the SUFU research network. *Neurourol. Urodyn.* **2022**, *41*, 662–671. [CrossRef] [PubMed]
35. Liao, C.H.; Kuo, H.C. Increased risk of large post-void residual urine and decreased long-term success rate after intravesical onabotulinumtoxinA injection for refractory idiopathic detrusor overactivity. *J. Urol.* **2013**, *189*, 1804–1810. [CrossRef]
36. Manns, K.; Khan, A.; Carlson, K.V.; Wagg, A.; Baverstock, R.J.; Trafford Crump, R. The use of onabotulinumtoxinA to treat idiopathic overactive bladder in elderly patients is in need of study. *Neurourol. Urodyn.* **2022**, *41*, 42–47. [CrossRef] [PubMed]
37. Kuo, H.C.; Liao, C.H.; Chung, S.D. Adverse events of intravesical botulinum toxin A injections for idiopathic detrusor overactivity: Risk factors and influence on treatment outcome. *Eur. Urol.* **2010**, *58*, 919–926. [CrossRef]
38. Abrar, M.; Pindoria, N.; Malde, S.; Chancellor, M.; DeRidder, D.; Sahai, A. Predictors of poor response and adverse events following botulinum toxin A for refractory idiopathic overactive bladder: A systematic review. *Eur. Urol. Focus* **2021**, *7*, 1448–1467. [CrossRef]
39. Shawer, S.; Khunda, A.; Waring, G.J.; Ballard, P. Impact of intravesical onabotulinumtoxinA (Botox) on sexual function in patients with overactive bladder syndrome: A systematic review and meta-analysis. *Int. Urogynecol. J.* **2022**, *33*, 235–243. [CrossRef]
40. Dykstra, D.D.; Sidi, A.A.; Scott, A.B.; Pagel, J.M.; Goldish, G.D. Effects of botulinum A toxin on detrusor-sphincter dyssynergia in spinal cord injury patients. *J. Urol.* **1988**, *139*, 919–922. [CrossRef]

41. Schurch, B.; de Sèze, M.; Denys, P.; Chartier-Kastler, E.; Haab, F.; Everaert, K.; Plante, P.; Perrouin-Verbe, B.; Kumar, C.; Fraczek, S.; et al. Botulinum toxin type a is a safe and effective treatment for neurogenic urinary incontinence: Results of a single treatment, randomized, placebo controlled 6-month study. *J. Urol.* **2005**, *174*, 196–200. [CrossRef]
42. Kalsi, V.; Apostolidis, A.; Popat, R.; Gonzales, G.; Fowler, C.J.; Dasgupta, P. Quality of life changes in patients with neurogenic versus idiopathic detrusor overactivity after intradetrusor injections of botulinum neurotoxin type A and correlations with lower urinary tract symptoms and urodynamic changes. *Eur. Urol.* **2006**, *49*, 528–535. [CrossRef]
43. Conte, A.; Giannantoni, A.; Proietti, S.; Giovannozzi, S.; Fabbrini, G.; Rossi, A.; Porena, M.; Berardelli, A. Botulinum toxin A modulates afferent fibers in neurogenic detrusor overactivity. *Eur. J. Neurol.* **2012**, *19*, 725–732. [CrossRef]
44. Gamé, X.; Castel-Lacanal, E.; Bentaleb, Y.; Thiry-Escudié, I.; De Boissezon, X.; Malavaud, B.; Marque, P.; Rischmann, P. Botulinum toxin A detrusor injections in patients with neurogenic detrusor overactivity significantly decrease the incidence of symptomatic urinary tract infections. *Eur. Urol.* **2008**, *53*, 613–618. [CrossRef] [PubMed]
45. Hori, S.; Patki, P.; Attar, K.H.; Ismail, S.; Vasconcelos, J.C.; Shah, P.J.R. Patients' perspective of botulinum toxin-A as a long-term treatment option for neurogenic detrusor overactivity secondary to spinal cord injury. *Br. J. Urol.* **2009**, *104*, 216–220. [CrossRef] [PubMed]
46. Cruz, F.; Herschorn, S.; Aliotta, P.; Brin, M.; Thompson, C.; Lam, W.; Daniell, G.; Heesakkers, J.; Haag-Molkenteller, C. Efficacy and safety of onabotulinumtoxinA in patients with urinary incontinence due to neurogenic detrusor overactivity: A randomised, double-blind, placebo-controlled trial. *Eur. Urol.* **2011**, *60*, 742–750. [CrossRef] [PubMed]
47. Ginsberg, D.; Gousse, A.; Keppenne, V.; Sievert, K.D.; Thompson, C.; Lam, W.; Brin, M.F.; Jenkins, B.; Haag-Molkenteller, C. Phase 3 efficacy and tolerability study of onabotulinumtoxinA for urinary incontinence from neurogenic detrusor overactivity. *J. Urol.* **2012**, *187*, 2131–2139. [CrossRef]
48. Herschorn, S.; Gajewski, J.; Ethans, K.; Corcos, J.; Carlson, K.; Bailly, G.; Bard, R.; Valiquette, L.; Baverstock, R.; Carr, L.; et al. Efficacy of botulinum toxin A injection for neurogenic detrusor overactivity and urinary incontinence: A randomized, double-blind trial. *J. Urol.* **2011**, *185*, 2229–2235. [CrossRef]
49. Wang, C.C.; Chou, E.C.; Chuang, Y.C.; Lin, C.C.; Hsu, Y.C.; Liao, C.H.; Kuo, H.C. Effectiveness and safety of intradetrusor onabotulinumtoxinA injection for neurogenic detrusor overactivity and overactive bladder patients in Taiwan—A phase IV prospective, iterventional, Mmultiple-center study (rstore Sstudy). *Toxins* **2021**, *13*, 911. [CrossRef]
50. Cheng, T.; Shuang, W.B.; Jia, D.D.; Zhang, M.; Tong, X.N.; Yang, W.D.; Jia, X.M.; Li, S. Efficacy and safety of onabotulinumtoxinA in ptients with Nnurogenic detrusor overactivity: A systematic review and meta-analysis of randomized controlled trials. *PLoS ONE* **2016**, *11*, e0159307.
51. Krebs, J.; Pannek, J.; Rademacher, F.; Wöllner, J. Are 200 units of onabotulinumtoxin A sufficient for the suppression of neurogenic detrusor overactivity in individuals with established 300-unit botulinum toxin treatment? A retrospective cohort study. *World J. Urol.* **2021**, *39*, 543–547. [CrossRef] [PubMed]
52. Mackay, A.; Sosland, R.; Tran, K.; Stewart, J.; Boone, T.; Khavari, R. Prospective Evaluation of intradetrusor injections of onabotulinumtoxinA in adults with spinal dysraphism. *Urology* **2022**, *161*, 146–152. [CrossRef] [PubMed]
53. Honda, M.; Yokoyama, O.; Takahashi, R.; Matsuda, T.; Nakayama, T.; Mogi, T. Botulinum toxin injections for Japanese patients with urinary incontinence caused by neurogenic detrusor overactivity: Clinical evaluation of onabotulinumtoxinA in a randomized, placebo-controlled, double-blind trial with an open-label extension. *Int. J. Urol.* **2021**, *28*, 906–912. [CrossRef]
54. Hebert, K.P.; Klarskov, N.; Bagi, P.; Biering-Sørensen, F.; Elmelund, M. Long term continuation with repeated Botulinum toxin A injections in people with neurogenic detrusor overactivity after spinal cord injury. *Spinal Cord* **2020**, *58*, 675–681. [CrossRef] [PubMed]
55. Ni, J.; Wang, X.; Cao, N.; Si, J.; Gu, B. Is repeat botulinum toxin A injection valuable for neurogenic detrusor overactivity—A systematic review and meta-analysis. *Neurourol. Urodyn.* **2018**, *37*, 542–553. [CrossRef]
56. O'Connor, R.C.; Johnson, D.P.; Guralnick, M.L. Intradetrusor botulinum toxin injections (300 units) for the treatment of poorly compliant bladders in patients with adult neurogenic lower urinary tract dysfunction. *Neurourol. Urodyn.* **2020**, *39*, 2322–2328. [CrossRef]
57. Lee, C.L.; Jhang, J.F.; Jiang, Y.H.; Kuo, H.C. Real-world data regarding satisfaction to botulinum toxin A injection into the urethral sphincter and further bladder management for voiding dysfunction among patients with spinal cord injury and voiding dysfunction. *Toxins* **2022**, *14*, 30. [CrossRef]
58. Lin, C.C.; Kuo, H.C. Video-urodynamic characteristics and predictors of switching from botulinum neurotoxin A injection to augmentation enterocystoplasty in spinal cord injury patients. *Toxins* **2022**, *14*, 47. [CrossRef]
59. Michel, F.; Ciceron, C.; Bernuz, B.; Boissier, R.; Gaillet, S.; Even, A.; Chartier-Kastler, E.; Denys, P.; Gamé, X.; Ruffion, A.; et al. Botulinum toxin type A injection after failure of augmentation enterocystoplasty performed for neurogenic detrusor overactivity: Preliminary results of a salvage strategy. The ENTEROTOX Study. *Urology* **2019**, *129*, 43–47. [CrossRef]
60. Baron, M.; Peyronnet, B.; Aublé, A.; Hascoet, J.; Castel-Lacanal, E.; Miget, G.; Le Doze, S.; Prudhomme, T.; Manunta, A.; Cornu, J.N.; et al. Long-term discontinuation of botulinum toxin A intradetrusor injections for neurogenic detrusor overactivity: A multicenter study. *J. Urol.* **2019**, *201*, 769–776. [CrossRef]
61. Chen, S.F.; Jiang, Y.H.; Jhang, J.F.; Kuo, H.C. Satisfaction with detrusor onabotulinumtoxinA injections and cnversion to other badder management in patients with chronic spinal cord injury. *Toxins* **2022**, *14*, 35. [CrossRef] [PubMed]
62. Nickle, J.C. Interstitial cystitis: A chronic pelvic pain syndrome. *Med. Clin. N. Am.* **2004**, *88*, 467–481. [CrossRef]

63. Nickel, J.C.; Shoskes, D.; Irvine-Bird, K. Clinical phenotyping of women with interstitial cystitis/painful bladder syndrome: A key to classification and potentially improved management. *J. Urol.* **2009**, *182*, 155–160. [CrossRef]
64. Tripp, D.A.; Nickel, J.C.; Wong, J.; Pontari, M.; Moldwin, R.; Mayer, R.; Carr, L.K.; Doggweiler, R.; Yang, C.C.; Mishra, N.; et al. Mapping of pain phenotypes in female patients with bladder pain syndrome/interstitial cystitis and controls. *Eur. Urol.* **2012**, *62*, 1188–1194. [CrossRef] [PubMed]
65. Slobodov, G.; Feloney, M.; Gran, C.; Kyker, K.D.; Hurst, R.E.; Culkin, D.J. Abnormal expression of molecular markers for bladder impermeability and differentiation in the urothelium of patients with interstitial cystitis. *J. Urol.* **2004**, *171*, 1554–1558. [CrossRef] [PubMed]
66. Daha, L.K.; Riedl, C.R.; Lazar, D.; Simak, R.; Pflüger, H. Effect of intravesical glycosaminoglycan substitution therapy on bladder pain syndrome/interstitial cystitis, bladder capacity and potassium sensitivity. *Scand. J. Urol. Nephrol.* **2008**, *42*, 369–372. [CrossRef] [PubMed]
67. Hurst, R.E.; Roy, J.B.; Min, K.W.; Veltri, R.W.; Marley, G.; Patton, K.; Shackelford, D.L.; Stein, P.; Parsons, C.L. A deficit of chondroitin sulfate proteoglycans on the bladder uroepithelium in interstitial cystitis. *Urology* **1996**, *48*, 817–821. [CrossRef]
68. Shim, S.R.; Cho, Y.J.; Shin, I.S.; Kim, J.H. Efficacy and safety of botulinum toxin injection for interstitial cystitis/bladder pain syndrome: A systematic review and meta-analysis. *Int. Urol. Nephrol.* **2016**, *48*, 1215–1227. [CrossRef]
69. Smith, C.P.; Radziszewski, P.; Borkowski, A.; Somogyi, G.T.; Boone, T.B.; Chancellor, M.B. Botulinum toxin A has antinociceptive effects in treating interstitial cystitis. *Urology* **2004**, *64*, 871–875. [CrossRef]
70. Giannantoni, A.; Porena, M.; Costantini, E.; Zucchi, A.; Mearini, L.; Mearini, E. Botulinum A toxin intravesical injection in patients with painful bladder syndrome: 1-year followup. *J. Urol.* **2008**, *179*, 1031–1034. [CrossRef]
71. Giannantoni, A.; Cagini, R.; Del Zingaro, M.; Proietti, S.; Quartesan, R.; Porena, M.; Piselli, M. Botulinum A toxin intravesical injections for painful bladder syndrome: Impact upon pain, psychological functioning and quality of Life. *Curr. Drug. Deliv.* **2010**, *7*, 442–446. [CrossRef]
72. Kuo, H.C.; Chancellor, M.B. Comparison of intravesical botulinum toxin type A injections plus hydrodistention with hydrodistention alone for the treatment of refractory interstitial cystitis/painful bladder syndrome. *BJU. Int.* **2009**, *104*, 657–661. [CrossRef] [PubMed]
73. Shie, J.H.; Liu, H.T.; Wang, Y.S.; Kuo, H.C. Immunohistochemical evidence suggests repeated intravesical application of botulinum toxin A injections may improve treatment efficacy of interstitial cystitis/bladder pain syndrome. *BJU. Int.* **2013**, *111*, 638–646. [CrossRef] [PubMed]
74. Kuo, H.C.; Jiang, Y.H.; Tsai, Y.C.; Kuo, Y.C. Intravesical botulinum toxin-A injections reduce bladder pain of interstitial cystitis/bladder pain syndrome refractory to conventional treatment—A prospective, multicenter, randomized, double-blind, placebo-controlled clinical trial. *Neurourol. Urodyn.* **2016**, *35*, 609–614. [CrossRef]
75. Chen, C.L.; Meng, E. Can botulinum toxin A play a role In treatment of chronic pelvic pain syndrome in fmale patients?—Clinical and animal evidence. *Toxins* **2020**, *12*, 110. [CrossRef]
76. Chuang, F.C.; Yang, T.H.; Kuo, H.C. Botulinum toxin A injection in the treatment of chronic pelvic pain with hypertonic pelvic floor in women: Treatment techniques and results. *Low. Urin. Tract Symptoms* **2021**, *13*, 5–12. [CrossRef] [PubMed]
77. Lee, C.L.; Kuo, H.C. Intravesical botulinum toxin a injections do not benefit patients with ulcer type interstitial cystitis. *Pain Physician* **2013**, *16*, 109–116. [PubMed]
78. Lee, C.L.; Kuo, H.C. Long-term efficacy and safety of repeated intravescial onabotulinumtoxinA injections plus hydrodistention in the treatment of interstitial cystitis/badder pain syndrome. *Toxins* **2015**, *7*, 4283–4293. [CrossRef]
79. Jiang, Y.H.; Jhang, J.F.; Lee, C.L.; Kuo, H.C. Comparative study of efficacy and safety between bladder body and trigonal intravesical onabotulinumtoxina injection in the treatment of interstitial cystitis refractory to conventional treatment—A prospective, randomized, clinical trial. *Neurourol. Urodyn.* **2018**, *37*, 1467–1473. [CrossRef]
80. Wang, H.J.; Yu, W.R.; Ong, H.L.; Kuo, H.C. Predictive factors for a satisfactory treatment outcome with intravesical botulinum toxin A injection in patients with interstitial cystitis/badder pain syndrome. *Toxins* **2019**, *11*, 676. [CrossRef]
81. Dobberfuhl, A.D.; van Uem, S.; Versi, E. Trigone as a diagnostic and therapeutic target for bladder-centric interstitial cystitis/bladder pain syndrome. *Int. Urogynecol. J.* **2021**, *32*, 3105–3111. [CrossRef] [PubMed]
82. Pinto, R.; Lopes, T.; Frias, B.; Silva, A.; Silva, J.A.; Silva, C.M.; Cruz, C.; Cruz, F.; Dinis, P. Trigonal injection of botulinum toxin A in patients with refractory bladder pain syndrome/interstitial cystitis. *Eur. Urol.* **2010**, *58*, 360–365. [CrossRef] [PubMed]
83. Evans, R.J.; Overholt, T.; Colaco, M.; Walker, S.J. Injection location does not impact botulinum toxin A efficacy in interstitial cystitis/bladder pain syndrome patients. *Can. J. Urol.* **2020**, *27*, 10125–10129. [PubMed]
84. Yunfeng, G.; Fei, L.; Junbo, L.; Dingyuan, Y.; Chaoyou, H. An indirect comparison meta-analysis of noninvasive intravesical instillation and intravesical injection of botulinum toxin-A in bladder disorders. *Int. Urol. Nephrol.* **2022**, *54*, 479–491. [CrossRef]
85. Jhang, J.F.; Kuo, H.C. Novel applications of onabotulinumtoxinA in lower urinary tract dysfunction. *Toxins* **2018**, *10*, 260. [CrossRef]
86. Schulte-Baukloh, H.; Michael, T.; Schobert, J.; Stolze, T.; Knispel, H.H. Efficacy of botulinum-a toxin in children with detrusor hyperreflexia due to myelomeningocele: Preliminary results. *Urology* **2002**, *59*, 325–328. [CrossRef]
87. Riccabona, M. Botulinum-A toxin injection into the detrusor: A safe alternative in the treatment of children with myelomeningocele with detrusor hyperreflexia. *J. Urol.* **2004**, *171*, 845–848. [CrossRef]

88. Kajbafzadeh, A.M.; Moosavi, S.; Tajik, P.; Arshadi, H.; Payabvash, S.; Salmasi, A.H.; Akbari, H.R.; Nejat, F. Intravesical injection of botulinum toxin type A: Management of neuropathic bladder and bowel dysfunction in children with myelomeningocele. *Urology* **2006**, *68*, 1091–1097. [CrossRef]
89. Safari, S.; Jamali, S.; Habibollahi, P.; Arshadi, H.; Nejat, F.; Kajbafzadeh, A.M. Intravesical injections of botulinum toxin type A for management of neuropathic bladder: A comparison of two methods. *Urology* **2010**, *76*, 225–230. [CrossRef]
90. Marte, A.; Borrelli, M.; Sabatino, M.D.; Balzo, B.D.; Prezioso, M.; Pintozzi, L.; Nino, F.; Parmeggiani, P. Effectiveness of botulinum-A toxin for the treatment of refractory overactive bladder in children. *Eur. J. Pediatr. Surg.* **2010**, *20*, 153–157. [CrossRef]
91. Lahdes-Vasama, T.T.; Anttila, A.; Wahl, E.; Taskinen, S. Urodynamic assessment of children treated with botulinum toxin A injections for urge incontinence: A pilot study. *Scand. J. Urol. Nephrol.* **2011**, *45*, 397–400. [CrossRef] [PubMed]
92. McDowell, D.T.; Noone, D.; Tareen, F.; Waldron, M.; Quinn, F. Urinary incontinence in children: Botulinum toxin is a safe and effective treatment option. *Pediatr. Surg. Int.* **2012**, *28*, 315–320. [CrossRef] [PubMed]
93. Gamé, X.; Mouracade, P.; Chartier-Kastler, E.; Viehweger, E.; Moog, R.; Amarenco, G.; Denys, P.; De Seze, M.; Haab, F.; Karsenty, G.; et al. Botulinum toxin-A (Botox) intradetrusor injections in children with neurogenic detrusor overactivity/neurogenic overactive bladder: A systematic literature review. *J. Pediatr. Urol.* **2009**, *5*, 156–164. [CrossRef] [PubMed]
94. Austin, P.F.; Franco, I.; Dobremez, E.; Kroll, P.; Titanji, W.; Geib, T.; Jenkins, B.; Hoebeke, P.B. OnabotulinumtoxinA for the treatment of neurogenic detrusor overactivity in children. *Neurourol. Urodyn.* **2021**, *40*, 493–501. [CrossRef] [PubMed]
95. Softness, K.A.; Thaker, H.; Theva, D.; Rajender, A.; Cilento, B.G., Jr.; Bauer, S.B. Onabotulinumtoxin A (Botox): A reasonable alternative for refractory neurogenic bladder dysfunction in children and young adults. *Neurourol. Urodyn.* **2021**, *40*, 1981–1988. [CrossRef]
96. Lambregts, A.P.; Nieuwhof-Leppink, A.J.; Klijn, A.J.; Schroeder, R.P.J. Intravesical botulinum-A toxin in children with refractory non-neurogenic overactive bladder. *J. Pediatr. Urol.* **2022**, *18*, 351.e1–351.e8. [CrossRef]
97. Tan, D.J.Y.; Weninger, J.; Goyal, A. Mirabegron in overactive bladder and its role in exit strategy after botulinum toxin treatment in children. *Front. Pediatr.* **2022**, *9*, 801517. [CrossRef]
98. Greer, T.; Abbott, J.; Breytenbach, W.; McGuane, D.; Barker, A.; Khosa, J.; Samnakay, N. Ten years of experience with intravesical and intrasphincteric onabotulinumtoxinA in children. *J. Pediatr. Urol.* **2016**, *12*, 94.e1–94.e6. [CrossRef]
99. Sekerci, C.A.; Tanidir, Y.; Garayev, A.; Akbal, C.; Tarcan, T.; Simsek, F. Clinical and urodynamic results of repeated intradetrusor onabotulinum toxin A injections in refractory neurogenic dtrusor overactivity: Up to 5 injections in a cohort of children with myelodysplasia. *Urology* **2018**, *111*, 168–175. [CrossRef]
100. Joussain, C.; Popoff, M.; Phé, V.; Even, A.; Bosset, P.O.; Pottier, S.; Falcou, L.; Levy, J.; Vaugier, I.; Kastler, E.C.; et al. Long-term outcomes and risks factors for failure of intradetrusor onabotulinumtoxin A injections for the treatment of refractory neurogenic detrusor overactivity. *Neurourol. Urodyn.* **2018**, *37*, 799–806. [CrossRef]
101. Madec, F.X.; Suply, E.; Forin, V.; Chamond, O.; Lalanne, A.; Irtan, S.; Audry, G.; Lallemant, P. Repeated detrusor injection of botulinum toxin A for neurogenic bladder in children: A long term option? *Prog. Urol.* **2022**, *32*, 319–325. [CrossRef]
102. Kuo, H.C.; Liu, H.T. Investigation of dysfunctional voiding in children with urgency frequency syndrome and urinary incontinence. *Urol. Int.* **2006**, *76*, 72–76. [CrossRef] [PubMed]
103. Mokhless, I.; Gaafar, S.; Fouda, K.; Shafik, M.; Assem, A. Botulinum A toxin urethral sphincter injection in children with nonneurogenic neurogenic bladder. *J. Urol.* **2006**, *176*, 1767–1770. [CrossRef]
104. Vricella, G.J.; Campigotto, M.; Coplen, D.E.; Traxel, E.J.; Austin, P.F. Long-term efficacy and durability of botulinum-A toxin for refractory dysfunctional voiding in children. *J. Urol.* **2014**, *191*, 1586–1591. [CrossRef] [PubMed]
105. Franco, I.; Landau-Dyer, L.; Isom-Batz, G.; Collett, T.; Reda, E.F. The use of botulinum toxin A injection for the management of external sphincter dyssynergia in neurologically normal children. *J. Urol.* **2007**, *178*, 1775–1780. [CrossRef] [PubMed]
106. Dykstra, D.D.; Sidi, A.A. Treatment of detrusor-sphincter dyssynergia with botulinum A toxin: A double-blind study. *Arch. Phys. Med. Rehabil.* **1990**, *71*, 24–26.
107. Kuo, H.C. Botulinum A toxin urethral injection for the treatment of lower urinary tract dysfunction. *J. Urol.* **2003**, *170*, 1908–1912. [CrossRef]
108. Smith, C.P.; Chancellor, M.B. Emerging role of botulinum toxin in the treatment of voiding dysfunction. *J. Urol.* **2004**, *171*, 2128–2137. [CrossRef]
109. de Sèze, M.; Petit, H.; Gallien, P.; de Sèze, M.P.; Joseph, P.A.; Mazaux, J.M.; Barat, M. Botulinum a toxin and detrusor sphincter dyssynergia: A double-blind lidocaine-controlled study in 13 patients with spinal cord disease. *Eur. Urol.* **2002**, *42*, 56–62. [CrossRef]
110. Mehta, S.; Hill, D.; Foley, N.; Hsieh, J.; Ethans, K.; Potter, P.; Baverstock, R.; Teasell, R.W.; Wolfe, D. Spinal Cord Injury Rehabilitation Evidence Research Team. A meta-analysis of botulinum toxin sphincteric injections in the treatment of incomplete voiding after spinal cord injury. *Arch. Phys. Med. Rehabil.* **2012**, *93*, 597–603. [CrossRef]
111. Smith, C.P.; Nishiguchi, J.; O'Leary, M.; Yoshimura, N.; Chancellor, M.B. Single-institution experience in 110 patients with botulinum toxin A injection into bladder or urethra. *Urology* **2005**, *65*, 37–41. [CrossRef] [PubMed]
112. Chen, Y.H.; Kuo, H.C. Botulinum A toxin treatment of urethral sphincter pseudodyssynergia in patients with cerebrovascular accidents or intracranial lesions. *Urol. Int.* **2004**, *73*, 156–161. [CrossRef] [PubMed]
113. Huang, Y.H.; Chen, S.L. Concomitant detrusor and external urethral sphincter botulinum toxin-A injections in male spinal cord injury patients with detrusor overactivity and detrusor sphincter dyssynergia. *J. Rehabil. Med.* **2022**, *54*, jrm00264. [CrossRef]

114. Goel, S.; Pierce, H.; Pain, K.; Christos, P.; Dmochowski, R.; Chughtai, B. Use of botulinum toxin A (BoNT-A) in detrusor external sphincter dyssynergia (DESD): A systematic review and meta-analysis. *Urology* **2020**, *140*, 7–13. [CrossRef]
115. Haylen, B.T.; de Ridde, D.; Freeman, R.M.; Swift, S.E.; Berghmans, B.; Lee, J.; Monga, A.; Petri, E.; Rizk, D.E.; Sand, P.K.; et al. An International Urogynecological Association (IUGA)/International Continence Society (ICS) joint report on the terminology for female pelvic floor dysfunction. *Neurourol. Urodyn. Off. J. Int. Cont. Soc.* **2010**, *29*, 4–20. [CrossRef] [PubMed]
116. Kaplan, W.; Firlit, C.F.; Schoenberg, H.W. The female urethral syndrome: External sphincter spasm as etiology. *J. Urol.* **1980**, *124*, 48–49. [CrossRef]
117. Hinman, F. Nonneurogenic neurogenic bladder (the Hinmann syndrome)—15 years later. *J. Urol.* **1986**, *136*, 769–777. [CrossRef]
118. Kuo, H.C. Dysfunctional voiding in women with lower urinary tract symptoms. *Tzu. Chi. Med. J.* **2000**, *12*, 217–223.
119. Jiang, Y.H.; Lee, C.L.; Chen, S.F.; Kuo, H.C. Therapeutic effects of urethral sphincter botulinum toxin A injection on dysfunctional voiding with different videourodynamic characteristics in non-neurogenic women. *Toxins* **2021**, *13*, 362. [CrossRef]
120. Ou, Y.-C.; Huang, K.-H.; Jan, H.-C.; Kuo, H.-C.; Kao, Y.-L.; Tsai, K.-J. Therapeutic efficacy of urethral sphincteric botulinum toxin injections for female sphincter dysfunctions and a search for predictive factors. *Toxins* **2021**, *13*, 398. [CrossRef]
121. Lee, Y.K.; Kuo, H.C. Therapeutic effects of botulinum toxin A, via urethral sphincter injection on voiding dysfunction due to different bladder and urethral sphincter dysfunctions. *Toxins* **2019**, *11*, 487. [CrossRef] [PubMed]
122. Kuo, H.C. Prostate botulinum A toxin injection–an alternative treatment for benign prostatic obstruction in poor surgical candidates. *Urology* **2005**, *65*, 670–674. [CrossRef] [PubMed]
123. Chuang, Y.C.; Chiang, P.H.; Yoshimura, N.; De Miguel, F.; Chancellor, M.B. Sustained beneficial effects of intraprostatic botulinum toxin type A on lower urinary tract symptoms and quality of life in men with benign prostatic hyperplasia. *BJU. Int.* **2006**, *98*, 1033–1037. [CrossRef]
124. Hamidi Madani, A.; Enshaei, A.; Heidarzadeh, A.; Mokhtari, G.; Farzan, A.; Mohiti Asli, M.; Esmaeili, S. Transurethral intraprostatic Botulinum toxin-A injection: A novel treatment for BPH refractory to current medical therapy in poor surgical candidates. *World J. Urol.* **2013**, *31*, 235–239. [CrossRef] [PubMed]
125. El-Dakhakhny, A.S.; Gharib, T.; Issam, A.; El-Karamany, T.M. Transperineal intraprostatic injection of botulinum neurotoxin A vs. transurethral resection of prostate for management of lower urinary tract symptoms secondary to benign prostate hyperplasia: A prospective randomised study. *Arab. J. Urol.* **2019**, *17*, 270–278. [CrossRef] [PubMed]
126. Totaro, A.; Pinto, F.; Pugliese, D.; Vittori, M.; Racioppi, M.; Foschi, N.; Bassi, P.F.; Sacco, E. Intraprostatic botulinum toxin type "A" injection in patients with benign prostatic hyperplasia and unsatisfactory response to medical therapy: A randomized, double-blind, controlled trial using urodynamic evaluation. *Neurourol. Urodyn.* **2018**, *37*, 1031–1038. [CrossRef] [PubMed]
127. Moussa, A.S.; Ragheb, A.M.; Abdelbary, A.M.; Ibrahim, R.M.; El Adawy, M.S.; Aref, A.; Assem, A.; Elfayoumy, H.; Elzawy, F. Outcome of botulinum toxin-A intraprostatic injection for benign prostatic hyperplasia induced lower urinary tract symptoms: A prospective multicenter study. *Prostate* **2019**, *79*, 1221–1225. [CrossRef]
128. Marberger, M.; Chartier-Kastler, E.; Egerdie, B.; Lee, K.S.; Grosse, J.; Bugarin, D.; Zhou, J.; Patel, A.; Haag-Molkenteller, C. A randomized double-blind placebo-controlled phase 2 dose-ranging study of onabotulinumtoxinA in men with benign prostatic hyperplasia. *Eur. Urol.* **2013**, *63*, 496–503. [CrossRef]
129. Shim, S.R.; Cho, Y.J.; Shin, I.S.; Kim, J.H. Efficacy and safety of botulinum toxin injection for benign prostatic hyperplasia: A systematic review and meta-analysis. *Int. Urol. Nephrol.* **2016**, *48*, 19–30. [CrossRef]
130. Chen, J.L.; Chen, C.Y.; Kuo, H.C. Botulinum toxin A injection to the bladder neck and urethra for medically refractory lower urinary tract symptoms in men without prostatic obstruction. *J. Formos. Med. Assoc.* **2009**, *108*, 950–956. [CrossRef]
131. Chuang, Y.C.; Chiang, P.H.; Huang, C.C.; Yoshimura, N.; Chancellor, M.B. Botulinum toxin type A improves benign prostatic hyperplasia symptoms in patients with small prostates. *Urology* **2005**, *66*, 775–779. [CrossRef] [PubMed]
132. Sacco, E.; Bientinesi, R.; Marangi, F.; Totaro, A.; D'Addessi, A.; Racioppi, M.; Pinto, F.; Vittori, M.; Bassi, P. Patient-reported outcomes in men with lower urinary tract symptoms (LUTS) due to benign prostatic hyperplasia (BPH) treated with intraprostatic OnabotulinumtoxinA: 3-month results of a prospective single-armed cohort study. *BJU. Int.* **2012**, *110*, E837-44. [CrossRef] [PubMed]
133. Kuo, H.C.; Liu, H.T. Therapeutic effects of add-on botulinum toxin A on patients with large benign prostatic hyperplasia and unsatisfactory response to combined medical therapy. *Scand. J. Urol. Nephrol.* **2009**, *43*, 206–211. [CrossRef] [PubMed]
134. Jiang, Y.H.; Chen, S.F.; Jhang, J.F.; Kuo, H.C. Therapeutic effect of urethral sphincter onabotulinumtoxinA injection for urethral sphincter hyperactivity. *Neurourol. Urodyn.* **2018**, *37*, 2651–2657. [CrossRef] [PubMed]
135. Krishnappa, P.; Sinha, M.; Krishnamoorthy, V. A prospective study to evaluate the efficacy of botulinum toxin-A in the management of dysfunctional voiding in women. *Clin. Med. Insights Womens Health* **2018**, *11*, 1179562X18811340. [CrossRef] [PubMed]
136. Arnouk, R.; Suzuki Bellucci, C.H.; Benatuil Stull, R.; de Bessa, J., Jr.; Malave, C.A.; Mendes Gomes, C. Botulinum neurotoxin type A for the treatment of benign prostatic hyperplasia: Randomized study comparing two doses. *Sci. World J.* **2012**, *2012*, 463574. [CrossRef] [PubMed]
137. Wu, S.Y.; Jiang, Y.H.; Jhang, J.F.; Hsu, Y.H.; Ho, H.C.; Kuo, H.C. Inflammation and barrier function deficits in the bladder urothelium of ptients with chronic spinal cord injury and recurrent urinary tract infections. *Biomedicines* **2022**, *10*, 220. [CrossRef]
138. Traini, C.; Del Popolo, G.; Lazzeri, M.; Mazzaferro, K.; Nelli, F.; Calosi, L.; Vannucchi, M.G. γEpithelial Na(+) Channel (γENaC) and the Acid-Sensing Ion Channel 1 (ASIC1) expression in the urothelium of patients with neurogenic detrusor overactivity. *BJU. Int.* **2015**, *116*, 797–804. [CrossRef]

139. Ke, Q.S.; Lee, C.L.; Kuo, H.C. Recurrent urinary tract infection in women and overactive bladder—Is there a relationship? *Tzu. Chi. Med. J.* **2020**, *33*, 13–21.
140. Banakhar, M.; Yamani, A. In patients with neurogenic detrusor overactivity and Hinman's syndrome: Would intravesical botox injections decrease the incidence of symptomatic urinary tract infections. *Res. Rep. Urol.* **2021**, *13*, 659–663. [CrossRef]
141. Bickhaus, J.A.; Bradley, M.S.; Amundsen, C.L.; Visco, A.G.; Truong, T.; Li, Y.J.; Siddiqui, N.Y. Does a recent urinary tract infection increase the risk of postprocedure urinary tract infection after onabotulinum toxin A? *Female Pelvic Med. Reconstr. Surg.* **2021**, *27*, 121–125. [CrossRef] [PubMed]
142. Elmer-Lyon, C.G.; Streit, J.A.; Takacs, E.B.; Ten Eyck, P.P.; Bradley, C.S. Urinary tract infection and drug-resistant urinary tract infection after intradetrusor onabotulinumtoxinA injection versus sacral neuromodulation. *Int. Urogynecol. J.* **2020**, *31*, 871–879. [CrossRef]
143. Chang, S.C.; Zeng, S.; Tsai, S.J. Outcome of different approaches to reduce urinary tract infection in patients with spinal cord lesions: A systematic review. *Am. J. Phys. Med. Rehabil.* **2020**, *99*, 1056–1066. [CrossRef] [PubMed]
144. Mouttalib, S.; Khan, S.; Castel-Lacanal, E.; Guillotreau, J.; De Boissezon, X.; Malavaud, B.; Marque, P.; Rischmann, P.; Gamé, X. Risk of urinary tract infection after detrusor botulinum toxin A injections for refractory neurogenic detrusor overactivity in patients with no antibiotic treatment. *BJU. Int.* **2010**, *106*, 1677–1680. [CrossRef] [PubMed]
145. Chen, G.; Liao, L.; Zhang, F. Efficacy and safety of botulinum toxin a injection into urethral sphincter for underactive bladder. *BMC Urol.* **2019**, *19*, 60. [CrossRef]
146. Chen, S.F.; Jhang, J.F.; Jiang, Y.H.; Kuo, H.C. Treatment outcomes of detrusor underactivity in women based on clinical and videourodynamic characteristics. *Int. Urol. Nephrol.* **2022**, *54*, 1215–1223. [CrossRef]
147. Jiang, Y.H.; Jhang, J.F.; Chen, S.F.; Kuo, H.C. Videourodynamic factors predictive of successful onabotulinumtoxinA urethral sphincter injection for neurogenic or non-neurogenic detrusor underactivity. *Low. Urin. Tract Symptoms* **2019**, *11*, 66–71. [CrossRef]
148. Kuo, H.C. Botulinum toxin paves the way for the treatment of functional lower urinary tract dysfunction. *Toxins* **2020**, *12*, 394. [CrossRef]

toxins

MDPI

Review

Role of Urological Botulinum Toxin-A Injection for Overactive Bladder and Voiding Dysfunction in Patients with Parkinson's Disease or Post-Stroke

Ju-Chuan Hu [1], Lin-Nei Hsu [2], Wei-Chia Lee [3,*], Yao-Chi Chuang [3,4] and Hung-Jen Wang [3,4]

1 Division of Urology, Department of Surgery, Taichung Veterans General Hospital, Taichung 407, Taiwan
2 Department of Urology, An Nan Hospital, China Medical University, Tainan City 833, Taiwan
3 Division of Urology, Kaohsiung Chang Gung Memorial Hospital, Chang Gung University College of Medicine, Kaohsiung 807, Taiwan
4 Center for Shock Wave Medicine and Tissue Engineering, Kaohsiung Chang Gung Memorial Hospital, Kaohsiung 807, Taiwan
* Correspondence: dinor666@ms32.hinet.net; Tel.: +886-7-7317123 (ext. 8094); Fax: +886-7-7318762

Abstract: Botulinum toxin A (BoNT-A) paralyzes muscle by blocking acetylcholine release at the synaptic junction. BoNT-A has shown its therapeutic effects in neurological disorders such as Parkinson's disease (PD) and post-stroke spasticity. A high proportion of patients with PD and post-stroke develop neurogenic detrusor overactivity (nDO) and then develop urinary incontinence and overactive bladder (OAB) symptoms. This study aimed to disclose the safety and efficacy of BoNT-A injection in treating bladder and voiding dysfunction in PD and post-stroke patients by reviewing the current evidence. At present, intradetrusor injection of BoNT-A is a Food and Drug Administration (FDA)-approved third-line therapy for nDO and idiopathic OAB. Although intradetrusor injection of onaBoNT-A 200 U is already approved for nDO treatment, most researchers would like to manage PD and post-stroke patients by using onaBoNT-A 100 U intradetrusor injection to achieve long-term efficacy and reduce adverse effects. However, in contrast to its inclusion in the International Continence Society guidelines for PD treatment, the clinical use of BoNT-A for post-stroke patients is limited to experimental use due to the development of urinary retention in about one-fifth of patients. For treating urethral pseudodyssynergia, half of patients may respond to onaBoNT-A 100 U urethral injection. However, refinement is needed to reduce unwanted urinary incontinence.

Keywords: botulinum toxin A; incontinence; Parkinson's disease; stroke; dyssynergia

Key Contribution: Patients with upper motor neuron syndrome (i.e., patients with Parkinson's disease and post-stroke) may develop urinary incontinence and voiding difficulty because of disturbances in the brain–bladder circuit. Despite the rationale for and efficacy of using BoNT-A injection in other neurological and urological disorders, the application of urological injection of BoNT-A for voiding dysfunction originating from chronic brain lesions has only reached barely satisfactory results, especially for post-stroke patients. Results of this review demonstrate the safety and efficacy of BoNT-A, suggesting that intradetrusor injection of 100 U BoNT-A should be the standard third-line treatment for bladder dysfunction associated with Parkinson's disease.

Citation: Hu, J.-C.; Hsu, L.-N.; Lee, W.-C.; Chuang, Y.-C.; Wang, H.-J. Role of Urological Botulinum Toxin-A Injection for Overactive Bladder and Voiding Dysfunction in Patients with Parkinson's Disease or Post-Stroke. *Toxins* **2023**, *15*, 166. https://doi.org/10.3390/toxins15020166

Received: 26 December 2022
Revised: 1 February 2023
Accepted: 11 February 2023
Published: 17 February 2023

Copyright: © 2023 by the authors. Licensee MDPI, Basel, Switzerland. This article is an open access article distributed under the terms and conditions of the Creative Commons Attribution (CC BY) license (https://creativecommons.org/licenses/by/4.0/).

1. Introduction

Botulinum toxin A (BoNT-A) is a neurotoxin derived from *Clostridium botulinum*. Its mechanism of action in treating overactive bladder (OAB) and urinary urgency incontinence (UUI) involves inducing flaccid paralysis via blockade of the acetylcholine release at the synaptic junction [1]. In addition, BoNT-A inhibits bladder afferent nerve firing and provides anti-inflammatory effects to manage bladder disorders. The United States Food and Drug Administration (FDA) first approved BoNT-A in 2011 for the treatment of neurogenic detrusor overactivity (nDO) and then approved it later in 2013 for refractory OAB.

The expectation for intradetrusor injection of BoNT-A for reducing urinary tract dysfunction (LUTD) would be to decrease detrusor contractility, reduce bladder hypersensitivity, and eliminate painful sensations [1]. Therefore, researchers investigated the application of BoNT-A to manage the detrusor hyperreflexia (i.e., nDO) and UUI, which both originated from upper motor neuron syndrome, as seen in patients with Parkinson's disease (PD), post-stroke, and early dementia [2].

Chronic brain disorders such as PD and stroke lead to a high proportion of LUTD in the affected patients [3]. The majority of these patients may have nDO in the cystometrography and experience UUI in their daily activity [4,5]. The occurrence of urinary incontinence (UI) in such patients may result from either nDO or impaired cognition and immobilization. Proper evaluation of micturition dysfunction in these patients is dependent on urodynamic diagnosis combined with imaging and pressure flow studies. Some patients may have concurrent detrusor underactivity, bladder neck dysfunction, and pseudodyssynergia (delay in striated sphincter relaxation or unrelaxing) [2,4,5]. Effective management of LUTD in these patients may benefit psychosocial and health-related quality of life and decrease social isolation, anxiety, depression, and fall risk.

Usually, intradetrusor injection of BoNT-A for OAB is classified as the third-line option among all OAB therapies [6]. Meanwhile, first-line management includes behavior therapies and lifestyle modifications followed by pharmacotherapy as second-line therapy [7]. Nevertheless, mainstream pharmacotherapy of OAB, which includes antimuscarinics and β3 agonists, is often problematic in older adults [6]. Constipation, dry mouth, blurred vision, and cognitive impairment are common adverse effects of antimuscarinics. Furthermore, researchers have reported a strong association between the use of antimuscarinics and risk of incident dementia [6]. Hence, of particular concern in elderly PD or post-stroke patients, procedural interventions (i.e., third-line therapies) must be optimized in older patients with motor symptoms, such as using BoNT-A injection, sacral neuromodulation (SNM), and percutaneous tibial nerve stimulation (PTNS).

2. Brain–Bladder Circuit

The lower urinary tract consists of the bladder and urethra, which are regulated by three micturition centers, including the sacral spinal center, subconscious structures (e.g., cerebellum, striate nucleus, and hypothalamus), and conscious structures (e.g., limbic cortex, frontal ascending, and parietal ascending circumduction) [4,5]. The brain–bladder circuit is illustrated in Figure 1.

Generally speaking, "urinary urgency" may be initiated by the "afferent noise" from an unstable bladder, including firing pain C-fibers, stretching Aδ/C afferents, chemical stimulating urothelium, and microcontraction of the detrusor. The afferent signals may pass through the spinal cord and medulla to the cortex [8]. The forebrain influences voluntary control of the human micturition switch and maintenance of incontinence. The prefrontal cortex receives input from the bladder pertaining to the "viscerosensory system" at the orbital prefrontal network, whereas the medial network serves as a "visceromotor system" that relays major cortical output to the hypothalamus and periaqueduct gray in the midbrain [5]. Then, the arc of the spinal cord/periaqueduct gray/pontine micturition center plays a suppressive role in activity of the urethral sphincter and bladder detrusor to maintain bladder control [5,8].

In the pathological conditions of upper motor neuron syndrome, nDO is a major cause of UUI. In lesions above the brain stem, the reflex arc of micturition is intact, whereas the existence of DO may exaggerate the micturition reflex [3–5]. For instance, the lesions in the basal ganglia (i.e., striatum, globus pallidus, substantia nigra, and subthalamic nucleus) play an important role in the development of neurogenic OAB [5,9]. The net effect of basal ganglia is inhibitory. The abnormal activation of putamen in functional neuroimaging has been reported in PD patients with DO [10], as well as hypersensitive bladder in ketamine-induced cystitis in a rat model [11].

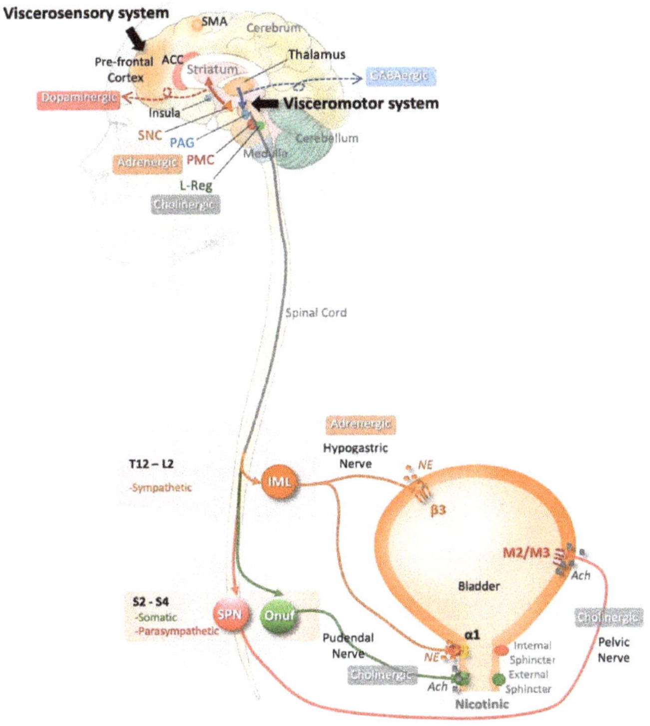

Figure 1. Brain–bladder circuit for micturition. The voiding switch is operated by the "viscerosensory system" and "visceromotor system." The viscerosensory system consists of the prefrontal lobe, thalamus, insula, SMA, ACC, and other associated regions, and helps to manage afferent signals from the lower urinary tract. The visceromotor system includes the hypothalamus and PAG in the midbrain and mediates the efferent signals from PMC to the spinal cord. The lower urinary tract, including the urinary bladder and its outlet, are controlled by the coordination of three neural systems. The sympathetic system controls the detrusor (via β3 receptor) and bladder neck (via α1 receptor). The somatic system works simultaneously with the sympathetic system and contributes to the urethral closure through the cholinergic pathway. Activating the parasympathetic motor system results in detrusor contraction via M_2 and M_3 receptors. Lesions at the brain or brainstem, as in stroke and Parkinson's disease, interfere with the brain–bladder neural circuity, resulting in lower urinary tract dysfunction. **Abbreviation: ACC**: anterior cingulate cortex; **Ach**, acetylcholine; **α1**, alpha-1 adrenergic receptor; **β3**, beta-3 adrenergic receptor; **GABA**, γ-aminobutyric acid; **IML**, intermediolateral cell column; **L**, lumbar; **L-reg**, L region (Pontine storage center); **M2/M3**, muscarinic acetylcholine receptor 2 and 3; **NE**, norepinephrine; **Onuf**, Onuf's nucleus; **PAG**, periaqueductal grey; **PMC**, pontine micturition center; **S**, sacral; **SMA**, supplementary motor area; **SNC**, substantia nigra pars compacta; **SPN**, sacral parasympathetic nucleus; **T**, thoracic.

3. Bladder Dysfunction in PD Patients

The prevalence of PD is around 0.1–0.2% in the population at any given time [12]. PD is a chronic, progressive, neurodegenerative disease characterized by the manifestation of motor symptoms such as bradykinesia, static tremor, and rigidity. These symptoms are caused by a loss of dopaminergic neurons in the substantia nigra. In addition, autonomic dysfunction is a classic non-motor phenotype of PD, including gastrointestinal malfunction, cardiovascular dysregulation, urination disturbances, sexual dysfunction, thermoregulatory aberrance, and tear abnormalities [13]. LUTD, which may present with storage and emptying symptoms, is a common non-motor sequela of PD [14] and has been reported to occur in 27–85% of PD patients during any stage of the disease [15]. In a recent meta-analysis, Li et al. [16] reported that the most prevalent storage symptom in PD patients is nocturia (59%), followed by frequency (52%), urgency (46%), and UUI (32%). One-third of PD patients may experience OAB. The emptying symptoms of PD patients may manifest as voiding difficulty, presenting symptoms of hesitancy, poor stream, and straining [15,16]. LUTS symptoms often occur five years after the onset of Parkinsonian motor symptoms [4]. Together these symptoms have substantial negative effects on patients' quality of life and are a major cause of hospitalization and dependence upon caregivers.

Most bladder disorders in PD patients are caused by PD itself [17,18] and the occurrence of LUTS is associated with progression of motor symptoms and cognitive dysfunction [18,19]. OAB is the major issue of bladder dysfunction in patients with PD [4]. Common diseases that may cause bladder dysfunction, including urological cancer, stone disease, and urinary tract infections, must be ruled out. Questionnaires (e.g., OAB symptom score and American Urological Association Symptom Index), bladder diary, uroflowmetry, and post-void residual estimate are especially useful for the initial evaluation of bladder function in patients with PD. Because the development of LUTS in PD patients may relate to nigrostriatal dopaminergic degeneration [17,18], the first line of LUTS treatment for PD patients is to provide levodopa or other dopaminergic drugs [9]. Although not addressing LUTS directly, treatment with levodopa has been shown to improve the storage symptoms in PD patients. The second line therapies may include antimuscarinic agents and β3 agonists (i.e., mirabegron). However, the adverse effects (e.g., constipation and cognitive impairment) of antimuscarinics remain of concern, particularly for oxybutynin [4,6,9]. In addition, desmopressin (an analogue of arginine vasopressin) for nocturnal polyuria and tamsulosin (an α1-blocker) for symptoms of bladder outlet obstruction are suggested for symptom relief in PD patients [4,9,14].

For some patients with PD who do not respond well to the initial treatment of LUTS, urodynamic studies are required to differentiate the voiding dysfunction in detail, particularly using pressure-flow and video-urodynamic studies [4,9,14]. For instance, the disease of multiple system atrophy (MSA) is also a progressive neurodegenerative disorder with glial cytoplasmic inclusion, which is possibly involved in cytoskeletal alterations and neuronal degeneration [4]. Patients with MSA may have Parkinson-like motor symptoms and similar symptoms of LUTS. However, those with MSA generally show little response to the dopamine medications used to treat PD [4]. In a urodynamic investigation, Shin et al. [20] reported that DO and associated UUI were dominant in PD patients. In contrast, MSA patients may have a lower maximal flow rate, decreased compliance, detrusor underactivity, and an increase in post-void residual urine. In addition, Vurture et al. [21] suggested that nDO is almost universal in PD patients complaining of OAB symptoms. However, bladder outlet obstruction, detrusor underactivity and increased post-void residual urine may also be observed in PD patients [21,22]. Following proper evaluation of bladder dysfunction, third-line therapies can be applied to patients who discontinued pharmacotherapy or in whom drug therapy has inadequate efficacy. However, the use of SNM and PTNS may have some inherent limitations in PD patients, such as the more invasive procedure of SNM or the need for frequent visits for receiving PTNS. Therefore, intradetrusor injection of BoNT-A may offer the advantages of long-term efficacy, appropriate cost, and a less invasive procedure.

4. UI in Post-Stroke Patients

With the increasing growth and aging of populations, it is expected that stroke events, their long-term sequelae, and the corresponding costs will increase dramatically [23,24]. Stroke is a leading cause of adult disability. Increases are estimated to be 1.1 million and 2 million new cases annually in Europe [23] and China [24]. Using stroke survivors as an indication of prevalent stroke cases, Wang et al. [25] reported that 1.5% of adult residents of China experienced stroke. Among stroke types, ischemic stroke constituted 77.8%, intracerebral hemorrhage 15.8%, and subarachnoid hemorrhage 4.4%. A large spectrum of post-stroke LUTS is also documented, varying from UI to urinary retention [26]. In the immediate post-stroke phase, device-based management of incontinence, such as indwelled catheters or urinary pads, is most common. UI affects around half of stroke survivors in the acute phase. After the acute period, OAB symptoms are the dominant LUTS symptoms in post-stroke patients. Akkoç et al. [27] reported that two-thirds of post-stroke patients presented with urgency at six-months follow-up. In post-stroke patients, UUI causes embarrassment and distress, adding to the disability and helplessness caused by neurological deficits. Therefore, clinicians need to develop formal plans to guide UI practice, and subsequently use individualized management strategies to improve patients' outcomes.

The exact mechanism of UI after a stroke is still unclear, but it may be a sign of patients' poor prognosis in later life. Researchers suggest that UI presenting at 30 days after a stroke may increase the risk of one-year mortality of continent stroke survivors by four times [28]. Post-stroke UI was also associated with a negative functional outcome [29]. Hemorrhage stroke, chronic cough, aphasia, cognitive impairments, upper limb dysfunction, and fecal impaction were predictors of post-stroke UI [30,31]. However, the lesion sites of stroke seem not to correlate with patients' urodynamic presentations [32]. At one month after stroke, Pizzi et al. [33] reported that 30% of patients with UI may present with normal functional bladder, and 48% will present with nDO; DO with impaired contractility is reported in 6%, and detrusor underactivity in 6%. Nevertheless, nDO is the most prevalent urodynamic finding and the major cause of UUI in post-stroke patients. In addition, around 10% of stroke patients may have sphincter pseudodyssynergia after stroke [5]. Therefore, urodynamic studies are necessary in the management of difficult cases of post-stroke UUI.

After the recovery period, post-stroke patients may still exhibit bladder dysfunction and UUI. Behavior therapies are the first-line treatment of such patients with OAB, including bladder training and fluid management [5]. Second-line therapies include antimuscarinics and β3 agonists. Intradetrusor BoNT-A injection may be the choice for third-line therapy for more difficult patients in order to avoid the adverse effects of medication, as well as to reach long-term efficacy and improve patients' quality of life.

5. Application of BoNT-A in LUTD

The use of BoNT-A for LUTD was first described by Dykstra et al. [34] in 1988 for the treatment of patients with detrusor external sphincter dyssynergia. Following the successful demonstration of BoNT-A efficacy and safety, clinical trials were conducted for treating voiding dysfunction, especially for neurogenic DO in spinal cord injury and multiple sclerosis [2]. Generally, BoNT is classified into seven distinct neurotoxins (i.e., types A-G) that inhibit acetylcholine release at the presynaptic cholinergic neuromuscular junction to paralyze muscles [35]. Although little to no evidence supported the effects of other types, clinicians concentrated on the use of BoNT-A, including onaBoNT-A (Botox®, Allergan, Westport County Mayo, Ireland) and aboBoNT-A (Dysport®, Ipsen Ltd., Boulogne-Billancourt, France) to manage LUTD. On the other hand, serving as a powerful muscle relaxant, BoNT-A is widely used in treating the sequelae of Parkinsonism [36] and post-stroke muscle spasticity [37]. Particularly, the use of BoNT-A in urological dysfunctions of patients suffering from PD has been summarized [38].

5.1. Structure and Function of BoNT-A

BoNT-A is a synthesized inactive protein with a 50 kDa light chain and a 100 kDa heavy chain linked by disulfide and noncovalent bonds [39]. The major cell surface receptor of BoNT-A is synaptic vesicle protein-2 (SV2). The heavy chain binds to SV2 on the surface of the nerve ending. BoNT-A is cleaved to leave the light chain as its true active moiety due to endocytic internalization of the toxin within the nerve terminal. Then, the light chain of BoNT-A cleaves synaptosome-associated protein 25 (SNAP-25), a protein essential to the binding of synaptic vesicles to the cell membrane, to prevent neurotransmitter-containing vesicles' exocytosis at the nerve terminal (Figure 2). SV2-immunoreactive and SNAP-25-immuoreactive nerve fibers may be distributed within the suburothelium and muscle layer in the human bladder [39].

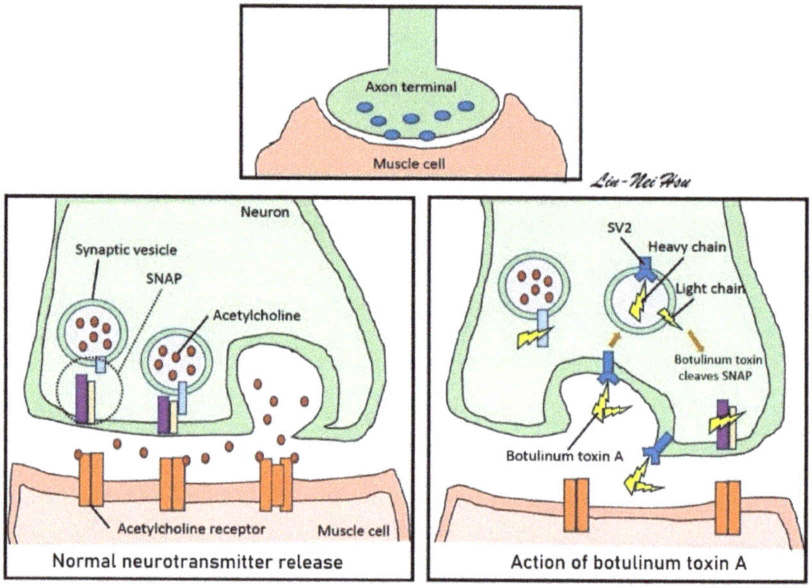

Figure 2. Simplified mechanisms of BoNT-A to paralyze the detrusor muscle. In physiology, synaptic vesicles interact with SNAP to release acetylcholine at the nerve terminals. However, via binding with SV2, the BoNT-A is endocytosed to cleave the SNAP-25 by its light chain and prevent the release of acetylcholine. **Abbreviation: BoNT-A,** botulinum toxin A; **SNAP**, synaptosomal-associated protein; **SV2**, synaptic vesicle associated protein-2.

5.2. Biological Effects

BoNT-A may have motor effects, sensory effects, and anti-inflammatory effects that will improve LUTD by inducing chemical denervation. BoNT-A can temporarily inactivate cholinergic transmission at the neuromuscular junction in both bladder detrusor and sphincter muscle [40]. In the bladder, BoNT-A may play a complex role in micturition reflex. For the sympathetic system, BoNT-A can inhibit the release of vesicular adrenaline and inactivate the α-adrenoceptors and β3-adrenoceptors, and theoretically facilitate the excretion of urine. In fact, BoNT-A injection mainly inhibits the parasympathetic system of the bladder by inactivation of the M2 and M3 muscarinic receptors and subsequently ameliorates the urinary storage [39]. The intradetrusor injection of BoNT-A has analgesic properties through retrograde axonal transport to decrease $P2X_3$ and TRPV1 expression in the suburothelial C-fibers of the human bladder [41]. Moreover, BoNT-A accumulates in the urothelium layer to inhibit ATP release [42]. The duration of BoNT-A effects on sensory bladder disorders is typically 6–9 months [39]. In rat models, BoNT-A showed its ability to inhibit the release of calcitonin gene-related peptide and substance P from afferent nerve terminals, suggesting a potential role of BoNT-A as a treatment for neurogenic inflammation occurring in patients with nDO [43,44].

6. Urological Injection Techniques of BoNT-A

6.1. Dosage

Differences in dosing are shown for each condition and in brand models by different urological studies. The only FDA-approved doses for OnaBoNT-A BOTOX® are 100 U for idiopathic OAB and 200 U for nDO treatments [45]. However, this has not limited ongoing research on dosage (e.g., 300 and 500 U) and effects of aboBoNT-A (Dysport®) or in off-labeled use. The units between BOTOX® and Dysport® preparations are not the same nor are they interchangeable. In general, 1 U of BOTOX® is equivalent approximately to 3 U Dysport® [46]. Moreover, dilution of the toxin, the amount of liquid injected, and the number of injection sites have varied between studies and in clinical use.

6.2. The Technique in Bladder Injection

The BoNT-A solution can be injected directly into the detrusor muscle, submucosal space, and trigone [47] (Figure 3). During the injection of BoNT-A, a thin layer of bladder wall may simultaneously receive and contain the BoNT-A in the area of the detrusor and submucosal area. The trigone in the bladder base contains rich sensory fibers, which may have a role in eliciting urgency and DO. Clinically, the injection of BoNT-A into the trigone area could itself fulfill OAB treatment without inducing vesicoureteral reflux [48,49].

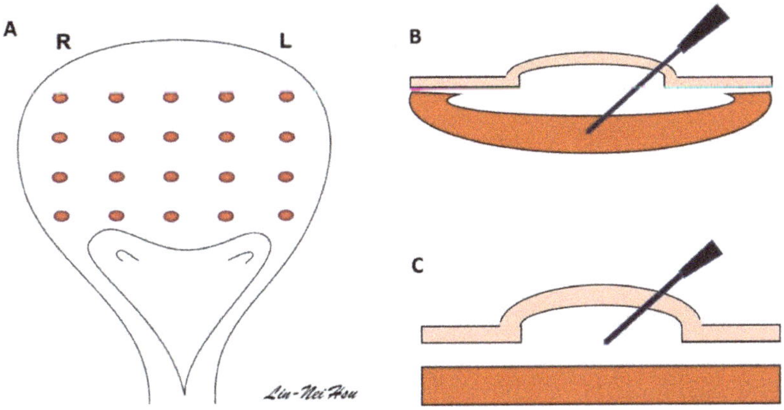

Figure 3. Regular BoNT-A injection of the bladder. (**A**) Usually, urologists mapped twenty injection sites over the bladder. (**B**) Intradetrusor method: BoNT-A solution was injected directly into the trabeculation or detrusor muscle of the bladder. (**C**) Submucosal method: Using a needle to inject and retain solution in the submucosal layer, a balloon formation was observed in the bladder after direct injection of the BoNT-A solution.

Usually, we prepare 100 U of BOTOX® into 10 mL with dilution by normal saline. This volume is delivered to between 10 and 20 different sites of the bladder, which is typically kept at a capacity of 150–200 mL. A submucosal injection can be performed by inserting a needle into the submucosal area and observing a balloon formation in the bladder. A rigid or flexible cystoscope is able to deliver BoNT-A solution under general or local anesthesia [39,47,50].

6.3. The Technique in Urethral Sphincter Injection

For injection of BoNT-A into the external sphincter of the urethra, a bottle of 100 U of BOTOX® is reconstituted to 4 mL with normal saline. At the 3, 6, 9, and 12 o'clock positions (Figure 4), 1 mL of BoNT-A solution in 25 U/mL was injected into the sphincter four times [51]. The cystoscope is a suitable instrument by which to perform the urethral injection in both sexes. Nevertheless, some doctors would like to inject the BoNT-A solution along the female urethra using a 23 G 1-mL syringe at the 3, 6, 9, and 12 o'clock areas of the meatus side. The BoNT-A solution can be injected in men at the circumferential sites of the urethral sphincter. For an extensive treatment of sphincter dysfunction, some may choose to inject the divided dosage of BoNT-A into the trigone, superficial prostate urethra, and external sphincter (Figure 4C) [52].

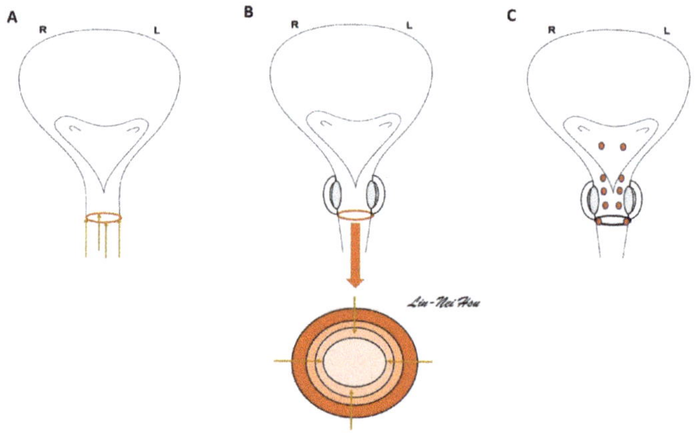

Figure 4. BoNT-A injection for relaxation of the urethra. (**A**) For female patients, it is convenient to use a 23 G 1-mL syringe and inject BoNT-A solution along the urethra at the 3, 6, 9, and 12 o'clock positions from the meatus side. (**B**) For male patients, cystoscopic injection of BoNT-A solution at the 3, 6, 9, and 12-o'clock areas of the external sphincter is common in routine urology practice. (**C**) For an extensive treatment for sphincter dysfunction, the divided dosage of BoNT-A may be injected into the trigone, superficial prostate urethra, and external sphincter for patients unresponsive to the regular injection [52].

7. Clinical Efficacy of BoNT-A Treatment in PD

At present, intradetrusor injection using 100 U onaBoNT-A is a rational choice for treating bladder dysfunction of PD, which has proven to be a safe and effective procedure for the treatment of nDO, particularly for patients with inadequate response to antimuscarinic medications [14]. In 2009, Giannantoni et al. [53] reported four patients with PD and two patients with MSA, who received 200 U BoNT-A intradetrusor injection in 20 sites under cystoscopic guidance. The authors showed that BoNT-A injection was an effective and safe treatment for PD-related OAB symptoms and DO. Only one patient with MSA required intermittent catheterization because of an increase in post-void residual urine. In the following study by the same research team [54], 100 U BoNT-A intradetrusor injection was administered to manage eight patients with PD who were refractory to antimuscarinics. The clinical and urodynamic improvements in OAB symptoms of these PD patients lasted for at least 6 months. In 2010, Kulaksizoglu and Parman [55] reported positive results in 16 PD patients by using the flexible cystoscopic injection of 500 IU aboBoNT-A at 30 sites (trigone spared), including the improvement of urinary symptoms and incontinence and the relief of caregivers' burden through nine months of observation.

In another comprehensive study, Anderson et al. [56] treated 20 clinic patients with PD with incontinence using 100 U onaBONT-A injection of the bladder under local anesthesia. The authors used a flexible cystoscopic instrument to disperse the solution of onaBONT-A (10 U/mL) into 10–20 submucosal/detrusor sites of the bladder, including the trigone. Results of that study showed that intradetrusor injection of BoNT-A can be safely utilized in male patients with PD who also have benign prostatic hypertrophy. Moreover, Vurture et al. [57] reported that the success rate was approximately 80% in the intradetrusor injection of onaBoNT-A 100 U for DO-driven storage symptoms of PD patients. Additionally, a repeat injection can increase the success rate to 87.5%. The rate of urinary retention requiring clean intermittent catheterization was 12.5%. In 2021, Atamian et al. [58] reported their treatment results of intradetrusor BoNT-A injection in 16 PD patients with UUI. Among these patients, 60% achieved improvement and 28% needed intermittent self-catheterization.

Urethral sphincter dysfunction may be an issue of voiding dysfunction in PD patients, including pseudodyssynergia or delay in striated sphincter relaxation [3]. Despite the rationale and success of chemical sphincterotomy in the first BoNT-A sphincter injection for detrusor sphincter dyssynergia in a patient with spinal cord injury [34], this procedure has yet to be widely utilized among patients with spinal cord injury. Regardless of whether injections are performed transperineally or transurethrally, previous studies have confirmed treatment efficacy [2]. About 50% of patients can achieve successful treatment with a decrease in urinary tract infections, nDO, and post-void residual urine [59]. However, nearly half of such cases developed UI and persistent incomplete bladder emptying, limiting the utility of urethral injection of BoNT-A [60,61]. Jiang et al. [62] reported that 100 U onaBoNT-A urethral sphincter injection is suitable to treat urethral sphincter hyperactivity, including in PD patients. The authors reported that two of three PD patients experienced satisfactory outcomes. Clearly, the BoNT-A urethral sphincter injection of PD does need some refinement, in light of the previous studies [60–62]. For example, a videourodynamic study may aid in the accurate diagnosis of dysfunctional voiding patterns in PD patients. Lee et al. [63] suggested that patients who were found to have a tight bladder neck during the videourodynamic study had less favorable therapeutic outcomes from BoNT-A urethral injections.

8. Clinical Role of BoNT-A Treatment in Post-Stroke

The ability to urinate independently is an important issue associated with human dignity [64]. Direct stroke-induced damage to the neuromicturition pathway causes involuntary leakage of urine accompanied by urgency in 40% to 60% of people admitted to hospital after a stroke [64]. First-line behavioral therapy may increase independent voiding behavior to control LUTS [64,65]. Second-line therapies of antimuscarinics and mirabegron also may improve OAB symptoms and not affect cognitive function during short-term observation [64,66]. However, post-stroke incontinence may last for a long time and not recover spontaneously. Third-line therapies may have a role in treating post-stroke incontinence. Evidence has shown that PTNS has little or no difference in the continence of participants after treatment [64]. SNM requires a surgical procedure with implantation of the InterStim® device for bladder and bowel control (Medtronic, Minneapolis, MN, USA), providing continuous stimulation through close nerve contact. Despite a high success rate in treatment, SNM may have adverse effects such as pain (15–42%) and infection (3.4–6.1%) at the implant site. Moreover, the surgical revision rate of SNM may be as high as 33% [67,68].

Theoretically, BoNT-A injection in the lower urinary tract may be a third-line adjuvant therapy for post-stroke incontinence. However, only a few studies have demonstrated successful outcomes of BoNT-A treatment in these patients. In 2006, Kuo [69] reported that 12 post-stroke patients with nDO received bladder submucosal injection of 200 U onaBoNT-A, in which only 50% of participants benefited from improvement of incontinence. Another 25% of patients developed transient urinary retention in the first postoperative week. The therapeutic effect declined gradually after 3 months and symptoms relapsed at month 6. In 2014, Jiang et al. [70] reported their experience in treating post-stroke bladder dysfunction by using 100 U onaBoNT-A intradetrusor injection, in which 17.4% of post-stroke patients developed acute urinary retention. Additionally, the therapeutic duration of these post-stroke patients is similar to those of control patients with OAB. Results of that study suggest that using 100 U onaBoNT-A intradetrusor injection for post-stroke patients is a rational dosage to reach a proper therapeutic effect and to avoid adverse effects. For treating pseudodyssynergia of post-stroke patients with difficult urination, Chen and Kuo [71] applied 100 U onaBoNT-A to external sphincter injections in 12 patients, of whom, 91% resumed spontaneous voiding.

As illustrated in Table 1, sufficient evidence has shown the beneficial effects of intradetrusor injection of BoNT-A in treating the UUI of PD patients. In contrast to the guidelines of PD treatment [14], urological BoNT-A injection for post-stroke patients remains an experimental entity in clinical practice. Further selection of suitable patients and refinements of technique may help to promote the usage of BoNT-A injection in treating voiding dysfunction in post-stroke patients.

Table 1. Characteristics among studies of botulinum injection in patients with CVA and PD.

Etiology	Author (Year)	Group/ Botulinum Brand	Patient Number (Male/Female)	Mean Age (SD)	Mean Duration of Disease (SD)	Injection Site	Dosage (Sites)	Anesthesia	Post-Injection Outcome			Adverse Events (Events/All Cases)
									Urodynamics	Clinical Outcome	Response Rate	
PD	Giannantoni (2009) [53]	Botox	4 (0/4)	76.3 (4.8)	9 years (3.5)	Detrusor (Trigone including)	200 U in saline 20 mL (20 sites)	IVGA	**IDC volume**: Significantly increased (+234 mL) at 3rd month **CMG capacity**: Significantly increased (+225.5 mL) at 3rd month **Pdet.Qmax**: Significantly reduced (−3.5 cm H_2O) at 3rd month **Qmax**: Significant reduced (−11.3 mL/s) at 3rd month **PVR**: Significantly increased (+88.8 mL) at 3rd month	Significantly improved daytime and nighttime Frequency Completely resolved daily UI (100%) Significantly improved I-QOL(+52.5)	4/4 (100%)	0/4 (0%) UTI 3/4 (75%) Dysuria 3/4 (75%) Voiding difficulty
	Kulaksizoglu (2010) [55]	Dysport	16	67.2 (5.1)	6 years	Detrusor	500 U in saline 30 mL (30 sites)	LA	**CMG capacity**: Significantly increased (+136 mL at 3rd month,+180 mL at 6th month, +183 mL at 9th month, +76.5 mL at 12th month) **Pdet at IDC**: Reduced (−28 cm H_2O in men, −12 cm H_2O in women) **Persistent urodynamic UI**: None after injection	Significantly reduced SEAPI score at 3rd, 6th, 9th and 12th month 6 incontinent patients at baseline: all with reduced UUI episode	16/16 (100%)	0/20 (0%) AUR need catheterization
	Giannantoni (2011) [54]	Botox	8 (1/7)	66 (3)	NA	Detrusor (Trigone including)	100 U in saline 10 mL (10 sites)	IVGA	**Complete resolution of IDC**: 3/8 (37.5%) **CMG capacity**: Significantly increased at 1st, 3rd, and 6th month **PVR**: increased at 1st month, markedly decreased at 3rd and 6th month **Qmax**: No significant change **Pdet.Qmax**: No significant change	Significantly decreased frequency (daytime and nighttime) and UI Significantly improved I-QOL (+43) and VAS (+3.5) at 6th month	NA	2/8 (25%) AUR need catheterization 0/8 (0%) UTI
	Jiang (2014) [70]	Botox	9	73.6 (11.2)	NA	Detrusor	100 U in saline 10 mL (20 sites)	IVGA	**CMG capacity**: Increased (+17 mL at 3rd month) **Qmax**: No significant change **Pdet.Qmax**: No significant change **PVR**: Significantly increased (+77.3 mL at 3rd month)	Significantly improved USS (−1.28) Improved urgency (−13 times) Improved UUI (−1.1 times)	NA	1/9(11.1%) AUR need catheterization 3/9(33.3%) PVR > 150 mL 1/9(11.1%) Voiding difficulty need strain 1/9(11.1%) Hematuria 2/9(22.2%) UTI
	Anderson (2014) [56]	Botox	20(12/8)	70.4	10.6 years	Detrusor(Trigone including)	100 U in saline 10 mL (10–20 sites)	LA	**VV**: No significant change at 1st, 3rd, and 6th month **Qmax**: Significant reduced (−4.7 mL/s) at 1st month, but not in 3rd and 6th month **PVR**: Significantly increased at 1st month (+106 mL) and 3rd month(+40 mL), but not in 6th month	Significantly improved UUI at 1st, 3rd, and 6th month Significantly improved AUA symptom scores at 1st, 3rd, and 6th month	20/20 (100%)	0/20 (0%) AUR need catheterization 2/20 (10%) UTI 0/20 (0%) Significant hematuria
	Knüpfer (2016) [72]	Botox	10 (6/4)	67.9 (5.4)	9.2 years (8.2)	Detrusor (Trigone including)	200 U in saline 20 mL (20 sites)	NA	**CMG capacity**: Significantly increased (+136 mL) **Pdet.Max at voiding**: Significantly reduced (−40 cm H_2O) **Compliance**: Increased (+11.1 mL/cm H_2O) **VV**: Significantly increased (+115 mL) **PVR**: scantly increased (+16 mL) **Urodynamic DO**: Markedly reduced (90% to 20%) **Qmax**: No significant change	Significantly improved frequency, nocturia and daily pad Significantly improved ICIQ score	10/10 (100%)	0/10 (0%) AUR need catheterization 0/10 (0%) UTI 0/10 (0%) Hematuria
	Vurture (2018) [57]	Botox	24 (17/7)	77.2 (7.5)	9.8 years (5.7)	Detrusor (Trigone including)	100 U in saline 10 mL (20 sites)	LA	**PVR**: Significantly increased (+108 mL)	Significantly decreased daily pad amount and UUI	19/24 (79.2%)	3/24 (12.5%) AUR need catheterization 6/24 (25%) UTI

Table 1. *Cont.*

Etiology	Author (Year)	Group/ Botulinum Brand	Patient Number (Male/Female)	Mean Age (SD)	Mean Duration of Disease (SD)	Injection Site	Dosage (Sites)	Anesthesia	Post-Injection Outcome			Adverse Events (Events/All Cases)
									Urodynamics	Clinical Outcome	Response Rate	
CVA	Chen (2004) [71]	Botox	11 (5/6)	66.5 (14.7)	NA	Sphincter	100 U in saline 4 mL (4 sites)	IVGA	**Pdet.Qmax**: Significantly reduced (−24 cmH_2O) **Qmax**: Significantly increased (+3.1 mL/s)	Significantly improved IPSS and QoL index in Botox group IPSS −13.6 in Botox vs. −4 in Control QoL Index −2.4 in Botox vs. −1.2 in Control	10/11 (91%)	0/11 (0%)
		Control	10	65.4 (15.5)		None	None	None	NA	NA	4/10 (40%)	0/10 (0%)
	Kuo (2006) [69]	Botox	12 (6/6)	72.4 (5.7)	NA	Detrusor	200 U in saline 20 mL (40 sites)	IVGA	**IDC volume**: Significantly Increased at 1st month (+139.9 cm H_2O) but not at 3rd month (+56.3 mL) **CMG capacity**: Significantly increased at 1st month (+144.9 mL) but not at 3rd month (+56.2 mL) **Pdet.Max at voiding**: Reduced (−5.4 cm H_2O at 1st month and −7.5 Cm H_2O at 3rd month) **PVR**: Significantly increased at 1st month (+123 mL) but not at 3rd month (+31.5 mL)	Improved incontinence grade (−1.3 at 1st month and −0.9 at 3rd month) Significantly increased grade of voiding difficulty (+1.5 at 1st month and +0.7 at 3rd month) 7/12 (58%) voiding difficulty	6/12 (50%)	3/12 (25%) AUR need catheterization 21% Mild hematuria 25% UTI
	Jiang (2014) [70]	Botox	23	73.6 (7.5)	NA	Detrusor	100 U in saline 10 mL (20 sites)	IVGA	**CMG capacity**: Significantly increased (+160 mL at 3rd month) **Qmax**: No significant change **Pdet.Qmax**: No significant change **PVR**: Significantly increased (+112.5 mL at 3rd month)	Improved USS (−0.57) Improved urgency (−8.3 times) Significantly improved UUI (−7.8 times)	NA	4/23 (17.4%) AUR need catheterization 12/23 (52.2%) PVR > 150 mL 17/23 (73.9%) Voiding difficulty need strain 2/23 (8.7%) Hematuria 1/23 (4.3%) UTI

Abbreviation: AUA symptom score, American Urological Association symptom score questionnaire; **AUR**, Acute urine retention; **CVA**, Cerebrovascular accident; **CMG**, cystometry; **DO**, Detrusor overactivity; **ICIQ**, International Consultation on Incontinence Questionnaire; **IDC**, Involuntary detrusor contraction; **IPSS**, International Prostate Symptom Score; **I-QoL**, Incontinence quality of life; **IVGA**, Intravenous anesthesia; **LA**, Local anesthesia; **NA**, No available data in the published paper; **PD**, Parkinson disease; **Pdet**, Detrusor pressure; **Pdet.Max**, Maximum detrusor pressure during voiding; **Pdet.Qmax**, Detrusor pressure at peak flow rate; **PVR**, Post-voiding residual volume; **Qmax**, Maximum flow rate; **QoL**, Quality of life; **SEAPI**, stress, emptying, anatomy, protection, inhibition Incontinence Quality of Life Assessment questionnaire; **UI**, Urinary incontinence; **USS**, Urgency severity score; **UTI**, Urinary tract infection; **UUI**, Urge urinary incontinence; **VAS**, Visual analogue scale; **VV**, Voiding volume.

Author Contributions: J.-C.H., L.-N.H. and W.-C.L. wrote the manuscript and figures, Y.-C.C. supervised and revised the paper, H.-J.W. collected information and references. All authors have read and agreed to the published version of the manuscript.

Funding: This work is supported by Grants MOST 104-2314-B-182A-081 and MOST 111-2314-B-182A-081-MY3 from the Ministry of Science and Technology of the Republic of China, and CMRPG8M0741, and CMRPG8K1431 from Chang Gung Medical Foundation and Chang Gung Memorial Hospital.

Institutional Review Board Statement: Not applicable.

Informed Consent Statement: Not applicable.

Data Availability Statement: Not applicable.

Conflicts of Interest: The authors declare no conflict of interest.

References

1. Kuo, H.C. Clinical application of botulinum neurotoxin in lower-urinary-tract disease and dysfunctions: Where are we now and what more can we do? *Toxins* **2022**, *14*, 498. [CrossRef]
2. Jiang, Y.H.; Chen, S.F.; Kuo, H.C. Frontiers in the clinical applications of botulinum toxin A as treatment for neurogenic lower urinary tract dysfunction. *Int. Neurourol. J.* **2020**, *24*, 301–312. [CrossRef]
3. Chiang, C.H.; Chen, S.F.; Kuo, H.C. Video-urodynamic characteristics of lower urinary tract dysfunction in patients with chronic brain disorders. *Neurourol. Urodyn.* **2022**, *41*, 255–263. [CrossRef]
4. Ogawa, T.; Sakakibara, R.; Kuno, S.; Ishizuka, O.; Kitta, T.; Yoshimura, N. Prevalence and treatment of LUTS in patients with Parkinson disease or multiple system atrophy. *Nat. Rev. Urol.* **2017**, *14*, 79–89. [CrossRef] [PubMed]
5. Chou, Y.C.; Jiang, Y.H.; Harnod, T.; Lee, H.T.; Kuo, H.C. Stroke and lower urinary tract symptoms: A neurosurgical view. *Urol. Sci.* **2019**, *30*, 8–13.
6. Zillioux, J.; Slopnick, E.A.; Vasavada, S.P. Third-line therapy for overactive bladder in the elderly: Nuances and considerations. *Neurourol. Urodyn.* **2022**, *41*, 1967–1974. [CrossRef] [PubMed]
7. Lightner, D.J.; Gomelsky, A.; Souter, L.; Vasavada, S.P. Diagnosis and treatment of overactive bladder (non-neurogenic) in adults: AUA/SUFU guideline Amendment 2019. *J. Urol.* **2019**, *202*, 558–563. [CrossRef] [PubMed]
8. Gillespie, J.I.; van Koeveringe, G.A.; de Wachter, S.G.; de Vente, J. On the origins of the sensory output from the bladder: The concept of afferent noise. *BJU Int.* **2009**, *103*, 1324–1333. [CrossRef]
9. Sakakibara, R.; Tateno, F.; Nagao, T.; Yamamoto, T.; Uchiyama, T.; Yamanishi, T.; Yano, M.; Kishi, M.; Tsuyusaki, Y.; Aiba, Y. Bladder function of patients with Parkinson's disease. *Int. J. Urol.* **2014**, *21*, 638–646. [CrossRef]
10. Kitta, T.; Kakizaki, H.; Furuno, T.; Moriya, K.; Tanaka, H.; Shiga, T.; Tamaki, N.; Yabe, I.; Sasaki, H.; Nonomura, K. Brain activation during detrusor overactivity in patients with Parkinson's disease: A PET study. *J. Urol.* **2006**, *175*, 994–998. [CrossRef]
11. Huang, Y.C.; Lee, W.C.; Chuang, Y.C.; Tsai, C.N.; Yu, C.C.; Wang, H.J.; Su, C.H. Using a rat model to translate and explore the pathogenesis of ketamine-induced cystitis. *Urol. Sci.* **2022**, *33*, 176–181.
12. Tysnes, O.B.; Storstein, A. Epidemiology of Parkinson's disease. *J. Neural. Transm.* **2017**, *124*, 901–905. [CrossRef] [PubMed]
13. Chen, Z.; Li, G.; Liu, J. Autonomic dysfunction in Parkinson's disease: Implication for pathophysiology, diagnosis, and treatment. *Neurobiol. Dis.* **2020**, *134*, 104700. [CrossRef] [PubMed]
14. Sakakibara, R.; Panicker, J.; Finazzi-Agro, E.; Iacovelli, V.; Bruschini, H.; Parkinson's Disease Subcomittee. A guideline for the management of bladder dysfunction in Parkinson's disease and other gait disorders. *Neurourol. Urodyn.* **2016**, *35*, 551–563. [CrossRef]
15. McDonald, C.; Winge, K.; Burn, D.J. Lower urinary tract symptoms in Parkinson's disease: Prevalence, aetiology and management. *Park. Relat. Disord.* **2017**, *35*, 8–16. [CrossRef]
16. Li, F.F.; Cui, Y.S.; Yan, R.; Cao, S.S.; Feng, T. Prevalence of lower urinary tract symptoms, urinary incontinence and retention in Parkinson's disease: A systematic review and meta-analysis. *Front. Aging Neurosci.* **2022**, *14*, 977572. [CrossRef]
17. Wang, J.; Cao, R.; Huang, T.; Liu, C.; Fan, Y. Urinary dysfunction is associated with nigrostriatal dopaminergic degeneration in early and untreated patients with Parkinson's disease. *Park. Dis.* **2020**, *2020*, 4981647. [CrossRef]
18. Mito, Y.; Yabe, I.; Yaguchi, H.; Takei, T.; Terae, S.; Tajima, Y. Relation of overactive bladder with motor symptoms and dopamine transporter imaging in drug-naïve Parkinson's disease. *Park. Relat. Disord.* **2018**, *50*, 37–41. [CrossRef] [PubMed]
19. Tkaczynska, Z.; Pilotto, A.; Becker, S.; Gräber-Sultan, S.; Berg, D.; Liepelt-Scarfone, I. Association between cognitive impairment and urinary dysfunction in Parkinson's disease. *J. Neural. Transm.* **2017**, *124*, 543–550. [CrossRef]
20. Shin, J.H.; Park, K.W.; Heo, K.O.; Chung, S.J.; Choo, M.S. Urodynamic study for distinguishing multiple system atrophy from Parkinson disease. *Neurology* **2019**, *93*, e946–e953. [CrossRef]
21. Vurture, G.; Peyronnet, B.; Palma, J.A.; Sussman, R.D.; Malacarne, D.R.; Feigin, A.; Palmerola, R.; Rosenblum, N.; Frucht, S.; Kaufmann, H.; et al. Urodynamic mechanisms underlying overactive bladder symptoms in patients with Parkinson disease. *Int. Neurourol. J.* **2019**, *23*, 211–218. [CrossRef] [PubMed]

22. Xing, T.; Ma, J.; Ou, T. Evaluation of neurogenic bladder outlet obstruction mimicking sphincter bradykinesia in male patients with Parkinson's disease. *BMC Neurol.* **2021**, *21*, 125. [CrossRef] [PubMed]
23. Wafa, H.A.; Wolfe, C.D.; Emmett, E.; Roth, G.A.; Johnson, C.O.; Wang, Y. Burden of stroke in Europe: Thirty-year projections of incidence, prevalence, deaths, and disability-adjusted life year. *Stroke* **2020**, *51*, 2418–2427. [CrossRef] [PubMed]
24. Wu, S.; Wu, B.O.; Liu, M.; Chen, Z.; Wang, W.; Anderson, C.S.; Sandercock, P.; Wang, Y.; Huang, Y.; Cui, L.; et al. Stroke in China: Advances and challenges in epidemiology, prevention, and management. *Lancet Neurol.* **2019**, *18*, 394–405. [CrossRef]
25. Wang, W.; Jiang, B.; Sun, H.; Ru, X.; Sun, D.; Wang, L.; Wang, L.; Jiang, Y.; Li, Y.; Wang, Y.; et al. Prevalence, incidence, and mortality of stroke in China: Results from a nationwide population-based survey of 480687 adults. *Circulation* **2017**, *135*, 759–771. [CrossRef]
26. Holroyd, S. Urinary incontinence after stroke. *Br. J. Community Nurs.* **2019**, *24*, 590–594. [CrossRef]
27. Akkoç, Y.; Yıldız, N.; Bardak, A.N.; Ersöz, M.; Tunç, H.; Köklü, K.; Alemdaroğlu, E.; Güler, A.; Şaşmaz, E.; Doğan, A.; et al. The course of post-stroke bladder problems and their relation with functional and mental status and quality of life: A six-month, prospective, multicenter study. *Turk. J. Phys. Med. Rehabil.* **2019**, *65*, 335–342. [CrossRef]
28. Chohan, S.A.; Venkatesh, P.K.; How, C.H. Long-term complications of stroke and secondary prevention: An overview for primary care physicians. *Singap. Med. J.* **2019**, *60*, 616–620. [CrossRef]
29. Turhan, N.; Atalay, A.; Atabek, K. Impact of stroke etiology, lesion location and aging on post-stroke urinary incontinence as a predictor of functional recovery. *Int. J. Rehabil. Res.* **2006**, *29*, 335–338. [CrossRef]
30. Cai, W.; Wang, J.; Wang, L.; Wang, J.; Guo, L. Prevalence and risk factors of urinary incontinence for the post-stroke inpatients in Southern China. *Neurol. Urodyn.* **2015**, *34*, 231–235. [CrossRef]
31. Bizovičar, N.; Mali, B.; Goljar, N. Clinical risk factors for the post-stroke urinary incontinence during rehabilitation. *Int. J. Rehabil. Res.* **2020**, *43*, 310–315. [CrossRef] [PubMed]
32. Gupta, A.; Taly, A.B.; Srivastava, A.; Thyloth, M. Urodynamics post stroke in patients with urinary incontinence: Is there correlation between bladder type and site of lesion? *Ann. Indian Acad. Neurol.* **2009**, *12*, 104–107. [CrossRef] [PubMed]
33. Pizzi, A.; Falsini, C.; Martini, M.; Rossetti, M.A.; Verdesca, S.; Tosto, A. Urinary incontinence after ischemia stroke: Clinical and urodynamic studies. *Neurol. Urodyn.* **2014**, *33*, 420–425. [CrossRef] [PubMed]
34. Dykstra, D.D.; Sidi, A.A.; Scott, A.B.; Pagel, J.M.; Goldish, G.D. Effects of botulinum A toxin on detrusor-sphincter dyssynergia in spinal cord injury patients. *J. Urol.* **1988**, *139*, 919–922. [CrossRef]
35. Aoki, K.R.; Guyer, B. Botulinum toxin type A and other botulinum toxin serotypes: A comparative review of biochemical and pharmacological actions. *Eur. J. Neurol.* **2001**, *8* (Suppl. S5), 21–29. [CrossRef]
36. Anandan, C.; Jankovic, J. Botulinum toxin in movement disorder: An update. *Toxins* **2021**, *13*, 42. [CrossRef]
37. Francisco, G.E.; Balbert, A.; Bavikatte, G.; Bensmail, D.; Carda, S.; Deltombe, T.; Draulans, N.; Escaldi, S.; Gross, R.; Jacinto, J.; et al. A practical guide to optimizing the benefits of post-stroke spasticity interventions with botulinum toxin A: An international group consensus. *J. Rehabil. Med.* **2021**, *53*, 2715. [CrossRef]
38. Jocson, A.; Lew, M. Use of botulinum toxin in Parkinson's disease. *Park. Relat. Disord.* **2019**, *59*, 57–64. [CrossRef]
39. Jiang, Y.H.; Liao, C.C.; Kuo, H.C. Current and potential urological applications of botulinum toxin A. *Nat. Rev. Urol.* **2015**, *12*, 519–533. [CrossRef]
40. Cruz, F. Targets for botulinum toxin in the lower urinary tract. *Neurourol. Urodyn.* **2014**, *33*, 31–38. [CrossRef]
41. Apostolidis, A.; Popat, R.; Yiangou, Y.; Cockayne, D.; Ford, A.P.D.W.; Davis, J.B.; Dasgupta, P.; Fowler, C.J.; Anand, P. Decreased sensory receptor P2X3 and TRPV1 in suburothelial nerve fibers following intradetrsuor injections of botulinum toxin for human detrusor overactivity. *J. Urol.* **2005**, *174*, 977–983. [CrossRef]
42. Khera, M.; Somogyi, G.T.; Kiss, S.; Boone, T.B.; Smith, C.P. Botulinum toxin A inhibits ATP release from the bladder urothelium after chronic spinal cord injury. *Neurochem. Int.* **2004**, *45*, 987–993. [CrossRef] [PubMed]
43. Rapp, D.E.; Turk, K.W.; Bales, G.T.; Cook, S.P. Botulinum toxin type a inhibits calcitonin gene-related peptide release from isolated rat bladder. *J. Urol.* **2006**, *175*, 1138–1142. [CrossRef] [PubMed]
44. Lucioni, A.; Bales, G.T.; Lotan, T.L.; McGehee, D.S.; Cook, S.P.; Rapp, D.E. Botulinum toxin type A inhibits sensory neuropeptide release in rat bladder models of acute injury and chronic inflammation. *BJU Int.* **2008**, *101*, 366–370. [CrossRef] [PubMed]
45. US Food & Drug Administration. BOTOX Label. Highlights of Prescribing Information. 2018. Available online: https://www.accessdata.fda.gov/drugsatfda_docs/label/2018/103000s5307lbl.pdf (accessed on 10 February 2023).
46. Wohlfarth, K.; Schwandt, I.; Wegner, F.; Jürgens, T.; Gelbrich, G.; Wagner, A.; Bogdahn, U.; Schulte-Mattler, W. Biological activity of two botulinum toxin type A complex (Dysport and Botox) in volunteers: A double-blind, randomized, dose-ranging study. *J. Neurol.* **2008**, *255*, 1932–1939. [CrossRef]
47. Kuo, H.C. Comparison of effectiveness of detrusor, suburothelial and bladder base injections of botulinum toxin a for idiopathic detrusor overactivity. *J. Urol.* **2007**, *178*, 1359–1363. [CrossRef]
48. Karsenty, G.; Elzayat, E.; Delapparent, T.; St-Denis, B.; Lemieux, M.C.; Corcos, J. Botulinum toxin type a injections into the trigone to treat idiopathic overactive bladder do not induce vesicoureteral reflux. *J. Urol.* **2007**, *177*, 1011–1014. [CrossRef]
49. Mascarenhas, F.; Cocuzza, M.; Gomes, C.M.; Leao, N. Trigonal injection of botulinum toxin-A does not cause vesicoureteral reflux in neurogenic patients. *Neurourol. Urodyn.* **2008**, *27*, 311–314. [CrossRef]
50. Giannantoni, A.; Costantini, E.; Di Stasi, S.M.; Tascini, M.C.; Bini, V.; Porena, M. Botulinum A toxin intravesical injections in the treatment of painful bladder syndrome: A pilot study. *Eur. Urol.* **2006**, *49*, 704–709. [CrossRef]

51. Kuo, H.C. Effectiveness of urethral injection of botulinum A toxin in the treatment of voiding dysfunction after radical hysterectomy. *Urol. Int.* **2005**, *75*, 247–251. [CrossRef]
52. Chen, J.L.; Chen, C.Y.; Kuo, H.C. Botulinum toxin A injection to the bladder neck and urethra for medically refractory lower urinary tract symptoms in men without prostatic obstruction. *J. Formos. Med. Assoc.* **2009**, *108*, 950–956. [CrossRef]
53. Giannantoni, A.; Rossi, A.; Mearini, E.; Del Zingaro, M.; Porena, M.; Berardelli, A. Botulinum toxin A for overactive bladder and detrusor muscle overactivity in patients with Parkinson's disease and multiple system atrophy. *J. Urol.* **2009**, *182*, 1453–1457. [CrossRef]
54. Giannantoni, A.; Conte, A.; Proietti, S.; Giovannozzi, S.; Rossi, A.; Fabbrini, G.; Porena, M.; Berardelli, A. Botulinum toxin type A in patients with Parkinson's disease and refractory overactive bladder. *J. Urol.* **2011**, *186*, 960–964. [CrossRef]
55. Kulaksizoglu, H.; Parman, Y. Use of botulinum toxin-A for the treatment of overactive bladder symptoms in patients with Parkinson's disease. *Park. Relat. Disord.* **2010**, *16*, 531–534. [CrossRef]
56. Anderson, R.U.; Orenberg, E.K.; Glowe, P. OnabotulinumtoxinA office treatment for neurogenic bladder incontinence in Parkinson's disease. *Urology* **2014**, *83*, 22–27. [CrossRef] [PubMed]
57. Vurture, G.; Peyronnet, B.; Feigin, A.; Biagioni, M.C.; Gilbert, R.; Rosenblum, N.; Frucht, S.; Di Rocco, A.; Nitti, V.W.; Brucker, B.M. Outcomes of intradetrusor onabotulinum toxin A injection in patients with Parkinson's disease. *Neurourol. Urodyn.* **2018**, *37*, 2669–2677. [CrossRef]
58. Atamian, A.; Sichez, P.C.; Michel, F.; Bandelier, Q.; Fall, M.; Gaillet, S.; Azoulay, J.P.; Lechevallier, E.; Karsenty, G. Intradetrusor injections of botulinum toxin A to treat urinary incontinence due to bladder overactivity during idiopathic Parkinson's disease. *Prog. Urol.* **2021**, *31*, 430–438. [CrossRef]
59. Mehta, S.; Hill, D.; Foley, N.; Hsieh, J.; Ethans, K.; Potter, P.; Baverstock, R.; Teasell, R.W.; Wolfe, D.; Spinal Cord Injury Rehabilitation Evidence Research Team. A meta-analysis of botulinum toxin sphincter injections in the treatment of incomplete voiding after spinal cord injury. *Arch. Phys. Med. Rehabil.* **2012**, *93*, 597–603. [CrossRef] [PubMed]
60. Kuo, H.C. Satisfaction with urethral injection of botulinum toxin A for detrusor sphincter dyssynergia in patients with spinal cord lesion. *Neurourol. Urodyn.* **2008**, *27*, 793–796. [CrossRef] [PubMed]
61. Kuo, H.C. Therapeutic outcome and quality of life between urethral and detrusor botulinum toxin treatment for patients with spinal cord lesions and detrusor sphincter dyssynergia. *Int. J. Clin.* **2013**, *67*, 1044–1049. [CrossRef]
62. Jiang, Y.H.; Chen, S.F.; Jhang, J.F.; Kuo, H.C. Therapeutic effect of urethral sphincter onabotulinumtoxinA injection for urethral sphincter hyperactivity. *Neurourol. Urodyn.* **2018**, *37*, 2651–2657. [CrossRef] [PubMed]
63. Lee, Y.K.; Kuo, H.C. Therapeutic effects of botulinum toxin A, via urethral sphincter injection on voiding dysfunction due to different bladder and urethral sphincter dysfunctions. *Toxins* **2019**, *11*, 487. [CrossRef] [PubMed]
64. Thomas, L.H.; Coupe, J.; Cross, L.D.; Tan, A.L.; Watkins, C.L. Interventions for treating urinary incontinence after stroke in adults. *Cochrane Database Syst. Rev.* **2019**, *2*, CD004462. [PubMed]
65. Shogenji, M.; Yoshida, M.; Sumiya, K.; Shimada, T.; Ikenaga, Y.; Ogawa, Y.; Hirako, K.; Sai, Y. Association of a continuous continence self-management program with independence in voiding behavior among stroke patients: A retrospective cohort study. *Neurourol. Urodyn.* **2022**, *41*, 1109–1120. [CrossRef]
66. Vasudeva, P.; Kumar, A.; Yadav, S.; Kumar, N.; Chaudhry, N.; Prasad, V.; Nagendra Rao, S.; Yadav, P.; Patel, S. Neurological safety and efficacy of darifenacin and mirabegron for the treatment of overactive bladder in patients with history of cerebrovascular accident. *Neurourol. Urodyn.* **2021**, *40*, 2041–2047. [CrossRef]
67. Lee, C.; Pizarro-Berdichevsky, J.; Clifton, M.M.; Vasavada, S.P. Sacral neuromodulation implant infection: Risk factor and prevention. *Curr. Urol. Rep.* **2017**, *18*, 16. [CrossRef]
68. Tutoto, M.; Ammirati, E.; Van der Aa, F. What is new in meuromodulation for overactive bladder? *Eur. Urol. Focus* **2018**, *4*, 49–53. [CrossRef]
69. Kuo, H.C. Therapeutic effects of suburothelial injection of botulinum A toxin for neurogenic detrusor overactivity due to chronic cerebrovascular accident and spinal cord lesions. *Urology* **2006**, *67*, 232–236. [CrossRef]
70. Jiang, Y.H.; Liao, C.H.; Tang, D.L.; Kuo, H.C. Efficacy and safety of intravesical onabotulinumtoxinA injection on elderly patients with chronic central nervous system lesions and overactive bladder. *PLoS ONE* **2014**, *9*, e105989. [CrossRef]
71. Chen, Y.H.; Kuo, H.C. Botulinum A toxin treatment of urethral sphincter pseudodyssynergia in patients with cerebrovascular accidents or intracranial lesions. *Urol. Int.* **2004**, *73*, 156–161. [CrossRef]
72. Knüpfer, S.C.; Schneider, S.A.; Averhoff, M.M.; Naumann, C.M.; Deuschl, G.; Jünemann, K.P.; Hamann, M.F. Preserved micturition after intradetrusor onabotulinumtoxinA injection for treatment of neurogenic bladder dysfunction in Parkinson's disease. *BMC Urol.* **2016**, *16*, 55. [CrossRef] [PubMed]

Disclaimer/Publisher's Note: The statements, opinions and data contained in all publications are solely those of the individual author(s) and contributor(s) and not of MDPI and/or the editor(s). MDPI and/or the editor(s) disclaim responsibility for any injury to people or property resulting from any ideas, methods, instructions or products referred to in the content.

toxins

MDPI

Review

Intravesical Injection of Botulinum Toxin Type A in Men without Bladder Outlet Obstruction and Post-Deobstructive Prostate Surgery

Hsiang-Ying Lee [1,2,3,4] and Hann-Chorng Kuo [5,6,*]

1 Department of Urology, Kaohsiung Medical University Hospital, Kaohsiung 80756, Taiwan; ashum1009@hotmail.com
2 Department of Urology, School of Medicine, College of Medicine, Kaohsiung Medical University, Kaohsiung 80756, Taiwan
3 Graduate Institute of Clinical Medicine, College of Medicine, Kaohsiung Medical University, Kaohsiung 80756, Taiwan
4 Center for Cancer Research, Kaohsiung Medical University, Kaohsiung 80756, Taiwan
5 Department of Urology, School of Medicine, Tzu Chi University, Hualien 970473, Taiwan
6 Department of Urology, Hualien Tzu Chi Hospital, Buddhist Tzu Chi Medical Foundation, Hualien 970473, Taiwan
* Correspondence: hck@tzuchi.com.tw

Abstract: Purpose: A significant proportion of men without bladder outlet obstruction (BOO) have been reported to have overactive bladders (OAB). This article aimed to review the specific group of reports on the use of botulinum toxin type A (BTX-A) injections into the bladder wall. Materials and methods: Original articles reporting men with small prostates without BOO were identified through a literature search using the PubMed and EMBASE databases. Finally, we included 18 articles that reviewed the efficacy and adverse effects of BTX-A injections in men. Results: Of the 18 articles screened, 13 demonstrated the therapeutic efficacy and adverse effects of BTX-A injections in men. Three studies compared BTX-A injection response between patients without prior prostate surgery and those undergoing prior prostate surgery, including transurethral resection of the prostate and radical prostatectomy (RP). Patients with prior RP experienced better efficacy and had a low risk of side effects. Two studies focused on patients who had undergone prior surgery for stress urinary incontinence, including male sling and artificial urethral sphincter surgery. The BTX-A injection was a safe and effective procedure for this specific group. OAB in men was found to have a different pathophysiology mechanism from that in female patients, which may decrease the efficacy of BTX-A injection in men. However, patients with small prostates and low prostate-specific antigen levels demonstrated better efficacy and tolerability after BTX-A injection. Conclusions: Although intravesical injection of BTX-A was a good option for controlling refractory OAB in men, the evidence-based guidelines are still limited. Further research is necessary to better understand the role of BTX-A injections on various aspects and histories. Therefore, treating patients using strategies tailored to their individual conditions is important.

Keywords: botulinum toxin; overactive bladder; men

Key Contribution: In men with small prostates and overactive bladder syndrome, intravesical injection of BTX-A had a similar efficacy compared with female patients. BTX-A injection is also feasible without severe adverse effects in men who ever received prostate surgery or stress urinary incontinence surgery.

Citation: Lee, H.-Y.; Kuo, H.-C. Intravesical Injection of Botulinum Toxin Type A in Men without Bladder Outlet Obstruction and Post-Deobstructive Prostate Surgery. *Toxins* **2023**, *15*, 221. https://doi.org/10.3390/toxins15030221

Received: 16 January 2023
Revised: 16 February 2023
Accepted: 9 March 2023
Published: 15 March 2023

Copyright: © 2023 by the authors. Licensee MDPI, Basel, Switzerland. This article is an open access article distributed under the terms and conditions of the Creative Commons Attribution (CC BY) license (https://creativecommons.org/licenses/by/4.0/).

1. Introduction

Lower urinary tract symptoms (LUTS) are common in male patients with bladder outlet obstruction (BOO) [1]. Subsequent detrusor physiological alterations, including hypertrophy, denervation caused by ischemia, and changes in neuronal mechanisms resulting from obstruction may lead to overactive bladder (OAB) [2]. OAB is a bothersome condition defined as a symptom complex of urinary urgency. Usually, it is accompanied by frequent urination, nocturia, and urinary incontinence. The prevalence of OAB in men has been reported to be approximately 26–33% in the United States, which increases with age, such that 73.9% of men over 60 years report urinary storage symptoms [3,4]. In the EPIC study, 10.8% of the male population were shown to have OAB [5]. However, a significant proportion of male individuals had OAB symptoms even without obstruction. In a total of 128 young men who underwent a urodynamic study (UDS) by Manohar et al., 18% had OAB without BOO [6].

Intervention for OAB in male patients is similar to that in female patients, usually beginning with behavioral treatment and medication management, including antimuscarinic agents and β3 agonists. However, in patients with persistent OAB symptoms despite conservative and medication treatment, defined as refractory OAB, more aggressive and invasive interventions are required, including intravesical injection of onabotulinum toxin A (BTX-A). BTX-A injections were approved by the US Food and Drug Administration for treatment in patients with non-neurogenic OAB in 2013 [7]. Most previous studies have evaluated the efficacy and adverse effects of BTX-A injections in female patients. However, there is a paucity of data on male patients with OAB. In a study by Rahnama'I et al., the success rate of intravesical BTX-A injection in men was 21%, with a mean follow-up of approximately 69 months. The most common reasons for discontinuing BTX-A injections were insufficient efficacy and side effects [8]. A recent systematic review that discussed BTX-A injections in men with OAB concluded that BTX-A injections could induce therapeutic response and have an impact on urodynamic parameters. Although the review article enrolled <1000 men, the available evidence was heterogeneous and limited [9].

The pathophysiology of OAB with or without BOO may differ. This review focuses on BTX-A injections in men with a small prostate size or history of prostate surgery. Studying the effect of BTX-A in this subgroup of patients would help clinicians better understand the response and adverse effects, and whether patients with small prostates were more likely to respond favorably to BTX-A injection compared to those with obstructed urethra due to large prostates.

2. Evidence Acquisition

A literature search of PubMed and EMBASE databases was conducted in October 2022, screening all topics on intravesical BTX-A injection in male patients without BOO who had refractory OAB after medication treatment. The search strategy included the following keywords/mesh terms: "Botox injection" and "overactive bladder". The searches were pooled with the limitations of men and language (English). Thereafter, animal model studies and review articles were excluded. Children and patients with neurogenic bladder were excluded from the study. Congress abstracts and book chapters were not considered for discussion in this review article.

After removing duplicates, we screened titles and abstracts to select appropriate studies and exclude unrelated articles. Initially, 99 related original articles retrieved from PubMed and EMBASE were included. Additionally, full-text articles were further assessed. Many studies have included both sexes but have not evaluated them separately. To focus on the male population, we only used studies in which data could be identified as results from men without BOO. We finally included 18 articles for our narrative review. Most of the articles were retrospective, single-center studies. A flowchart of this process is shown in Figure 1.

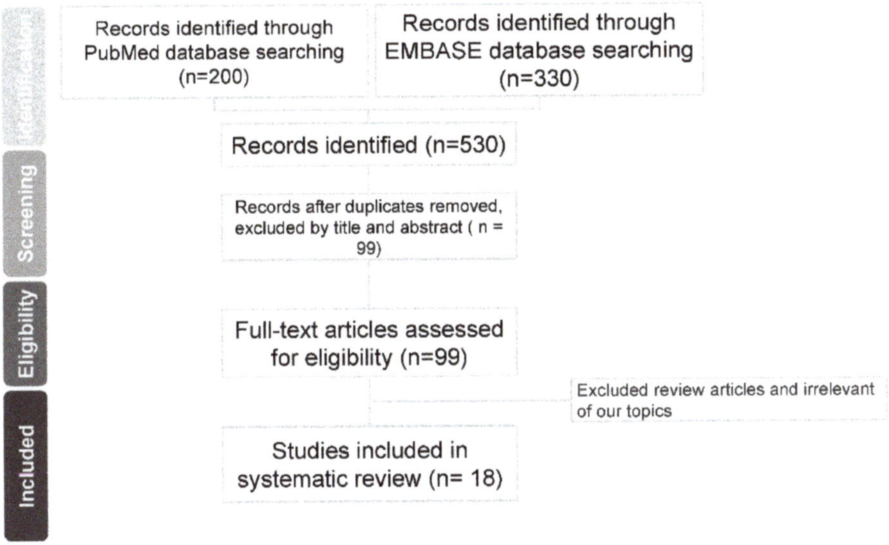

Figure 1. Flowchart of included articles for review.

3. Therapeutic Effectiveness and Adverse Events after BTX-A Injection

BTX-A intravesical injection focusing on male patients without BOO is presented in Table 1.

Regarding the mechanism underlying BTX-A, it inhibits signal transmission at the neuromuscular junction by inhibiting acetylcholine release, which interferes with the binding of neurotransmitters to postsynaptic receptors. Wang et al. [10], in Taiwan, reported a post-marketing survey of intradetrusor BTX-A injections in patients with OAB, including 62 male individuals. There was a significant improvement in OAB symptoms according to the Patient Perception of Bladder Condition and OAB Symptom Score questionnaires at 4 and 12 weeks after intervention compared with baseline. In terms of adverse events, although increased post-voiding residual urine (PVR) was found at 4 and 12 weeks, the PVR at 12 weeks declined compared with that at 4 weeks. Moreover, there were no patients with de novo acute urine retention (AUR). The incidence of urinary tract infection (UTI) was low (4.6%). Acceptance of BTX-A injections among patients was high owing to its acceptable efficacy and safety. BTX-A has been shown to be effective in patients with and without urinary incontinence. Grishin et al. [11] divided enrolled patients, including men and women, into OAB without imperative urinary incontinence (Group 1) and OAB with imperative urinary incontinence (Group 2). After 200 units of BTX-A injection, a decrease in the number of urinary incontinence episodes by 1.59 times ($p < 0.05$) in Group 1 and 2.75 times ($p < 0.05$) in Group 2 was found. The quality of life (QoL) also improved according to the SF-36.

The pathophysiology of OAB has been suggested to differ between men with and without BOO. Regarding antimuscarinic treatment, previous research demonstrated that patients with OAB with smaller prostates might benefit from antimuscarinic agents alone without adding σ-adrenergic agents to relieve OAB symptoms. Men with OAB due to primary bladder conditions may respond well to antimuscarinic therapy alone [12]. A positive correlation between prostate-specific antigen (PSA) levels and prostate size was confirmed before high PSA levels could be translated to a large prostate volume [13]. Similarly, Roehrborn et al. demonstrated that among patients with PSA level < 1.3 ng/mL, tolterodine ER alone significantly improved the frequency and International Prostate Symptom Score storage scores compared with placebo [14]. Theoretically, patients with OAB with a small prostate size would likely benefit from intravesical BTX-A injections. In a phase III randomized controlled phase (RCT) study, Yokoyama et al. [15] compared BTX-A injection and placebo groups, dividing participants into lower PSA levels (<1.5 ng/mL) and higher PSA levels (≥1.5 ng/mL). The cut-off value was according to previous research in which PSA ≥ 1.5 ng/mL could be considered an enlarged prostate (>30 mL) [16]. BTX-A injection was effective, with tolerable adverse effects in patients with lower PSA levels. Urinary incontinence episodes showed a greater decline compared with the placebo in patients with small prostates. However, no significant improvement in OAB symptoms was observed in the subgroup with higher PSA levels. The risk of urine retention in patients with lower PSA levels was low, owing to a small elevated PVR.

Men with higher PSA levels were considered to have larger prostate volume, which might worsen OAB symptoms due to BOO [17]. Abrar et al. [18] demonstrated that male sex was a significant predictor of poor response in patients with LUTS and associated with a higher risk of clean intermittent self-catheterization (CISC) after BTX-A injection compared with female sex. Although men with BOO were excluded from this study, prostate enlargement may still be a possible reason why OAB symptoms might partially result from voiding resistance. However, the treatment response rate in men was 62% in a study conducted by Mateu Arrom et al. [19], which showed that the efficacy of BTX-A injection was similar to that in the female population. Based on urodynamic results, in terms of objective outcome evaluation, decreased detrusor pressure, maximum flow rate, and impaired voiding efficiency were observed 3 months after injection. In this study, 13% of the patients required CISC, which may be slightly higher than that in female patients. Although male patients without BOO may experience similar benefits to those in the female population after receiving Botox injections, the extent of prostate urethral resistance is still the main reason for the worsening efficacy, with a higher risk of complications. The authors observed that the BOO index (BOOI) was related to the BTX-A injection response and development of complications after treatment. Careful evaluation of BOOI before BTX-A intervention may be useful for predicting efficacy and adverse effects. Since only 30–50% of patients with OAB could have detrusor overactivity (DO) [20], Kanagarajah et al. [21] included only patients with OAB without DO. Both sexes showed similar improvements in the urogenital distress inventory-6 questionnaire and visual analog scale scores at week 12 post-injection. A study by Walker et al. [22] indicated that some men developed de novo CISC after receiving a BTX-A injection, even with BOOI < 20. However, according to the results of a questionnaire in a real-life clinical setting in men, BTX-A injection could objectively improve QoL. Patients with good detrusor function in terms of bladder contractility index value > 150 were less likely to require de novo CISC.

Table 1. Therapeutic effectiveness and adverse events after BTX-A injection.

Study	Design	Population Number of Men	Dose/Units	Technique	Comparator	Outcomes	Follow-Up Schedule
Wang et al. [10]	Prospective cohort study	62 men Treatment-naïve to Botox injection	100 units	Injection into the detrusor at 10 points	NA	Improving PPBC and OABSS at 4 and 12 weeks	1 week 4 weeks 12 weeks
Yokoyama et al. [15]	RCT, phase III	62 men Patients with BOO were excluded	100 units	Injection into the detrusor at 20 points	BTX-A vs. Placebo	Greater decrease in UI episodes in men with lower PSA levels	2 weeks 6 weeks 12 weeks
Abrar M et al. [18]	Retrospective cohort study	24 men	10 units/mL/ injection site	NA	NA	Men had worse responses and required CISC more than women	4–6 weeks
Mateu Arrom L et al. [19]	Retrospective cohort study	146 men	100 units	20 points excluding the trigone	Pretreatment vs. posttreatment	62% response rate	3 months

Table 1. *Cont.*

Study	Design	Population Number of Men	Dose/Units	Technique	Comparator	Outcomes	Follow-Up Schedule
Kanagarajah P et al. [21]	Prospective cohort study	5 men	100 or 150 units	10 points	Baseline UDI-6 and VAS score vs. postinjection UDI-6 and VAS score	Both genders showed improvements in UDI-6 and VAS score in patients without DOA	12 weeks
Faure Walker NA et al. [22]	Retrospective comparative study	65 men	Initial 200 → start at 100 units	10–20 points	Men vs. women	Improving QoL	4–12 weeks
Hsiao SM et al. [23]	Retrospective cohort study	46 men	100 units	20 points excluding the trigone	Men vs. women	Male gender was associated with worse therapeutic efficacy	6 months
Hsiao SM et al. [24]	Retrospective cohort study	148 men	100 units	20 points excluding the trigone	NA	Men had shorter persistent PVR > 150 mL intervals than women	6 months
Jiang YH et al. [25]	Retrospective cohort study	148 men	100 units	20–40 points excluding the trigone	AUR vs. large PVR vs. UTI	Men had more AUR postinjection than women	6 months
Kuo HC et al. [26]	Prospective cohort study	112 men	100–200 units	20 points including the trigone	NA	Men had more AUR postinjection than women	12 months
Liao CH et al. [27]	Retrospective cohort study	93 men	100 units	40 points excluding the trigone	Frail elderly vs. elderly without frailty vs. people younger than 65 years	Men did not have an increased risk of PVR greater than 150 mL	12 months
Osborn DJ et al. [28]	Retrospective cohort study	38 men	100 or 200 units	NA	No retention vs. retention	Gender was not associated with postoperative urinary retention	40 weeks
Makovey I et al. [29]	Retrospective cohort study	17 men	150–200 units	20 points including the trigone	Lack of efficacy vs. intolerable side effects	Lack of anticholinergic efficacy had less success in Botox injections	11 months

NA: Not available.

Hsiao et al. [23] evaluated the factors affecting therapeutic efficacy after BTX-A injection. They found that symptoms could improve six months after injection in both sexes. However, male sex was associated with worse therapeutic efficacy compared with female sex. The success rate was 63.8% (male and female). In a further study by the same research group [24], they assessed if the urodynamic factors could predict large PVR urine volume after BTX-A injection. A total of 44% of male patients experienced large PVR (>200 mL) during follow-up. Daytime frequency episodes and voiding efficiency were significant predictors of a large PVR. They discovered that sex was not one of the causative factors, and both sexes may have induced large PVR during the 6-month follow-up period. However, male patients showed a shorter persistent PVR (>150 mL) interval than did women in terms of faster recovery from a large PVR.

The adverse effects of BTX-A injections were discussed in a study by Jiang et al. [25]. Male patients (14.2%) experienced AUR and 28.4% had large PVR (≥200 mL) in one month. The initial greater increase in PVR in male patients than in female ones was not significant after one month. UTIs developed in 8.8% of male patients. The incidence of AUR was significantly higher in male patients than in female ones. However, female patients had a higher incidence of UTI compared with male patients. Similarly, Kuo et al. [26] revealed that male patients had a higher risk of AUR after BTX-A injection using both univariate and multivariate analyses and a higher incidence of UTI adverse events than female patients. When selecting male patients with OAB to receive BTX-A injections, even without BOO, the possibility of AUR should be considered. However, the success rate in male patients was 67%, which was not significantly different from that in female patients (66%). Specifically, male patients with a history of prior transurethral resection of the prostate (TURP) had a higher success rate (74%) compared with no TURP history cohort, without a statistically significant difference. Male patients without TURP history had higher incidence of hematuria and UTI, which may have resulted from prostate-related adverse effects. According to baseline UDS variables, detrusor pressure during voiding was not related to adverse event occurrence after BTX-A injection in male patients. In contrast, Liao et al. [27] evaluated the impact of BTX-A injections on refractory idiopathic detrusor overactivity. They found that the success rate at 12 months in frail older patients was lower than that in older patients without frailty and younger patients (6.82%, 22.3%, and 23.1%, respectively). Sex was not a factor inducing a higher risk of PVR > 150 mL. However, frail older patients were at greater risk for a large PVR and a higher chance of requiring an indwelling catheter or CISC. Similarly, in a study by Osborn et al. [28], male patients did not have an increased risk of urinary retention after BTX-A injections. Postoperative urinary retention was defined as the requirement for a CISC or indwelling catheter. Therefore, the threshold postoperative PVR urine volume to initiate CISC could determine postoperative urinary retention rate.

Patients with refractory OAB required additional BTX-A injections for two reasons. One reason was the lack of medication efficacy. The other reason was the intolerable adverse effects of anticholinergic agents. Makovey et al. [29] reported that more men had a history of anticholinergic medication efficacy than of intolerable side effects. They further indicated that BTX-A injection had a higher success rate in patients with refractory idiopathic OAB due to anticholinergic intolerability than in those with poor medication efficacy.

4. The Impact of Injection Site, Dosage, and Numbers of BTX-A

Previous studies have assessed whether the injection site can affect the efficacy and adverse effects of BTX-A injections. The current guidelines recommend that BTX-A should not be injected over the trigone area, based on the results of early research that exhibited a potential risk of development of vesicoureteral reflux after trigone area injections [30]. However, further evidence did not support this risk. El-Hefnawy et al. [31] compared trigonal-sparing versus trigonal-involved BTX-A injections and found that improvement in all components of OAB symptoms occurred at both sites. Additionally, the response reached maximum efficacy in the third month. Significant improvements in episodes of urge incontinence and urinary frequency were observed in the trigonal-sparing group at six months. In contrast, higher UTI incidence rate and detrusor leak point pressure were found in the trigonal-involved injection group. The abundance of sensory fibers in the trigonal area, which is considered to play a role in bladder urgency sensation, is assumed to induce a better response after BTX-A injection. Kuo et al. [32] demonstrated that intravesical BTX-A injection was an effective treatment, regardless of the injection site. In addition, detrusor and suburothelial injection techniques showed similar efficacies in idiopathic detrusor overactivity (IDO). Various physiological mechanisms are related to urinary function within the suburothelial space, including sensory and solute transport. The effect of BTX-A injection generally diffuses from the detrusor muscle and suburothelial space [33]. The function of detrusor injection may be due to an effect on acetylcholine release in the neuromuscular junction. In contrast, suburothelial injection might affect the sensory receptor, which further mediates detrusor contractions. When performing BTX-A injections over the detrusor muscle, one should be cautious as BTX-A may be lost outside the bladder if the needle passes over the bladder wall. Suburothelial injection can retain

BTX-A within the suburothelium and it is easier to visualize the mucosal swelling, which has more precise toxin localization, if the injection site is appropriate.

Regarding idiopathic OAB, 100 units of intravesical BTX-A is recommended. Abdelwahab et al. [34] compared between 100- and 200-unit BTX-A intradetrusor injections. They revealed that the efficacy was similar regardless of the BTX-A dosage, and a higher incidence of adverse effects occurred in patients receiving 200 units of BTX-A after nine months of follow-up. Therefore, an injection of 100 units could be sufficient to achieve satisfactory outcomes in patients with idiopathic OAB with or without IDO [35]. In addition to the dosage of BTX-A, the number of injection sites did not affect treatment outcomes. A prospective randomized study compared patients receiving different numbers of intravesical 100-unit BTX-A injections in 10 mL (10, 20, and 40) into the bladder body. It has been demonstrated that 10 sites were adequate to achieve equal therapeutic effects to 20 and 40 sites [36]. The number of injections was less relevant by spreading the BTX-A solution across the suburothelial space. BTX-A injection is performed as an office-based procedure under local anesthesia. Therefore, a small number of injection sites might reduce adverse effects and uncomfortable experiences due to injection, such as bladder pain, hematuria, and possible UTI [36].

Repeated injections of BTX-A were as efficacious as the first injection, without resistance. The results showed improvements in OAB symptoms, urodynamic parameters, and QoL. The most common reason for dropping out was poor response or dislike of CISC. The interval between different injections was approximately 9–10 months. Additional evidence would eliminate the fear of toxin accumulation with repeated injections [37,38].

5. BTX-A Injection after Deobstructive Prostate Surgery

Intravesical BTX-A injection is a treatment option for relieving obstruction in men with persistent OAB after prostate surgery. However, studies involving male patients are limited. From a histopathological perspective, persistent DO following TURP may result from the increased resistance of bladder vessels and decreased perfusion [39]. Whether the histopathology differs between men who have undergone prostate surgery and those who have not remains unclear.

Habashy et al. [40] enrolled male patients who underwent prior prostate surgery, including radical prostatectomy (RP) and TURP, without undergoing surgery. Comparing prostate surgery with no surgery groups showed significant improvement in pad usage after BTX-A injection. However, there was no significant difference between the two groups in Patient Global Impression of Improvement (PGI-I) scores. In the subgroup analysis of patients who underwent prostate surgery, the RP group showed greater improvements in pad usage and PGI-I scores than did the TURP group. The reason for the different BTX-A injection efficacies is unclear. It is suggested that the TURP group had more severe detrusor dysfunction due to BOO, while the RP group had a relatively higher degree of sphincteric deficiency, which is the main reason for incontinence.

The long-term efficacy of BTX-A injections was demonstrated by Bels et al. [41] in subgroups based on prior prostate surgery. The discontinuation rate was 70.8% during the 23-month median follow-up. TURP, RP, and no-prior-prostate-surgery subgroups after BTX-A injection were compared. The results showed a higher incidence rate of necessary CISC and larger PVR volume in the no-prior-prostate-surgery subgroup than in the prior TURP or RP subgroups. The reason that patients without prior prostate surgery had a higher risk of adverse effects may be that BOO was more prominent in the subgroup without prior prostate surgery (50% of the enrolled patients). The RP subgroup had the lowest CISC rates in terms of a lower discontinuation rate with more tolerable BTX-A injections. This highlights the importance of evaluating the degree of obstruction and prostate size before BTX-A injection to minimize the possibility of de novo CISC.

Another study by Rahnama'I et al. [8] evaluated the long-term compliance and side effects of BTX-A injections in heterogeneous groups of male patients. The success rates of idiopathic OAB, TURP, and post-PCa treatments after a mean follow-up period of 69 months were 21%, 11%, and 29%, respectively. Similar to the studies by Habashy et al. and Bels et al. [39,40], patients with prior RP had better efficacy and a lower risk of side effects compared with patients with prior TURP. The insufficient effect of poor satisfaction after BTX-A injection in the post-TURP subgroup may be due to moderate detrusor dysfunction resulting from a history of long-term obstructed prostate.

6. BTX-A Injection after Stress Urinary Incontinency Surgery

Artificial urinary sphincters (AUS) and male slings are popular treatments for post-RP stress urinary incontinence (SUI). Preoperative OAB symptoms may persist after SUI surgery and 23–37.5% of patients develop de novo OAB after AUS implantation [42]. BTX-A injection is still considered an option for controlling refractory OAB symptoms after treatment. De Sallmard et al. showed that a significant number of male patients (90%) with an AUS implantation history had totally or partially improved OAB symptoms after injection. The discontinuation-free survival rate was 50% at 60 months. However, this was combined with the female results. Nevertheless, this study indicated that BTX-A injections were effective in patients undergoing AUS implantation. No significant BTX-A-related adverse effects were encountered after injection: two male patients experienced urethral erosion, which may have resulted from the temporarily necessary CISC. Therefore, the incidence of CISC may be related to the risk of AUS complications.

Mateu Arrom et al.'s study [43] enrolled patients with prior RP and TURP and a history of SUI surgery, including AUS and male sling implantation. At a median follow-up of 49 months, 66.7% of the patients showed subjective improvement in OAB symptoms after injection. All patients were confirmed to have DO before BTX-A injection using the UDS. There was a significant reduction in the proportion of patients with DO after BTX-A injections (from 100% to 53.3%). According to the UDS data, no significant change in voiding efficiency or PVR was noted three months after treatment. The results indicated a good response to treatment and a low complication rate in patients with prior SUI surgery. The authors mentioned that the procedure should be performed with caution to prevent urethral injury, which may increase the risk of further AUS cuff erosion. They recommended avoiding injection of BTX-A over the balloon side in cases of balloon perforation.

7. Conclusions

The available evidence regarding BTX-A injection for refractory OAB in male patients is limited. Furthermore, most studies have combined BTX-A injection in female patients to analyze the efficacy or adverse effects of BTX-A injection. Generally, the response rate in male patients was similar to that in female patients. However, some studies have indicated that female patients exhibited better therapeutic efficacy, considering that prostate-related OAB has a different pathophysiology. However, owing to the distinct pathophysiology between men with and without BOO, patients with a small prostate and without BOO or a history of prostate surgery could have a better response and fewer adverse effects after BTX-A injection. The degree of outlet resistance may determine the efficacy of BTX-A injections in OAB symptom control. Compared with prior prostate surgeries, patients receiving RP showed better improvement in OAB symptoms and the lowest CISC rates after BTX-A injection.

Male sling and AUS were surgical choices in patients with SUI after RP. Some patients showed persistent or de novo OAB symptoms after SUI surgery. It might be feasible for patients with prior SUI surgery to receive BTX-A injections, which could improve DO and was safe. However, caution should be observed about the possible complications, despite their rarity, such as balloon perforation and urethral erosion.

Author Contributions: Conceptualization, writing—review and editing: H.-C.K. Methodology, writing—original draft preparation: H.-Y.L. All authors have read and agreed to the published version of the manuscript.

Funding: This research was funded by the Buddhist Tzu Chi Medical Foundation grants TCMF-SP-108-01 and TCMF-MP-110-03-01.

Institutional Review Board Statement: Not applicable.

Informed Consent Statement: Not applicable.

Data Availability Statement: Not applicable.

Conflicts of Interest: The authors declare no conflict of interest.

References

1. Verhovsky, G.; Baberashvili, I.; Rappaport, Y.H.; Zilberman, D.E.; Neheman, A.; Gal, J.; Zisman, A.; Stav, K. Bladder Oversensitivity Is Associated with Bladder Outlet Obstruction in Men. *J. Pers. Med.* **2022**, *12*, 1675. [CrossRef]
2. Bosch, R.; Abrams, P.; Averbeck, M.A.; Agró, E.F.; Gammie, A.; Marcelissen, T.; Solomon, E. Do functional changes occur in the bladder due to bladder outlet obstruction?—ICI-RS 2018. *Neurourol. Urodyn.* **2019**, *38* (Suppl. S5), S56–S65. [CrossRef] [PubMed]
3. Irwin, D.E.; Milsom, I.; Kopp, Z.; Abrams, P.; Artibani, W.; Herschorn, S. Prevalence, severity, and symptom bother of lower urinary tract symptoms among men in the EPIC study: Impact of overactive bladder. *Eur. Urol.* **2006**, *50*, 1306–1314. [CrossRef]
4. Coyne, K.S.; Sexton, C.C.; Bell, J.A.; Thompson, C.L.; Dmochowski, R.; Bavendam, T.; Chen, C.-I.; Clemens, J.Q. The prevalence of lower urinary tract symptoms (LUTS) and overactive bladder (OAB) by racial/ethnic group and age: Results from OAB-POLL. *Neurourol. Urodyn.* **2012**, *32*, 230–237. [CrossRef]
5. Irwin, D.E.; Milsom, I.; Hunskaar, S.; Reilly, K.; Kopp, Z.; Herschorn, S.; Coyne, K.; Kelleher, C.; Hampel, C.; Artibani, W.; et al. Population-Based Survey of Urinary Incontinence, Overactive Bladder, and Other Lower Urinary Tract Symptoms in Five Countries: Results of the EPIC Study. *Eur. Urol.* **2006**, *50*, 1306–1315. [CrossRef] [PubMed]
6. Manohar, C.S.; Rajawat, M.S.; Keshavamurthy, R.; Chouhan, P.K.; Poonawala, A. Urodynamic profile of lower urinary tract symptoms in young men: A testimony of the truth? *Urol. Ann.* **2022**, *14*, 215–217.
7. Jambusaria, L.H.; Dmochowski, R.R. Intradetrusor onabotulinumtoxinA for overactive bladder. *Expert Opin. Biol. Ther.* **2014**, *14*, 721–727. [CrossRef]
8. Rahnama'i, M.S.; Marcelissen, T.A.; Brierley, B.; Schurch, B.; de Vries, P. Long-term compliance and results of intravesical botulinum toxin A injections in male patients. *Neurourol. Urodyn.* **2017**, *36*, 1855–1859. [CrossRef]
9. Truzzi, J.C.; Lapitan, M.C.; Truzzi, N.C.; Iacovelli, V.; Averbeck, M.A. Botulinum toxin for treating overactive bladder in men: A systematic review. *Neurourol. Urodyn.* **2022**, *41*, 710–723. [CrossRef] [PubMed]
10. Wang, C.C.; Chou, E.C.; Chuang, Y.C.; Lin, C.C.; Hsu, Y.C.; Liao, C.H.; Kuo, H.-C. Effectiveness and Safety of Intradetrusor OnabotulinumtoxinA Injection for Neurogenic Detrusor Overactivity and Overactive Bladder Patients in Taiwan-A Phase IV Prospective, Interventional, Multiple-Center Study (Restore Study). *Toxins* **2021**, *13*, 911. [CrossRef]
11. Grishin, A.; Spaska, A.; Kayumova, L. Correction of overactive bladder with botulinum toxin type A (BTX-A). *Toxicon* **2021**, *200*, 96–101. [CrossRef]
12. Roehrborn, C.G.; Kaplan, S.A.; Jones, J.S.; Wang, J.T.; Bavendam, T.; Guan, Z. Tolterodine Extended Release with or Without Tamsulosin in Men with Lower Urinary Tract Symptoms Including Overactive Bladder Symptoms: Effects of Prostate Size. *Eur. Urol.* **2009**, *55*, 472–481. [CrossRef]
13. Roehrborn, C.G.; Boyle, P.; Gould, A.; Waldstreicher, J. Serum prostate-specific antigen as a predictor of prostate volume in men with benign prostatic hyperplasia. *Urology* **1999**, *53*, 581–589. [CrossRef]
14. Roehrborn, C.G.; Kaplan, S.A.; Kraus, S.R.; Wang, J.T.; Bavendam, T.; Guan, Z. Effects of serum PSA on efficacy of tolterodine extended release with or without tamsulosin in men with LUTS, including OAB. *Urology* **2008**, *72*, 1061–1067. [CrossRef] [PubMed]
15. Yokoyama, O.; Honda, M.; Yamanishi, T.; Sekiguchi, Y.; Fujii, K.; Kinoshita, K.; Nakayama, T.; Ueno, A.; Mogi, T. Efficacy and safety of onabotulinumtoxinA in patients with overactive bladder: Subgroup analyses by sex and by serum prostate-specific antigen levels in men from a randomized controlled trial. *Int. Urol. Nephrol.* **2021**, *53*, 2243–2250. [CrossRef] [PubMed]
16. Gravas, S.; Cornu, J.N.; Gacci, M.; Gratzke, C.; Herrmann TR, W.; Mamoulakis, C.; Rieken, M.; Speakman, M.J.; Tikkinen, K.A.O. *Management of Nonneurogenic Male Lower Urinary Tract Symptoms (LUTS), Including Benign Prostatic Obstruction (BPO)*; European Association of Urology: Arnhem, The Netherlands, 2019.
17. Sharma, M.; Jamaiyar, A. Exploration of Serum Prostatic Specific Antigen Level in Enlarged Prostate with its Histopathological Correlation. *J. Pharm. Bioallied Sci.* **2022**, *14* (Suppl. S1), S880–S883. [CrossRef]
18. Abrar, M.; Stroman, L.; Malde, S.; Solomon, E.; Sahai, A. Predictors of Poor Response and Adverse Events Following Botulinum Toxin-A for Refractory Idiopathic Overactive Bladder. *Urology* **2020**, *135*, 32–37. [CrossRef] [PubMed]
19. Mateu Arrom, L.; Mayordomo Ferrer, O.; Sabiote Rubio, L.; Gutierrez Ruiz, C.; Martínez Barea, V.; Palou Redorta, J.; Smet, C.E. Treatment Response and Complications after Intradetrusor OnabotulinumtoxinA Injection in Male Patients with Idiopathic Overactive Bladder Syndrome. *J. Urol.* **2020**, *203*, 392–397. [CrossRef]
20. Ashok, K.; Wang, A. Detrusor overactivity: An overview. *Arch. Gynecol. Obstet.* **2010**, *282*, 33–41. [CrossRef]
21. Kanagarajah, P.; Ayyathurai, R.; Caruso, D.J.; Gomez, C.; Gousse, A.E. Role of botulinum toxin-A in refractory idiopathic overactive bladder patients without detrusor overactivity. *Int. Urol. Nephrol.* **2011**, *44*, 91–97. [CrossRef]

22. Faure Walker, N.A.; Syed, O.; Malde, S.; Taylor, C.; Sahai, A. Onabotulinum toxin a Injections in Men With Refractory Idiopathic Detrusor Overactivity. *Urology* **2019**, *123*, 242–246. [CrossRef]
23. Hsiao, S.-M.; Lin, H.-H.; Kuo, H.-C. Factors Associated with Therapeutic Efficacy of Intravesical OnabotulinumtoxinA Injection for Overactive Bladder Syndrome. *PLoS ONE* **2016**, *11*, e0147137. [CrossRef] [PubMed]
24. Hsiao, S.-M.; Lin, H.-H.; Kuo, H.-C. Urodynamic prognostic factors for large post-void residual urine volume after intravesical injection of onabotulinumtoxinA for overactive bladder. *Sci. Rep.* **2017**, *7*, srep43753. [CrossRef] [PubMed]
25. Jiang, Y.-H.; Ong, H.-L.; Kuo, H.-C. Predictive factors of adverse events after intravesical suburothelial onabotulinumtoxina injections for overactive bladder syndrome-A real-life practice of 290 cases in a single center. *Neurourol. Urodyn.* **2015**, *36*, 142–147. [CrossRef]
26. Kuo, H.-C.; Liao, C.-H.; Chung, S.-D. Adverse Events of Intravesical Botulinum Toxin a Injections for Idiopathic Detrusor Overactivity: Risk Factors and Influence on Treatment Outcome. *Eur. Urol.* **2010**, *58*, 919–926. [CrossRef]
27. Liao, C.-H.; Kuo, H.-C. Increased Risk of Large Post-Void Residual Urine and Decreased Long-Term Success Rate After Intravesical OnabotulinumtoxinA Injection for Refractory Idiopathic Detrusor Overactivity. *J. Urol.* **2013**, *189*, 1804–1810. [CrossRef] [PubMed]
28. Osborn, D.J.; Kaufman, M.R.; Mock, S.; Guan, M.J.; Dmochowski, R.R.; Reynolds, W. Urinary retention rates after intravesical onabotulinumtoxinA injection for idiopathic overactive bladder in clinical practice and predictors of this outcome. *Neurourol. Urodyn.* **2014**, *34*, 675–678. [CrossRef]
29. Makovey, I.; Davis, T.; Guralnick, M.L.; O'Connor, R.C. Botulinum toxin outcomes for idiopathic overactive bladder stratified by indication: Lack of anticholinergic efficacy versus intolerability. *Neurourol. Urodyn.* **2011**, *30*, 1538–1540. [CrossRef]
30. Karsenty, G.; Elzayat, E.; Delapparent, T.; St-Denis, B.; Lemieux, M.-C.; Corcos, J. Botulinum Toxin Type A Injections Into the Trigone to Treat Idiopathic Overactive Bladder do Not Induce Vesicoureteral Reflux. *J. Urol.* **2007**, *177*, 1011–1014. [CrossRef] [PubMed]
31. El-Hefnawy, A.S.; Elbaset, M.A.; Taha, D.; Wadie, B.S.; Kenawy, M.; Shokeir, A.A.; Badry, M.E. Trigonal-sparing versus trigonal-involved Botox injection for treatment of idiopathic overactive bladder: A randomized clinical trial. *Low Urin. Tract. Symptoms* **2020**, *13*, 22–30. [CrossRef]
32. Kuo, H.-C. Comparison of Effectiveness of Detrusor, Suburothelial and Bladder Base Injections of Botulinum Toxin A for Idiopathic Detrusor Overactivity. *J. Urol.* **2007**, *178*, 1359–1363. [CrossRef]
33. Apostolidis, A.; Popat, R.; Yiangou, Y.; Cockayne, D.; Ford, A.; Davis, J.; Dasgupta, P.; Fowler, C.; Anand, P. Decreased sensory receptors p2x 3 and trpv1 in suburothelial nerve fibers following intradetrusor injections of botulinum toxin for human detrusor overactivity. *J. Urol.* **2005**, *174*, 977–983. [CrossRef] [PubMed]
34. Abdelwahab, O.; Sherif, H.; Soliman, T.; Elbarky, I.; Eshazly, A. Efficacy of botulinum toxin type A 100 units versus 200 units for treatment of refractory idiopathic overactive bladder. *Int. Braz. J. Urol.* **2015**, *41*, 1132–1140. [CrossRef] [PubMed]
35. Jeffery, S.; Fynes, M.; Lee, F.; Wang, K.; Williams, L.; Morley, R. Efficacy and complications of intradetrusor injection with botulinum toxin A in patients with refractory idiopathic detrusor overactivity. *BJU Int.* **2007**, *100*, 1302–1306. [CrossRef]
36. Liao, C.-H.; Chen, S.-F.; Kuo, H.-C. Different number of intravesical onabotulinumtoxinA injections for patients with refractory detrusor overactivity do not affect treatment outcome: A prospective randomized comparative study. *Neurourol. Urodyn.* **2016**, *35*, 717–723. [CrossRef]
37. Dowson, C.; Watkins, J.; Khan, M.S.; Dasgupta, P.; Sahai, A. Repeated Botulinum Toxin Type A Injections for Refractory Overactive Bladder: Medium-Term Outcomes, Safety Profile, and Discontinuation Rates. *Eur. Urol.* **2012**, *61*, 834–839. [CrossRef] [PubMed]
38. Sahai, A.; Dowson, C.; Khan, M.S.; Dasgupta, P. Repeated Injections of Botulinum Toxin-A for Idiopathic Detrusor Overactivity. *Urology* **2010**, *75*, 552–558. [CrossRef]
39. Mitterberger, M.; Pallwein, L.; Gradl, J.; Frauscher, F.; Neuwirt, H.; Leunhartsberger, N.; Strasser, H.; Bartsch, G.; Pinggera, G.-M. Persistent detrusor overactivity after transurethral resection of the prostate is associated with reduced perfusion of the urinary bladder. *BJU Int.* **2007**, *99*, 831–835. [CrossRef]
40. Habashy, D.; Losco, G.; Tse, V.; Collins, R.; Chan, L. Botulinum toxin (OnabotulinumtoxinA) in the male non-neurogenic overactive bladder: Clinical and quality of life outcomes. *BJU Int.* **2015**, *116*, 61–65. [CrossRef]
41. Bels, J.; de Vries, P.; de Beij, J.; Marcelissen, T.; van Koeveringe, G.; Rademakers, K. Long-term Follow-up of Intravesical Onabotulinum Toxin-A Injections in Male Patients with Idiopathic Overactive Bladder: Comparing Surgery-naïve Patients and Patients After Prostate Surgery. *Eur. Urol. Focus* **2021**, *7*, 1424–1429. [CrossRef]
42. Ko, K.J.; Lee, C.U.; Kim, T.H.; Suh, Y.S.; Lee, K.-S. Predictive Factors of De Novo Overactive Bladder After Artificial Urinary Sphincter Implantation in Men with Postprostatectomy Incontinence. *Urology* **2018**, *113*, 215–219. [CrossRef] [PubMed]
43. Mateu-Arrom, L.; Gutiérrez-Ruiz, C.; Rubio, L.S.; Barea, V.M.; Redorta, J.P.; Errando-Smet, C. Efficacy and safety of onabotulinum-toxin A injection in male patients with detrusor overactivity after stress urinary incontinence surgery. *Actas Urol. Esp. (Engl. Ed).* **2021**, *46*, 22–27. [CrossRef] [PubMed]

Disclaimer/Publisher's Note: The statements, opinions and data contained in all publications are solely those of the individual author(s) and contributor(s) and not of MDPI and/or the editor(s). MDPI and/or the editor(s) disclaim responsibility for any injury to people or property resulting from any ideas, methods, instructions or products referred to in the content.

toxins

MDPI

Review

Treating Neurogenic Lower Urinary Tract Dysfunction in Chronic Spinal Cord Injury Patients—When Intravesical Botox Injection or Urethral Botox Injection Are Indicated

Po-Cheng Chen [1], Kau-Han Lee [2], Wei-Chia Lee [3], Ting-Chun Yeh [4], Yuh-Chen Kuo [5,6], Bing-Juin Chiang [7,8], Chun-Hou Liao [9,10], En Meng [11], Yao-Lin Kao [12], Yung-Chin Lee [13] and Hann-Chorng Kuo [14,*]

1 Urologic Department, En Chu Kong Hospital, New Taipei City 237414, Taiwan
2 Division of Urology, Department of Surgery, Chi Mei Medical Center, Tainan 71004, Taiwan
3 Department of Urology, Kaohsiung Chang Gung Memorial Hospital, College of Medicine, Chang Gung University, Taoyuan 33302, Taiwan
4 Division of Urology, Department of Surgery, Taiwan Adventist Hospital, Taipei City 10556, Taiwan
5 Department of Urology, Yangming Branch of Taipei City Hospital, Taipei 11146, Taiwan
6 Department of Exercise and Health Sciences, University of Taipei, Taipei 111036, Taiwan
7 College of Medicine, Fu-Jen Catholic University, New Taipei City 24205, Taiwan
8 Department of Urology, Cardinal Tien Hospital, New Taipei City 23148, Taiwan
9 Divisions of Urology, Department of Surgery, Cardinal Tien Hospital, New Taipei City 23148, Taiwan
10 School of Medicine, Fu Jen Catholic University, New Taipei City 242062, Taiwan
11 Division of Urology, Department of Surgery, Tri-Service General Hospital, National Defense Medical Center, Taipei 11490, Taiwan
12 Department of Urology, National Cheng Kung University Hospital, College of Medicine, National Cheng Kung University, Tainan 704, Taiwan
13 Department of Urology, Kaohsiung Municipal Siaogang Hospital, Kaohsiung 812, Taiwan
14 Department of Urology, Hualien Tzu Chi Hospital, Buddhist Tzu Chi Medical Foundation and Tzu Chi University, Hualien 97004, Taiwan
* Correspondence: hck@tzuchi.com.tw

Abstract: Lower urinary tract symptoms (LUTS), such as urgency, urinary incontinence, and/or difficulty voiding, hamper the quality of life (QoL) of patients with spinal cord injury (SCI). If not managed adequately, urological complications, such as urinary tract infection or renal function deterioration, may further deteriorate the patient's QoL. Botulinum toxin A (BoNT-A) injection within the detrusor muscle or urethral sphincter yields satisfactory therapeutic effects for treating urinary incontinence or facilitating efficient voiding; however, adverse effects inevitably follow its therapeutic efficacy. It is important to weigh the merits and demerits of BoNT-A injection for LUTS and provide an optimal management strategy for SCI patients. This paper summarizes different aspects of the application of BoNT-A injection for lower urinary tract dysfunctions in SCI patients and provides an overview of the benefits and drawbacks of this treatment.

Keywords: spinal cord injury; botulinum toxins; lower urinary tract symptoms

Key Contribution: This article offers a comprehensive review of using botulinum toxin-A injection within the detrusor muscle or the urethra for treating lower urinary tract dysfunction in patients with spinal cord injury in terms of therapeutic efficacy and adverse events.

Citation: Chen, P.-C.; Lee, K.-H.; Lee, W.-C.; Yeh, T.-C.; Kuo, Y.-C.; Chiang, B.-J.; Liao, C.-H.; Meng, E.; Kao, Y.-L.; Lee, Y.-C.; et al. Treating Neurogenic Lower Urinary Tract Dysfunction in Chronic Spinal Cord Injury Patients—When Intravesical Botox Injection or Urethral Botox Injection Are Indicated. *Toxins* **2023**, *15*, 288. https://doi.org/10.3390/toxins15040288

Received: 28 February 2023
Revised: 1 April 2023
Accepted: 11 April 2023
Published: 17 April 2023

Copyright: © 2023 by the authors. Licensee MDPI, Basel, Switzerland. This article is an open access article distributed under the terms and conditions of the Creative Commons Attribution (CC BY) license (https://creativecommons.org/licenses/by/4.0/).

1. Introduction

The annual incidence of traumatic spinal cord injury (SCI) in the United States is around 40 per million, with a reported prevalence of around 721 cases per million people [1]. In Taiwan, the reported annual incidence is about 56.1 per million in Hualien County and 14.6 per million in Taipei [1]. Patients sustaining a traumatic SCI may experience lower urinary tract symptoms (LUTS) of varying severity caused primarily by two mechanisms:

failure to store urine and failure to empty the bladder. Conventionally, alpha-blockers were used to improve bladder emptying, and antimuscarinic agents, or beta-3 agonists, were used for detrusor overactivity. However, some SCI patients were dissatisfied with the treatment effects or unable to tolerate the adverse events of oral medications [2–5]. Botulinum toxin A (BoNT-A) induces muscular paralysis by selectively regulating neurotransmitters (acetylcholine, substance P, and calcitonin gene-related peptides) from motor nerve endings. BoNT-A also could decrease pain and sensory disturbance by modulating sensory receptors and exerting an anti-inflammatory effect [6]. BoNT-A injections into the detrusor muscle, urethral sphincter, or both are used as an effective treatment for SCI patients with LUTS to facilitate urinary control and bladder emptying [6].

BoNT-A is a single-chain polypeptide comprising a 100 kDa heavy chain and a 50 kDa light chain [7]. The heavy chain binds to the nerve terminal, the toxin translocates into the cell cytoplasm through endocytosis, and the light chain cleaves synaptosomal-associated protein-25 (SNAP25), a part of the soluble N-ethylmaleimide-sensitive factor attachment protein receptor (SNARE) protein responsible for assisting the neurotransmitter-containing vesicles to fuse with the nerve terminal membrane, to block the neurotransmission. BoNT-A decreases neurogenic detrusor overactivity (NDO) by obstructing acetylcholine release and inhibiting detrusor contraction [8]. Other probable mechanisms include a decrease in the function of muscarinic receptors or the release of adenosine triphosphate (ATP) to the detrusor muscle from BoNT-A, resulting in decreased involuntary detrusor contraction [8]. The mediating sensory input of the bladder is another possible pathway to improve NDO. Reduction in purinergic receptors (P2X3, P2X2), or transient receptor potential vanilloid subfamily-1 (TRPV1) receptors on the urothelium has been observed in patients who received BoNT-A detrusor injection [8]. A similar mechanism possibly underlies the therapeutic effects of BoNT-A injection in the urethral sphincter for detrusor sphincter dyssynergia (DSD). Inhibiting neurotransmission to the urethral sphincter muscle can temporarily relax the sphincteric muscles to improve efficient urination in patients with both neurogenic and nonneurogenic voiding dysfunction [8].

Several commercial formulations of BoNT-A, namely onabotulinum toxin A, abobotulinum toxin A, incobotulinum toxin A, and rimabotulinum toxin B, are available [9] with varying potency [10]. Onatotulinum toxin A (trade name: "Botox") has been approved by the U.S. Food and Drug Administration for NDO and is widely used in clinical research [9]. The potency of 200 U of onabotulinum toxin A is equivalent to around 600–800 U of abobotulinum toxin A [11,12], and switching between formulations may be useful when one formulation is not clinically effective [10]. According to a systematic review, abobotulinum toxin A was found to be more effective than onabotulinum toxin A in reducing urge incontinence [12]. For the current review, we have used the dosage reported for Botox injections in the literature.

2. BoNT-A Detrusor Injection for Neurogenic Detrusor Overactivity and Urinary Incontinence in Chronic SCI Patients

BoNT-A was initially introduced in urology for treating patients with neurogenic lower urinary tract dysfunction (NLUTD) due to chronic SCI [13,14]. Detrusor BoNT-A injection reduces the incidence of NDO and lowers intravesical pressure, which improves urinary incontinence [15–17]. Subsequent studies proved the efficacy of BoNT-A on autonomic dysreflexia (AD) in patients with high-level SCI, in addition to treating NDO and urinary incontinence in pediatric patients with myelomeningocele or other NLUTDs [6].

The U.S. Food and Drug Administration and several European countries approved a 200 U BoNT-A detrusor injection as the standard treatment dose for urinary incontinence caused by NDO in SCI patients [11,12,18]; however, preliminary studies used 300 U to demonstrate its therapeutic effect of increasing maximal bladder capacity and compliance and decreasing reflux volume [19–22]. Compared with placebo, detrusor BoNT-A injection was effective in reducing NDO caused by SCI or multiple sclerosis [23]. Eventually, researchers compared the therapeutic efficacy of the 200 U and 300 U dosages and found that the former achieves comparable effects with possibly fewer adverse events (AEs), leading to the adoption of the 200 U dose by urologists [18]. Furthermore, repeat BoNT-A injections were found to have similar efficacy to the first one [24]. A pooled data analysis by Mangera et al. revealed detrusor BoNT-A injection in SCI patients could facilitate a decrease in the daily incontinence episodes (63%), the frequency of clean intermittent catheterization (CIC) (18%), and maximal detrusor pressure (42%) as well as an increase in the cystometric bladder capacity (68%) and reflux volume (61%) [6,25]. Detrusor BoNT-A injection can also significantly improve health-related quality of life (QoL) indexes [6,26] and decrease the rate of symptomatic urinary tract infection (UTI) in SCI patients [6,27]. The detrusor BoNT-A injection-induced improvement in bladder compliance and urinary continence can persist for up to nine months [16,28], and repeated injections can sustain improvement in continence and QoL [29].

However, symptom evaluation alone may not be sufficient. High intravesical pressure with potential upper urinary tract damage might be missed in some patients with urinary continence after detrusor BoNT-A injection [30]; therefore, a urodynamic examination might be necessary for some patients even with obvious symptomatic relief after detrusor BoNT-A injection [30]. Besides, detrusor BoNT-A injection usually impairs detrusor contractility, leading to a large postvoiding residual volume (PVR) or urinary retention in patients with NDO; hence, patients receiving detrusor BoNT-A injection may require CIC for large PVR and suffer from subsequent UTIs [15].

Several studies compared different BoNT-A injection methods for patients with NLUTD. Krhut et al. compared BoNT-A detrusor injection with submucosal injection in SCI patients with NDO and found no significant difference between the two groups regarding symptomatic improvement, change in urodynamic parameters, efficacy duration, and AEs [31]. Samal et al. also reported concurring findings as the two methods gave similar results in terms of urgency incontinence episodes, number of catheterizations, urodynamic profile, and efficacy duration [32]. Interestingly, Taha et al. compared a trigone-including injection with a trigone-sparing injection in SCI patients with refractory NDO and found that the former group had a significantly lower incontinence rate, higher complete dryness rate, and higher reflux volume [33]. No injection-related vesicoureteral reflux was found in either group. Another randomized control trial compared combined BoNT-A 160 U trigone-sparing and 40 U trigone-including injections with 200 U trigone-sparing BoNT-A injection for NDO in SCI patients [34]. Including the trigone resulted in superior outcomes for QoL, mean urinary incontinence episodes, complete dryness rate, mean voided volume, detrusor pressure, and involuntary detrusor contraction without any vesicoureteral reflux. In another randomized control trial, the effectiveness of combined BoNT-A injection (240 U into the detrusor and 60 U into the trigone) was compared to that of nontrigonal injection (300 U into the detrusor but not the trigone). The trial found that both methods had similar results, but the trigonal injection was found to be safer and more effective than the nontrigonal injection and did not increase the rate of vesicoureteral reflux [35]. The trigone has abundant sensory neural fibers and is highly sensitive to pressure changes, which possibly influences detrusor overactivity; therefore, the denervating effect of the trigone-including injection is more effective in inhibiting involuntary bladder contraction [36].

Treatment efficacy is a crucial factor for deciding whether SCI patients should receive a detrusor BoNT-A injection [37]. Certain pretreatment factors like higher maximum detrusor pressure and lower bladder compliance. Lower maximal cystometric capacity, and poor response after the first injection have been associated with higher treatment failure rates [38–40]. NDO patients with initially higher incontinence reduction rates after the first detrusor BoNT-A injection showed better outcomes for incontinence reduction and QoL during the subsequent treatment period [41]. Some NDO patients with poor response to the first dosage also reported gradually higher incontinence reduction after receiving subsequent BoNT-A therapy. Therefore, a second dose of detrusor BoNT-A injection must be given to patients who did not show a good response to the first injection before classifying them as poor responders.

3. Urethral Versus Detrusor BoNT-A Injection in SCI Patients with Urinary Incontinence and Incomplete Bladder Emptying

The presentation of NLUTD depends on the level of SCI—patients with a suprasacral cord injury might develop NDO with or without DSD, and symptoms of frequency, urgency, with or without urgency urinary incontinence, and incomplete voiding [42]. Patients with a sacral lesion might present with a poorly contracting detrusor with incomplete voiding and/or stress-related urinary incontinence associated with a weak sphincter, while a cauda equina lesion may develop detrusor areflexia and incompetent sphincter relaxation [42]. SCI patients commonly have both voiding and storage symptoms [43]; targeting the detrusor for urinary incontinence might worsen bladder emptying ability, whereas targeting the urethral sphincter for voiding dysfunction might aggravate the incontinence. It is a challenge for both the urologist and the patient to balance between being dry and complete bladder emptying.

While a detrusor BoNT-A injection of 200 U or 300 U can improve bladder compliance and restore urinary continence in SCI patients with NDO [16], this treatment usually hampers detrusor contractility. A large PVR or urinary retention might become bothersome, and about 70% of patients require periodic CIC and develop subsequent UTIs [15]. Therefore, a lower dose (200 U over 300 U) of BoNT-A is sufficient to produce similar improvements in urinary incontinence and urgency episodes without altering the spontaneous voiding function that is required [44,45].

Dykstra et al. first reported the use of urethral sphincter BoNT-A injection to improve bladder emptying in SCI patients with DSD [46]. This injection can decrease the mean maximal urethral pressure, duration of DSD, and PVR for three to nine months [13]. Improved voiding and reduced CIC frequency also improve the QoL [2]. However, a urethral sphincter injection would increase the severity of urinary incontinence and urgency or urge urinary incontinence episodes, which might lead to patient dissatisfaction [2,47]. Exacerbated incontinence and urgency episodes might compel the patient to select detrusor BoNT-A injection subsequently [48,49].

The optimal condition for chronic SCI patients is self-voiding without urinary incontinence or severe urgency. In order to achieve this goal of treatment result, concomitant BoNT-A detrusor and urethral sphincter injections might be adopted in patients craving less urinary incontinence and preservation of spontaneous voiding. Huang et al. reported that combined BoNT-A (200 U) detrusor and (100 U) urethral sphincter injections might induce a significant reduction in both detrusor and urethral pressure without increasing PVR, daily CIC frequency, or daily pad use [50]. Another study with the same BoNT-A dosage revealed that a combined injection could lower the detrusor and urethral pressures to improve the patient's QoL while protecting the upper urinary tract [51].

4. Long-Term Adherence to BoNT-A Injection and Patient Satisfaction

Sex-based differences are an important concern while treating patients with NDO or DSD. Male SCI patients can use an external urine collection device to prevent soiling and usually can do without being totally dry. On the other hand, female SCI patients tend to use a diaper and would rather prefer to be totally dry; if possible, be free of diapers and decrease the need for CIC to a minimum. A small dose of BoNT-A detrusor injection is adequate to increase bladder capacity and decrease urinary incontinence in this condition; Around 24% of patients can void by abdominal tapping (tapping the suprapubic area to induce reflex contraction of the bladder) without requiring CIC [52,53]. A dose–response study compared BoNT-A injections of 200 U, 100 U, and 50 U with placebo injections into the detrusor muscle [13]. The study found that the 50 U dose did not show any significant improvement over the placebo for any of the efficacy parameters. However, the 100 U dose showed some improvement over the placebo, although the observed magnitude of change was generally less favorable compared to that seen with the 200 U dose [13].

Before administering a BoNT-A detrusor injection in SCI patients, the following issues need to be considered:

1. Behavioral modifications should be the primary strategy.
2. BoNT-A injections could be considered in the case of failure of other treatments or intolerable adverse effects of oral medications, such as antimuscarinics or beta-3 agonists.
3. Most patients require CIC after BoNT-A detrusor injection. Patients unable to perform CIC might not be suitable for this treatment.
4. Regular monitoring is essential to check upper urinary tract function and prevent adverse effects and the occurrence of UTIs and large PVR.
5. Repeated injections are required to maintain therapeutic efficacy in SCI patients.

Repeat detrusor injections are required to sustain the therapeutic efficacy of BoNT-A on NDO. An estimated 67% of SCI patients, who received BoNT-A injections for NDO, continued with repeat injections during a five-year follow-up [54]. Of these patients, 90% reported high satisfaction and were willing to consider periodic BoNT-A injections as a long-term treatment option [6,17,54]. Herbert et al. conducted a retrospective chart review for SCI patients with NDO who received BoNT-A therapy and reported a 59.1% adherence rate at 5 years and 50% at 10 years [40]. Baron et al. also described similar adherence rates (5 years: 63.9%; 10 years: 49.1%) [55]. The most common reasons for discontinuation were lack of efficacy and AEs, such as UTI, urinary retention, and hematuria [37].

Adherence to detrusor BoNT-A injections in SCI patients is highly associated with the treatment outcome [54]. Repeated injections allow the maintenance of favorable effects and hence, greater patient satisfaction [37,54]. However, SCI patients with voiding dysfunction are not equally satisfied with long-term urethral sphincter BoNT-A injections as they are with detrusor injections [3]. Only 35.6% of patients in this study continued urethral sphincter BoNT-A injection therapy during a median follow-up of five years [3]. The low satisfaction rates after urethral sphincter injection were mainly caused by a high incontinence grade, inefficient therapeutic efficacy, and failure to help them wean off of CIC [3].

5. Adverse Events Related to BoNT-A Injections

The most common AEs with BoNT-A detrusor injections are symptomatic UTI, urinary retention, and hematuria [4]. BoNT-A detrusor injections are effective in reducing detrusor pressure and urinary incontinence and increasing maximal bladder capacity [4]. However, they also impair detrusor contractility leading to subsequent large PVR or urinary retention. Although BoNT-A urethral sphincter injection can facilitate bladder emptying and increase the flow rate (duration around three to nine months), it also enhances the risk of urinary incontinence, urgency sensation, and de novo frequency [3]; seldom, patients may be disappointed by the AEs that exceed the therapeutic effect. Largely, dissatisfaction with BoNT-A urethral sphincter injection is rooted in amplified urinary incontinence, whereas larger PVR requiring CIC is the primary reason for discontent with detrusor injection [52].

Intolerable AEs often cause patients to forsake repeat BoNT-A injections, although these patients can achieve complete dryness after detrusor injections. Chen et al. retrospectively reviewed 223 patients with chronic SCI who received BoNT-A detrusor injections for NDO and urinary incontinence; only 108 patients (48.4%) continued with repeat injections during the mean ten-year follow-up [17]. Among those discontinuing BoNT-A therapy, 41 patients (46.6%) discontinued due to UTIs, while 15 patients (17%) deferred due to the burden of CIC. Likewise, Hebert et al. reviewed 128 SCI patients receiving repeated detrusor BoNT-A injections for NDO, of which 58 discontinued therapy over a median follow-up of ten years [40]. Seventeen patients stopped therapy due to AEs despite the therapeutic efficacy of detrusor BoNT-A injection. Table 1 summarizes the therapeutic effects and AEs of the detrusor and urethral sphincter BoNT-A injection for patients with chronic SCI with NDO and/or DSD.

Table 1. A summary of therapeutic effects and adverse events related to detrusor and urethral BoNT-A injection in chronic SCI patients with NDO and/or DSD [2–5].

	Therapeutic Efficacy	Adverse Events
Detrusor injection	Maximal bladder capacity ↑ Voided volume ↑ Detrusor pressure ↓ Incidence of DO ↓ Involuntary detrusor contraction ↓ Urinary incontinence rate ↓ Diaper use ↓	Post-void residual volume ↑ Maximum flow rate ↓ Symptomatic UTI ↑ Urinary retention rate ↑ Hematuria ↑
Urethral sphincter injection	Urethral pressure ↓ Post-void residual volume ↓ Maximum flow rate ↑ Detrusor pressure ↓ Catheterization rate ↓	Urinary incontinence ↑ Urgency episode ↑ De novo frequency ↑

↓: decrease; ↑: increase; DO: detrusor overactivity; UTI: urinary tract infection.

6. Active Management of Chronic SCI Patients with Autonomic Dysreflexia

AD is an acute systemic disorienting autonomic response to specific stimuli, which may occasionally be potentially fatal. It typically develops in a complete SCI above the T6 level [56] and usually presents with pounding headaches, severe paroxysmal hypertension, bradycardia, flushing and sweating of the face and body above the level of the lesion, nasal congestion, blurred vision, and a sense of apprehension or anxiety. Some patients show irritability, combative behavior, or cognitive impairment [57]. AD commonly develops from a stimulus of bladder distention and stool impaction. UTI is also a potential cause of AD in SCI patients regardless of an indwelling urinary catheter [58]. In SCI, the reflex activity of the sympathetic nervous system, which responds to sensory stimuli, cannot be controlled by the brainstem. Therefore, an increase in blood pressure is maintained via sympathetic vasoconstriction; the baroreceptors sense the rise in blood pressure and trigger parasympathetic activity, which results in compensatory bradycardia [58].

Ke et al. reported that symptomatic AD resolved in 88.2% of SCI patients who underwent transurethral incision at the bladder neck (TUI-BN) with a significant increase in peak flow rate and decreased PVR [59]. Probably, sympathetic activity decreases either during bladder distention or when initiating voiding, which forms the therapeutic mechanism of the resolution of AD after TUI-BN. The authors also observed that 13 patients with impaired detrusor contractility at baseline retained effective and sustained detrusor contraction postoperatively after TUI-BN. An overactive sympathetic response might suppress detrusor contraction and result in low detrusor contractility and incomplete bladder emptying. TUI-BN might interrupt the sympathetic reflex circuit and activity and help these patients regain detrusor contractility.

BoNT-A detrusor or urethral sphincter injections are effective in ameliorating the severity and frequency of symptomatic AD in SCI patients [16,60–62]. BoNT-A injection in the detrusor or urethral sphincter possibly reduces the detrusor pressure during the bladder filling or voiding phase to reduce AD; additionally, the detrusor injection might inhibit the sensory afferent pathways that trigger AD. Walter et al. reported that AD severity decreased in 82% of SCI patients after BoNT-A detrusor injection, in addition to a reduction in both the total and bladder-related AD episodes [62]. Fougere et al. also reported that 59% of SCI patients receiving detrusor BoNT-A injections no longer experienced symptomatic AD, and the remaining 41% perceived a significant decrease in the severity [61]. The injections also reduced bladder-related AD events and improved AD-related QoL. A few case studies have also reported the role of urethral sphincter injection in reducing the degree and frequency of AD [60,63]. Therefore, BoNT-A injection (detrusor or urethral sphincter) is a viable option for effective AD control in SCI patients with refractory medical control, such as a selective alpha-1 blocker or a calcium channel blocker.

In contrast, AD might also occur during BoNT-A detrusor injection [4,48]. A study reported that 3.74% of SCI patients who received BoNT-A detrusor injections experienced AD compared to only 0.53% of patients in the placebo group [4]. Exacerbation of AD may result from injection-related bladder wall trauma, which induces acute suburothelial nerve plexus inflammation and sympathetic response activation.

7. Augmentation Enterocystoplasty Versus BoNT-A Detrusor Injection in SCI Patients

Augmentation enterocystoplasty (AEC) is an invasive surgery performed to increase bladder capacity and decrease detrusor pressure [64,65]. The bladder is opened, and an anastomosis is made to a detubularized bowel segment; the ileum is the most commonly used site [64,65]. Favorable outcomes have been reported for AEC in terms of improvement in the QoL, renal function preservation, and vesical ureteral reflux resolution in the neurogenic bladder [66]. Additionally, significant improvements in several urodynamic parameters, including increased bladder capacity, decreased maximum detrusor pressure, and detrusor overactivity, have been observed. Most people can become continent postoperatively, while the rate of CIC also increases after surgery [66]. A study reported high satisfaction (96.2%) in SCI patients undergoing augmentation ileocystoplasty, all of whom became completely continent [67].

However, there are certain contraindications for AEC, such as renal insufficiency, inflammatory bowel disease, congenital bowel anomalies, radiation enteritis, short bowel or previous bowel resection, bladder cancer, and inability to perform CIC postoperatively [65,68]. The reported mortality rate for AEC is around 0–3.2% [68]. Early postoperative complications include prolonged ileus, urinary fistula, wound infection, and bleeding requiring reoperation, whereas bacteriuria, UTI, bladder and kidney stone diseases, metabolic disturbances, vitamin B-12 deficiency, bowel complications, and bladder perforation are possible long-term complications [65,68]. Notably, AEC was also associated with an increased risk of malignancy [65,68]. Compared to AE, BoNT-A injection is less invasive with fewer complications and is reversible and easy to perform. In the United Kingdom, the number of AEC procedures decreased from 192 cases in 2000 to 120 in 2010, while that of BoNT-A injections increased from 50 in 2000 to 4088 cases in 2010 [57]. AEC was considered in chronic SCI patients only when conservative treatment, including BoNT-A injection, failed.

Padmanabhan et al. conducted a five-year cost analysis to compare BoNT-A detrusor injection with AEC [69]. Repeat BoNT-A injections are required to maintain clinical efficacy, while AEC is associated with higher long-term complication rates. The cost-analysis model revealed that BoNT-A injections were less when the injection duration was more than 5.1 months, and AEC was cheaper when the complication rate was <14% [69]. However, AEC was typically performed after failure of BoNT-A injection. Furthermore, a cross-sectional study compared the QoL in SCI patients who underwent AEC or BoNT-A detrusor injection and found that continence control and QoL scores were higher in the AEC group [70]. It is possible that the increase in incontinence episodes between consecutive BoNT-A detrusor injections may have caused this difference; accordingly, better re-injection timing might increase the QoL in SCI patients receiving BoNT-A injections [70].

BoNT-A detrusor injection is also a treatment of choice in patients with refractory symptoms after AEC. Toia et al. reported that 43% of SCI patients with failed AEC continued to receive regular BoNT-A detrusor injections (in the remnant native bladder avoiding trigone) with satisfactory symptomatic improvement [71]. Another study reported that 86% of patients with refractory urinary symptoms post-AEC had subjective improvement after receiving BoN-TA injections [72]. In this study, patients received either a detrusor-only injection or a combined detrusor + intestinal part injection, among which 80% of the former group and 91% of the latter reported subjective improvement.

8. BoNT-A Injection for Pediatric SCI Patients

Several studies have proved the clinical efficacy of BoNT-A detrusor injection for refractory pediatric neurogenic detrusor overactivity caused by congenital spinal dysraphism, such as myelomeningocele [24,73–78]. BoNT-A detrusor injection can also significantly reduce urinary incontinence and detrusor pressure and increase maximal bladder capacity and compliance in pediatric patients [24,73–78]. In a study including only pediatric SCI patients, BoNT-A detrusor injection significantly improved the clinical symptoms (decreased urge incontinence episodes and increased dryness rate) and urodynamic parameters (reduced detrusor pressure and duration of first detrusor overactivity during the study) [78]. Detrusor injection of 200 U was shown to be more effective. However, it is advised to avoid exceeding a dosage of 6 U/kg [78]. Furthermore, a trigone-including BoNT-A injection was effective without causing VUR. Concomitant detrusor and urethral sphincter injections have also been used in pediatric patients of NDO with DSD [76]. Compared to a detrusor-only injection, the combined injection can achieve comparable improvements in detrusor pressure, bladder capacity, and incontinence rate, along with significantly reduced PVR. Hence, the combined injection may be useful in pediatric NDO patients with DSD requiring a reduction in PVR. Repeated BoNT-A injections also demonstrated a persisting effect in the pediatric neurogenic bladder, with the treatment effect lasting for nine months in 84% of patients during a median follow-up of 4.5 years [18,66]. Low-compliant bladder and poor response to the first BoNT-A injection were risk factors for treatment failure [74,79].

9. Conclusions

Managing NLUTDs in patients with chronic SCI requires deliberating over several aspects of the condition, such as the level and severity of SCI, hand dexterity and walking ability, vocation and daily routine of the patient, abdominal muscle function and bladder sensation, clinical symptoms of voiding difficulty and urinary incontinence, bladder pressure, and upper urinary tract condition. Clinicians must review the pros and cons of the BoNT-A therapy with the patients before deciding on the site of injection (detrusor and/or urethral sphincter) to address their bladder emptying or storage problems. Regular urodynamic study and LUTS evaluation are essential for optimal adjustment of dosage and duration between BoNT-A injections. BoNT-A injections are a powerful tool for treating refractory NLUTDs in SCI patients. Despite the potential AEs, the effects typically wear off after six to nine months. Compared to other invasive treatments, the reversibility of BoNT-A injections is one of its major advantages.

Author Contributions: Methodology, T.-C.Y. and B.-J.C.; validation, E.M. and Y.-C.L.; investigation, Y.-L.K.; writing—original draft preparation, P.-C.C. and K.-H.L.; writing—review and editing, H.-C.K.; supervision, Y.-C.K.; project administration, W.-C.L. and C.-H.L. All authors have read and agreed to the published version of the manuscript.

Funding: This research was funded by the Buddhist Tzu Chi Medical Foundation grants TCMF-SP-108-01 and TCMF-MP-110-03-01.

Institutional Review Board Statement: Not applicable.

Informed Consent Statement: Not applicable.

Data Availability Statement: The data presented in this study are available this article.

Conflicts of Interest: The authors declare no conflict of interest.

Abbreviations

AD	autonomic dysreflexia
AE	adverse event
AEC	augmentation enterocystoplasty
BoNT-A	Botulinum toxin A
CIC	clean intermittent catheterization
DSD	detrusor sphincter dyssynergia
LUTS	lower urinary tract symptoms
NDO	neurogenic detrusor overactivity
NLUTD	neurogenic lower urinary tract dysfunction
PVR	postvoiding residual volume
QoL	quality of life
SCI	spinal cord injury
TUIBN	transurethral incision at the bladder neck
UTI	urinary tract infection

References

1. Singh, A.; Tetreault, L.; Kalsi-Ryan, S.; Nouri, A.; Fehlings, M.G. Global prevalence and incidence of traumatic spinal cord injury. *Clin. Epidemiol.* **2014**, *6*, 309–331. [CrossRef]
2. Kuo, H.C. Satisfaction with urethral injection of botulinum toxin A for detrusor sphincter dyssynergia in patients with spinal cord lesion. *Neurourol. Urodyn.* **2008**, *27*, 793–796. [CrossRef]
3. Lee, C.L.; Jhang, J.F.; Jiang, Y.H.; Kuo, H.C. Real-World Data Regarding Satisfaction to Botulinum Toxin A Injection into the Urethral Sphincter and Further Bladder Management for Voiding Dysfunction among Patients with Spinal Cord Injury and Voiding Dysfunction. *Toxins* **2022**, *14*, 30. [CrossRef]
4. Li, G.P.; Wang, X.Y.; Zhang, Y. Efficacy and Safety of OnabotulinumtoxinA in Patients With Neurogenic Detrusor Overactivity Caused by Spinal Cord Injury: A Systematic Review and Meta-analysis. *Int. Neurourol. J.* **2018**, *22*, 275–286. [CrossRef]
5. Mehta, S.; Hill, D.; Foley, N.; Hsieh, J.; Ethans, K.; Potter, P.; Baverstock, R.; Teasell, R.W.; Wolfe, D.; Spinal Cord Injury Rehabilitation Evidence Research, T. A meta-analysis of botulinum toxin sphincteric injections in the treatment of incomplete voiding after spinal cord injury. *Arch. Phys. Med. Rehabil.* **2012**, *93*, 597–603. [CrossRef]
6. Jiang, Y.H.; Chen, S.F.; Kuo, H.C. Frontiers in the Clinical Applications of Botulinum Toxin A as Treatment for Neurogenic Lower Urinary Tract Dysfunction. *Int. Neurourol. J.* **2020**, *24*, 301–312. [CrossRef]
7. Arnon, S.S.; Schechter, R.; Inglesby, T.V.; Henderson, D.A.; Bartlett, J.G.; Ascher, M.S.; Eitzen, E.; Fine, A.D.; Hauer, J.; Layton, M.; et al. Botulinum toxin as a biological weapon: Medical and public health management. *JAMA* **2001**, *285*, 1059–1070. [CrossRef]
8. Jhang, J.F.; Kuo, H.C. Botulinum Toxin A and Lower Urinary Tract Dysfunction: Pathophysiology and Mechanisms of Action. *Toxins* **2016**, *8*, 120. [CrossRef]
9. Romo, P.G.B.; Smith, C.P.; Cox, A.; Averbeck, M.A.; Dowling, C.; Beckford, C.; Manohar, P.; Duran, S.; Cameron, A.P. Non-surgical urologic management of neurogenic bladder after spinal cord injury. *World J. Urol.* **2018**, *36*, 1555–1568. [CrossRef]
10. Bottet, F.; Peyronnet, B.; Boissier, R.; Reiss, B.; Previnaire, J.G.; Manunta, A.; Kerdraon, J.; Ruffion, A.; Lenormand, L.; Perrouin Verbe, B.; et al. Switch to Abobotulinum toxin A may be useful in the treatment of neurogenic detrusor overactivity when intradetrusor injections of Onabotulinum toxin A failed. *Neurourol. Urodyn.* **2018**, *37*, 291–297. [CrossRef]
11. Kennelly, M.; Cruz, F.; Herschorn, S.; Abrams, P.; Onem, K.; Solomonov, V.K.; Del Rosario Figueroa Coz, E.; Manu-Marin, A.; Giannantoni, A.; Thompson, C.; et al. Efficacy and Safety of AbobotulinumtoxinA in Patients with Neurogenic Detrusor Overactivity Incontinence Performing Regular Clean Intermittent Catheterization: Pooled Results from Two Phase 3 Randomized Studies (CONTENT1 and CONTENT2). *Eur. Urol.* **2022**, *82*, 223–232. [CrossRef] [PubMed]
12. Cruz, F.; Danchenko, N.; Fahrbach, K.; Freitag, A.; Tarpey, J.; Whalen, J. Efficacy of abobotulinumtoxinA versus onabotulinumtoxinA for the treatment of refractory neurogenic detrusor overactivity: A systematic review and indirect treatment comparison. *J. Med. Econ.* **2023**, *26*, 200–207. [CrossRef] [PubMed]
13. Schurch, B.; Hauri, D.; Rodic, B.; Curt, A.; Meyer, M.; Rossier, A.B. Botulinum—A toxin as a treatment of detrusor-sphincter dyssynergia: A prospective study in 24 spinal cord injury patients. *J. Urol.* **1996**, *155*, 1023–1029. [CrossRef]
14. Dykstra, D.D.; Sidi, A.A. Treatment of detrusor-sphincter dyssynergia with botulinum A toxin: A double-blind study. *Arch. Phys. Med. Rehabil.* **1990**, *71*, 24–26.
15. Reitz, A.; Stohrer, M.; Kramer, G.; Del Popolo, G.; Chartier-Kastler, E.; Pannek, J.; Burgdorfer, H.; Gocking, K.; Madersbacher, H.; Schumacher, S.; et al. European experience of 200 cases treated with botulinum-A toxin injections into the detrusor muscle for urinary incontinence due to neurogenic detrusor overactivity. *Eur. Urol.* **2004**, *45*, 510–515. [CrossRef] [PubMed]
16. Schurch, B.; Stohrer, M.; Kramer, G.; Schmid, D.M.; Gaul, G.; Hauri, D. Botulinum-A toxin for treating detrusor hyperreflexia in spinal cord injured patients: A new alternative to anticholinergic drugs? Preliminary results. *J. Urol.* **2000**, *164*, 692–697. [CrossRef]

17. Chen, S.F.; Jiang, Y.H.; Jhang, J.F.; Kuo, H.C. Satisfaction with Detrusor OnabotulinumtoxinA Injections and Conversion to Other Bladder Management in Patients with Chronic Spinal Cord Injury. *Toxins* **2022**, *14*, 35. [CrossRef]
18. Cruz, F.; Herschorn, S.; Aliotta, P.; Brin, M.; Thompson, C.; Lam, W.; Daniell, G.; Heesakkers, J.; Haag-Molkenteller, C. Efficacy and safety of onabotulinumtoxinA in patients with urinary incontinence due to neurogenic detrusor overactivity: A randomised, double-blind, placebo-controlled trial. *Eur. Urol.* **2011**, *60*, 742–750. [CrossRef]
19. Apostolidis, A.; Thompson, C.; Yan, X.; Mourad, S. An exploratory, placebo-controlled, dose-response study of the efficacy and safety of onabotulinumtoxinA in spinal cord injury patients with urinary incontinence due to neurogenic detrusor overactivity. *World J. Urol.* **2013**, *31*, 1469–1474. [CrossRef]
20. Giannantoni, A.; Mearini, E.; Del Zingaro, M.; Porena, M. Six-year follow-up of botulinum toxin A intradetrusorial injections in patients with refractory neurogenic detrusor overactivity: Clinical and urodynamic results. *Eur. Urol.* **2009**, *55*, 705–711. [CrossRef]
21. Kennelly, M.; Dmochowski, R.; Ethans, K.; Karsenty, G.; Schulte-Baukloh, H.; Jenkins, B.; Thompson, C.; Li, D.; Haag-Molkenteller, C. Long-term efficacy and safety of onabotulinumtoxinA in patients with urinary incontinence due to neurogenic detrusor overactivity: An interim analysis. *Urology* **2013**, *81*, 491–497. [CrossRef]
22. Rovner, E.; Dmochowski, R.; Chapple, C.; Thompson, C.; Lam, W.; Haag-Molkenteller, C. OnabotulinumtoxinA improves urodynamic outcomes in patients with neurogenic detrusor overactivity. *Neurourol. Urodyn.* **2013**, *32*, 1109–1115. [CrossRef]
23. Schurch, B.; de Seze, M.; Denys, P.; Chartier-Kastler, E.; Haab, F.; Everaert, K.; Plante, P.; Perrouin-Verbe, B.; Kumar, C.; Fraczek, S.; et al. Botulinum toxin type a is a safe and effective treatment for neurogenic urinary incontinence: Results of a single treatment, randomized, placebo controlled 6-month study. *J. Urol.* **2005**, *174*, 196–200. [CrossRef]
24. Akbar, M.; Abel, R.; Seyler, T.M.; Bedke, J.; Haferkamp, A.; Gerner, H.J.; Mohring, K. Repeated botulinum-A toxin injections in the treatment of myelodysplastic children and patients with spinal cord injuries with neurogenic bladder dysfunction. *BJU Int.* **2007**, *100*, 639–645. [CrossRef]
25. Mangera, A.; Apostolidis, A.; Andersson, K.E.; Dasgupta, P.; Giannantoni, A.; Roehrborn, C.; Novara, G.; Chapple, C. An updated systematic review and statistical comparison of standardised mean outcomes for the use of botulinum toxin in the management of lower urinary tract disorders. *Eur. Urol.* **2014**, *65*, 981–990. [CrossRef]
26. Schurch, B.; Denys, P.; Kozma, C.M.; Reese, P.R.; Slaton, T.; Barron, R.L. Botulinum toxin A improves the quality of life of patients with neurogenic urinary incontinence. *Eur. Urol.* **2007**, *52*, 850–858. [CrossRef]
27. Game, X.; Castel-Lacanal, E.; Bentaleb, Y.; Thiry-Escudie, I.; De Boissezon, X.; Malavaud, B.; Marque, P.; Rischmann, P. Botulinum toxin A detrusor injections in patients with neurogenic detrusor overactivity significantly decrease the incidence of symptomatic urinary tract infections. *Eur. Urol.* **2008**, *53*, 613–618. [CrossRef] [PubMed]
28. Patki, P.S.; Hamid, R.; Arumugam, K.; Shah, P.J.; Craggs, M. Botulinum toxin-type A in the treatment of drug-resistant neurogenic detrusor overactivity secondary to traumatic spinal cord injury. *BJU Int.* **2006**, *98*, 77–82. [CrossRef] [PubMed]
29. Dowson, C.; Khan, M.S.; Dasgupta, P.; Sahai, A. Repeat botulinum toxin-A injections for treatment of adult detrusor overactivity. *Nat. Rev. Urol.* **2010**, *7*, 661–667. [CrossRef] [PubMed]
30. Koschorke, M.; Leitner, L.; Sadri, H.; Knupfer, S.C.; Mehnert, U.; Kessler, T.M. Intradetrusor onabotulinumtoxinA injections for refractory neurogenic detrusor overactivity incontinence: Do we need urodynamic investigation for outcome assessment? *BJU Int.* **2017**, *120*, 848–854. [CrossRef]
31. Krhut, J.; Samal, V.; Nemec, D.; Zvara, P. Intradetrusor versus suburothelial onabotulinumtoxinA injections for neurogenic detrusor overactivity: A pilot study. *Spinal Cord* **2012**, *50*, 904–907. [CrossRef] [PubMed]
32. Samal, V.; Mecl, J.; Sram, J. Submucosal administration of onabotulinumtoxinA in the treatment of neurogenic detrusor overactivity: Pilot single-centre experience and comparison with standard injection into the detrusor. *Urol. Int.* **2013**, *91*, 423–428. [CrossRef] [PubMed]
33. Abdel-Meguid, T.A. Botulinum toxin-A injections into neurogenic overactive bladder–to include or exclude the trigone? A prospective, randomized, controlled trial. *J. Urol.* **2010**, *184*, 2423–2428. [CrossRef] [PubMed]
34. Hui, C.; Keji, X.; Chonghe, J.; Ping, T.; Rubiao, O.; Jianweng, Z.; Xiangrong, D.; Liling, Z.; Maping, H.; Qingqing, L.; et al. Combined detrusor-trigone BTX-A injections for urinary incontinence secondary to neurogenic detrusor overactivity. *Spinal Cord* **2016**, *54*, 46–50. [CrossRef]
35. Chen, H.; Xie, K.; Jiang, C. A single-blind randomized control trial of trigonal versus nontrigonal Botulinum toxin-A injections for patients with urinary incontinence and poor bladder compliance secondary to spinal cord injury. *J. Spinal Cord Med.* **2021**, *44*, 757–764. [CrossRef]
36. Jo, J.K.; Kim, K.N.; Kim, D.W.; Kim, Y.T.; Kim, J.Y.; Kim, J.Y. The effect of onabotulinumtoxinA according to site of injection in patients with overactive bladder: A systematic review and meta-analysis. *World J. Urol.* **2018**, *36*, 305–317. [CrossRef]
37. Ni, J.; Wang, X.; Cao, N.; Si, J.; Gu, B. Is repeat Botulinum Toxin A injection valuable for neurogenic detrusor overactivity—A systematic review and meta-analysis. *Neurourol. Urodyn.* **2018**, *37*, 542–553. [CrossRef]
38. Alvares, R.A.; Araujo, I.D.; Sanches, M.D. A pilot prospective study to evaluate whether the bladder morphology in cystography and/or urodynamic may help predict the response to botulinum toxin a injection in neurogenic bladder refractory to anticholinergics. *BMC Urol.* **2014**, *14*, 66. [CrossRef]

39. Joussain, C.; Popoff, M.; Phe, V.; Even, A.; Bosset, P.O.; Pottier, S.; Falcou, L.; Levy, J.; Vaugier, I.; Chartier Kastler, E.; et al. Long-term outcomes and risks factors for failure of intradetrusor onabotulinumtoxin A injections for the treatment of refractory neurogenic detrusor overactivity. *Neurourol. Urodyn.* **2018**, *37*, 799–806. [CrossRef]
40. Hebert, K.P.; Klarskov, N.; Bagi, P.; Biering-Sorensen, F.; Elmelund, M. Long term continuation with repeated Botulinum toxin A injections in people with neurogenic detrusor overactivity after spinal cord injury. *Spinal Cord* **2020**, *58*, 675–681. [CrossRef]
41. Denys, P.; Dmochowski, R.; Aliotta, P.; Castro-Diaz, D.; Blok, B.; Ethans, K.; Aboushwareb, T.; Magyar, A.; Kennelly, M. Positive outcomes with first onabotulinumtoxinA treatment persist in the long term with repeat treatments in patients with neurogenic detrusor overactivity. *BJU Int.* **2017**, *119*, 926–932. [CrossRef]
42. Hamid, R.; Averbeck, M.A.; Chiang, H.; Garcia, A.; Al Mousa, R.T.; Oh, S.J.; Patel, A.; Plata, M.; Del Popolo, G. Epidemiology and pathophysiology of neurogenic bladder after spinal cord injury. *World J. Urol.* **2018**, *36*, 1517–1527. [CrossRef]
43. Weld, K.J.; Dmochowski, R.R. Association of level of injury and bladder behavior in patients with post-traumatic spinal cord injury. *Urology* **2000**, *55*, 490–494. [CrossRef]
44. Ginsberg, D.; Gousse, A.; Keppenne, V.; Sievert, K.D.; Thompson, C.; Lam, W.; Brin, M.F.; Jenkins, B.; Haag-Molkenteller, C. Phase 3 efficacy and tolerability study of onabotulinumtoxinA for urinary incontinence from neurogenic detrusor overactivity. *J. Urol.* **2012**, *187*, 2131–2139. [CrossRef]
45. Kuo, H.C. Therapeutic effects of suburothelial injection of botulinum a toxin for neurogenic detrusor overactivity due to chronic cerebrovascular accident and spinal cord lesions. *Urology* **2006**, *67*, 232–236. [CrossRef]
46. Dykstra, D.D.; Sidi, A.A.; Scott, A.B.; Pagel, J.M.; Goldish, G.D. Effects of botulinum A toxin on detrusor-sphincter dyssynergia in spinal cord injury patients. *J. Urol.* **1988**, *139*, 919–922. [CrossRef]
47. Smith, C.P.; Nishiguchi, J.; O'Leary, M.; Yoshimura, N.; Chancellor, M.B. Single-institution experience in 110 patients with botulinum toxin A injection into bladder or urethra. *Urology* **2005**, *65*, 37–41. [CrossRef] [PubMed]
48. Kuo, H.C. Therapeutic outcome and quality of life between urethral and detrusor botulinum toxin treatment for patients with spinal cord lesions and detrusor sphincter dyssynergia. *Int. J. Clin. Pract.* **2013**, *67*, 1044–1049. [CrossRef] [PubMed]
49. Mahfouz, W.; Karsenty, G.; Corcos, J. Injection of botulinum toxin type A in the urethral sphincter to treat lower urinary tract dysfunction: Review of indications, techniques and results: 2011 update. *Can. J. Urol.* **2011**, *18*, 5787–5795.
50. Huang, Y.H.; Chen, S.L. Concomitant Detrusor and External Urethral Sphincter Botulinum Toxin-A Injections in Male Spinal Cord Injury Patients with Detrusor Overactivity and Detrusor Sphincter Dyssynergia. *J. Rehabil. Med.* **2022**, *54*, jrm00264. [CrossRef] [PubMed]
51. Huang, M.; Chen, H.; Jiang, C.; Xie, K.; Tang, P.; Ou, R.; Zeng, J.; Liu, Q.; Li, Q.; Huang, J.; et al. Effects of botulinum toxin A injections in spinal cord injury patients with detrusor overactivity and detrusor sphincter dyssynergia. *J. Rehabil. Med.* **2016**, *48*, 683–687. [CrossRef]
52. Kuo, H.C. Therapeutic satisfaction and dissatisfaction in patients with spinal cord lesions and detrusor sphincter dyssynergia who received detrusor botulinum toxin a injection. *Urology* **2008**, *72*, 1056–1060. [CrossRef]
53. Dahlberg, A.; Perttila, I.; Wuokko, E.; Ala-Opas, M. Bladder management in persons with spinal cord lesion. *Spinal Cord* **2004**, *42*, 694–698. [CrossRef]
54. Hori, S.; Patki, P.; Attar, K.H.; Ismail, S.; Vasconcelos, J.C.; Shah, P.J. Patients' perspective of botulinum toxin-A as a long-term treatment option for neurogenic detrusor overactivity secondary to spinal cord injury. *BJU Int.* **2009**, *104*, 216–220. [CrossRef] [PubMed]
55. Baron, M.; Peyronnet, B.; Auble, A.; Hascoet, J.; Castel-Lacanal, E.; Miget, G.; Le Doze, S.; Prudhomme, T.; Manunta, A.; Cornu, J.N.; et al. Long-Term Discontinuation of Botulinum Toxin A Intradetrusor Injections for Neurogenic Detrusor Overactivity: A Multicenter Study. *J. Urol.* **2019**, *201*, 769–776. [CrossRef] [PubMed]
56. Valles, M.; Benito, J.; Portell, E.; Vidal, J. Cerebral hemorrhage due to autonomic dysreflexia in a spinal cord injury patient. *Spinal Cord* **2005**, *43*, 738–740. [CrossRef] [PubMed]
57. Khastgir, J.; Drake, M.J.; Abrams, P. Recognition and effective management of autonomic dysreflexia in spinal cord injuries. *Expert Opin. Pharm.* **2007**, *8*, 945–956. [CrossRef]
58. Karlsson, A.K. Autonomic dysreflexia. *Spinal Cord* **1999**, *37*, 383–391. [CrossRef]
59. Ke, Q.S.; Kuo, H.C. Transurethral incision of the bladder neck to treat bladder neck dysfunction and voiding dysfunction in patients with high-level spinal cord injuries. *Neurourol. Urodyn.* **2010**, *29*, 748–752. [CrossRef]
60. Tsai, S.J.; Ying, T.H.; Huang, Y.H.; Cheng, J.W.; Bih, L.I.; Lew, H.L. Transperineal injection of botulinum toxin A for treatment of detrusor sphincter dyssynergia: Localization with combined fluoroscopic and electromyographic guidance. *Arch. Phys. Med. Rehabil.* **2009**, *90*, 832–836. [CrossRef]
61. Fougere, R.J.; Currie, K.D.; Nigro, M.K.; Stothers, L.; Rapoport, D.; Krassioukov, A.V. Reduction in Bladder-Related Autonomic Dysreflexia after OnabotulinumtoxinA Treatment in Spinal Cord Injury. *J. Neurotrauma* **2016**, *33*, 1651–1657. [CrossRef]
62. Walter, M.; Kran, S.L.; Ramirez, A.L.; Rapoport, D.; Nigro, M.K.; Stothers, L.; Kavanagh, A.; Krassioukov, A.V. Intradetrusor OnabotulinumtoxinA Injections Ameliorate Autonomic Dysreflexia while Improving Lower Urinary Tract Function and Urinary Incontinence-Related Quality of Life in Individuals with Cervical and Upper Thoracic Spinal Cord Injury. *J. Neurotrauma* **2020**, *37*, 2023–2027. [CrossRef]

63. Chen, S.L.; Bih, L.I.; Chen, G.D.; Huang, Y.H.; You, Y.H.; Lew, H.L. Transrectal ultrasound-guided transperineal botulinum toxin a injection to the external urethral sphincter for treatment of detrusor external sphincter dyssynergia in patients with spinal cord injury. *Arch. Phys. Med. Rehabil.* **2010**, *91*, 340–344. [CrossRef]
64. Shreck, E.; Gioia, K.; Lucioni, A. Indications for Augmentation Cystoplasty in the Era of OnabotulinumtoxinA. *Curr. Urol. Rep.* **2016**, *17*, 27. [CrossRef] [PubMed]
65. Cheng, P.J.; Myers, J.B. Augmentation cystoplasty in the patient with neurogenic bladder. *World J. Urol.* **2020**, *38*, 3035–3046. [CrossRef] [PubMed]
66. Hoen, L.; Ecclestone, H.; Blok, B.F.M.; Karsenty, G.; Phe, V.; Bossier, R.; Groen, J.; Castro-Diaz, D.; Padilla Fernandez, B.; Del Popolo, G.; et al. Long-term effectiveness and complication rates of bladder augmentation in patients with neurogenic bladder dysfunction: A systematic review. *Neurourol. Urodyn.* **2017**, *36*, 1685–1702. [CrossRef]
67. Khastgir, J.; Hamid, R.; Arya, M.; Shah, N.; Shah, P.J. Surgical and patient reported outcomes of 'clam' augmentation ileocystoplasty in spinal cord injured patients. *Eur. Urol.* **2003**, *43*, 263–269. [CrossRef] [PubMed]
68. Cetinel, B.; Kocjancic, E.; Demirdag, C. Augmentation cystoplasty in neurogenic bladder. *Investig. Clin. Urol.* **2016**, *57*, 316–323. [CrossRef] [PubMed]
69. Padmanabhan, P.; Scarpero, H.M.; Milam, D.F.; Dmochowski, R.R.; Penson, D.F. Five-year cost analysis of intra-detrusor injection of botulinum toxin type A and augmentation cystoplasty for refractory neurogenic detrusor overactivity. *World J. Urol.* **2011**, *29*, 51–57. [CrossRef] [PubMed]
70. Anquetil, C.; Abdelhamid, S.; Gelis, A.; Fattal, C. Botulinum toxin therapy for neurogenic detrusor hyperactivity versus augmentation enterocystoplasty: Impact on the quality of life of patients with SCI. *Spinal Cord* **2016**, *54*, 1031–1035. [CrossRef] [PubMed]
71. Toia, B.; Pakzad, M.H.; Hamid, R.; Wood, D.N.; Greenwell, T.J.; Ockrim, J.L. The efficacy of onabotulinumtoxinA in patients with previous failed augmentation cystoplasty: Cohort series and literature review. *Neurourol. Urodyn.* **2020**, *39*, 1831–1836. [CrossRef]
72. Martinez, L.; Tubre, R.; Roberts, R.; Boone, T.; Griebling, T.L.; Padmanabhan, P.; Khavari, R. Refractory bladder dysfunction: A multi-institutional experience with intravesical botulinum toxin-a injection in adult patients who underwent previous augmentation cystoplasty. *Turk. J. Urol.* **2020**, *46*, 309–313. [CrossRef] [PubMed]
73. Riccabona, M.; Koen, M.; Schindler, M.; Goedele, B.; Pycha, A.; Lusuardi, L.; Bauer, S.B. Botulinum-A toxin injection into the detrusor: A safe alternative in the treatment of children with myelomeningocele with detrusor hyperreflexia. *J. Urol.* **2004**, *171*, 845–848; discussion 848. [CrossRef]
74. Altaweel, W.; Jednack, R.; Bilodeau, C.; Corcos, J. Repeated intradetrusor botulinum toxin type A in children with neurogenic bladder due to myelomeningocele. *J. Urol.* **2006**, *175*, 1102–1105. [CrossRef] [PubMed]
75. Safari, S.; Jamali, S.; Habibollahi, P.; Arshadi, H.; Nejat, F.; Kajbafzadeh, A.M. Intravesical injections of botulinum toxin type A for management of neuropathic bladder: A comparison of two methods. *Urology* **2010**, *76*, 225–230. [CrossRef] [PubMed]
76. Sharifiaghdas, F.; Narouie, B.; Rostaminejad, N.; Hamidi Madani, M.; Manteghi, M.; Rouientan, H.; Ahmadzade, M.; Dadpour, M. Intravesical Botulinum toxin-A injection in pediatric overactive neurogenic bladder with Detrusor overactivity: Radiologic and clinical outcomes. *Urologia* **2022**, 3915603221135681. [CrossRef]
77. Hui, C. Safety and efficacy of trigonal BTX-A injections for children with neurological detrusor overactivity secondary to spinal cord injury. *J. Pediatr. Surg.* **2020**, *55*, 2736–2739. [CrossRef]
78. Austin, P.F.; Franco, I.; Dobremez, E.; Kroll, P.; Titanji, W.; Geib, T.; Jenkins, B.; Hoebeke, P.B. OnabotulinumtoxinA for the treatment of neurogenic detrusor overactivity in children. *Neurourol. Urodyn.* **2021**, *40*, 493–501. [CrossRef]
79. Danacioglu, Y.O.; Keser, F.; Ersoz, C.; Polat, S.; Avci, A.E.; Kalkan, S.; Silay, M.S. Factors predicting the success of intradetrusor onabotulinum toxin-A treatment in children with neurogenic bladders due to myelomeningocele: The outcomes of a large cohort. *J. Pediatr. Urol.* **2021**, *17*, 520.e1–520.e7. [CrossRef]

Disclaimer/Publisher's Note: The statements, opinions and data contained in all publications are solely those of the individual author(s) and contributor(s) and not of MDPI and/or the editor(s). MDPI and/or the editor(s) disclaim responsibility for any injury to people or property resulting from any ideas, methods, instructions or products referred to in the content.

toxins

MDPI

Article

Effect of Intratrigonal Botulinum Toxin in Patients with Bladder Pain Syndrome/Interstitial Cystitis: A Long-Term, Single-Center Study in Real-Life Conditions

Pedro Abreu-Mendes [1,2,3,*], António Ferrão-Mendes [2], Francisco Botelho [1,4], Francisco Cruz [1,2,3] and Rui Pinto [1,2,3]

1 Department of Urology, São João Universitary Hospital Center, 4200-319 Porto, Portugal
2 Faculty of Medicine, University of Porto, 4099-002 Porto, Portugal
3 i3S—Instituto de Investigação e Inovação em Saúde, Universidade do Porto, 4200-135 Porto, Portugal
4 Life and Health Sciences Research Institute (ICVS), School of Medicine, University of Minho, 4710-057 Braga, Portugal
* Correspondence: pedromendes.uc@gmail.com

Abstract: The high percentage of treatment failures seen in patients with bladder pain syndrome/interstitial cystitis (BPS/IC) managed conservatively frequently demands invasive treatment options. We aimed to evaluate the long-term efficacy and adverse events of intratrigonal botulinum toxin injection in such circumstances, as well as to determine possible predictors of response to toxin treatment. A retrospective cohort study included 47 female BPS/IC patients treated with onabotulinum toxin A (OnabotA) in a tertiary hospital between the years 2009 and 2022. All patients received 100 U of OnabotA in ten injections limited to the trigonal area. Patients were divided into three groups based on their treatment response as responders, non-responders and lost to follow-up due to non-medical reasons. The clinical and surgical records of the individuals were retrieved, including the 10-point visual analogue scale (VAS), the number of treatments, the time between injections, and the age at the first injection. A total of 25 patients (>50% of the cohort) were long-term responders, but none of the evaluated parameters was a predictor for this circumstance: age, pain intensity, or duration of improvement following the injection. The time between injections was stable (around 1 year). No severe adverse events were registered. The intratrigonal injection of botulinum toxin in patients with BPS/IC was an effective and safe long-term treatment for patients' refractory to conservative forms of treatment. Age, basal pain intensity, and time to injection request did not predict long-term response to OnaBotA.

Keywords: botulinum toxin A; onabotulinum toxin A; bladder pain syndrome/interstitial cystitis; long-term treatment

Key Contribution: Long-term intravesical injection of OnaBotA is effective and safe for BPS/IC patients refractory to conservative treatments.

Citation: Abreu-Mendes, P.; Ferrão-Mendes, A.; Botelho, F.; Cruz, F.; Pinto, R. Effect of Intratrigonal Botulinum Toxin in Patients with Bladder Pain Syndrome/Interstitial Cystitis: A Long-Term, Single-Center Study in Real-Life Conditions. *Toxins* **2022**, *14*, 775. https://doi.org/10.3390/toxins14110775

Received: 18 October 2022
Accepted: 5 November 2022
Published: 10 November 2022

Publisher's Note: MDPI stays neutral with regard to jurisdictional claims in published maps and institutional affiliations.

Copyright: © 2022 by the authors. Licensee MDPI, Basel, Switzerland. This article is an open access article distributed under the terms and conditions of the Creative Commons Attribution (CC BY) license (https://creativecommons.org/licenses/by/4.0/).

1. Introduction

The European Society for the Study of Interstitial Cystitis (ESSIC) defines bladder pain syndrome/interstitial cystitis (BPS/IC) as a persistent or recurrent chronic pelvic pain, pressure or discomfort perceived to be related to the urinary bladder in the absence of any identifiable pathology which could explain this symptom [1]. It must be accompanied by at least one other urinary symptom, such as an urgent need to void or urinary frequency [1]. Therefore, BPS/IC diagnosis is still largely one of exclusion.

BPS/IC has no curative treatment as of yet [2]. Thus, symptom control, with the main focus on pain, represents a key part of BPS/IC management. The first line of treatment is centered on patient education and stress control to inform the patient about the uncertain evolution of the disease and to explain the importance of self-management by avoiding situations that may aggravate the symptoms [2]. When necessary, oral analgesic therapies and pharmacological agents intended to replenish the glycosaminoglycan layer and decrease urothelial permeability are used as the second-line treatment. When these measures are insufficient, surgical therapies may be introduced [3–5]. One option is the intratrigonal injection of onabotulinum toxin type A (OnaBotA) [6,7].

OnaBotA is a potent biological neurotoxin that accesses the neurons after binding the synaptic vesicle protein type 2C, a ubiquitous neuronal protein [6,8,9]. Once inside the neurons, the light chain of the toxin cleaves the proteins that are essential for the docking of the neuronal vesicles to the membrane in all types of neurons [9]. In sensory neurons, the trafficking of pain receptors from neuronal vesicles to the membrane of sensory neurons will be impaired and the release of CGRP and SP, two neuropeptides involved in neurogenic inflammation, will be substantially decreased [6,7,10]. In addition, a decrease of ATP release from urothelial cells occurs which may further impair bladder sensation [7,11,12]. The OnabotA-induced inhibition of the acetylcholine release from pre- and post-ganglionic parasympathetic neurons [13] is expected to have a limited role in BPS/IC, as this neurotransmitter is not involved in peripheral pain pathways and detrusor overactivity is a rare event associated with BPS/IC [9,14].

The application of OnabotA in the trigone is justified by the fact that this bladder region has the highest density of nociceptors [11,15,16]. Since 2004, multiple cohort studies and randomized placebo-controlled trials showed that OnaBotA was effective and safe in pain control in BPS/IC patients refractory to conservative treatment, in the dosage of 100 Units (U) [14,17–20]. In addition, trigonal injections of OnabotA also improve day and nighttime frequency, maximum functional bladder capacity, and overall quality of life, which are believed to result from less pain felt by patients during bladder filling [21].

One of the characteristics of OnabotA action is the limited duration of the effect, which, although variable, rarely extends for more than 12 months [7]. After this period of effect, BPS/IC symptoms tend to return, and repeated bladder injections are commonly requested by patients [21]. In previous prospective studies, overall, a statistically significant improvement in the pain as well as in other urinary symptoms has been reported, yet these results were mainly at short-term or after a few injection cycles [13,21–23]. Thus, information regarding the long-term effects and safety in real-life conditions is lacking.

We aim to report the results and safety of this intra-trigonal treatment in a real-life cohort of patients with a long-term follow-up. Differences between patients maintained in long-term therapy with intratrigonal OnaBotA treatment and those who stopped treatment, mainly for lack of response, were evaluated, looking for possible predictors of response. The rate of therapy maintenance was also assessed.

2. Results

2.1. Patients and Demographics

A total of 47 BPS/IC female patients available in the hospital records and that were refractory to lifestyle changes and oral/intravesical therapies (including non-opioid analgesics and anti-depressant drugs and anti-histaminics) were included. All patients received at least one intratrigonal injection of 100 U of OnaBotA. A total of 193 procedures were performed as depicted in Table 1, varying between 1 (10 patients) and 14 (one patient). The proportion of patients that received four or more treatments was 48% (see Table 1).

The mean age of the patients at the time of the first injection was 50.7 (±14.5) years. The mean initial VAS score of the cohort was 5.7 (±1.7), and the mean follow-up is 8.8 (±4.2) years. The cohort demographics are presented in Table 2.

Table 1. Number of patients by the number of treatments.

Number of Treatments	N (Patients)	%
1	10	21.3
2	8	17.0
3	7	14.9
4	3	6.4
5	7	14.9
6	3	6.4
7	2	4.3
8	3	6.4
9	2	4.3
11	1	2.1
14	1	2.1
	47	100%

Table 2. Cohort demographics.

	Cohort
N (%)	47 (100%)
Age at first treatment	50.7 (±14.5)
Initial VAS	5.7 (±1.7)
Time between injection and request for another treatment (days)	500 (350–581)
Time between first injection and the request for the second treatment (days)	390 (287–590)
Number of Treatments	4.1 (±2.9)
Follow-up (years)	8.8 (±4.2)

2.2. Duration of Effect per Injection

The median interval between the injection and the patient's request for a new injection is graphically shown in Figure 1, and it was 500.5 days (P25: 350; P75: 581), The duration of the effect of each treatment seems to be relatively stable during the follow-up. The median time between the first injection and the request for the second injection was the shortest with a median duration of 390 days (P25: 287; P75: 590). The median intervals for patients' requests for another treatment increased afterwards, ranging between 414 days and 669 days.

To investigate possible predictors of response, three groups of patients were defined. Group A comprised all patients currently in treatment, which included patients with the disease controlled confirmed at a visit or patients who already asked for a new injection). Group B comprised patients who were non-responders to OnaBotA (they could have shown treatment response at an initial phase of the OnabotA program but meanwhile the treatment lost efficacy). Group C included patients lost to follow-up due to non-therapeutic causes.

When comparing the duration of effect between responders and non-responders, no differences were found, as shown in Table 3. We omitted group C in this comparison given the low number of patients and since the loss to follow-up was not related to the response to the toxin injections.

The 10th treatment onward medians were not represented in Figure 1 and Table 3 since only two patients reached that number of procedures.

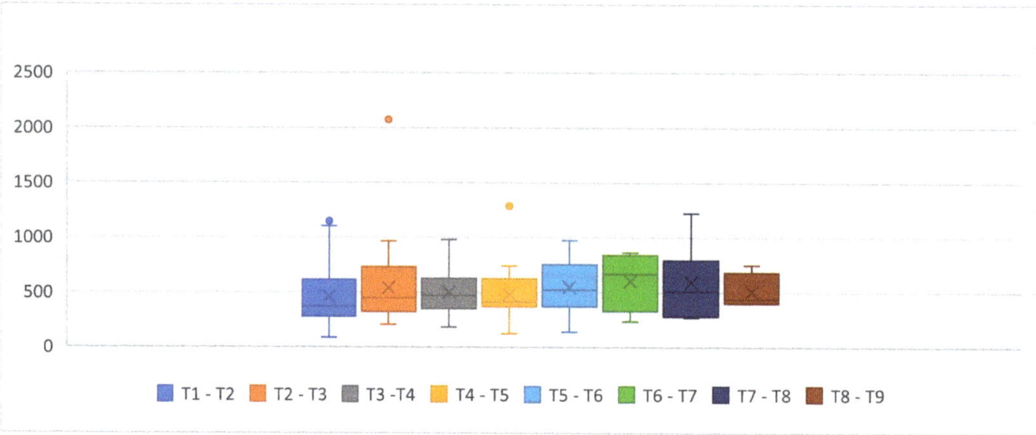

Figure 1. Median duration of effect between injections (*Y*-axis in days of effect duration counting time between an injection and the patient request for a new treatment).

Table 3. Median duration of the effect of each injection per injection, per group.

Treatment Response (in Days)	Group A	Group B	*p*-Value
After 1st treatment	447 (310–613)	337 (183–392)	0.57
After 2nd treatment	434 (308–553)	660 (327–1091)	0.64
After 3rd treatment	443 (343–622)	490 (279–673)	0.48
After 4th treatment	409 (377–647)	394 (184–571)	0.59
After 5th treatment	525 (405–845)	350 (140–562)	0.29
After 6th treatment	719 (399–848)		
After 7th treatment	543 (449–900)		
After 8th treatment	440 (403–681)		
After 9th treatment	450 (281–629)		

Interestingly, of the nine patients that had a response duration below the 25th percentile after the first injection, only two abandoned the OnabotA program due to a lack of response. The other seven are still in treatment, having more than five injections. Moreover, these patients had in the following injections a duration of effect within the median time. This suggests that the duration of the effect of the first injection should not be used as a predictor of long-term treatment success or failure.

2.3. Global Treatment Maintenance

Given that we could analyze the total number of patients treated with OnaBotA and identify which of them are still in treatment per each treatment, we were able to organize a Kaplan-Meier treatment maintenance graphic. The results are shown in Figure 2.

Notice that the graphic, which is not time-related, shows that more than half of the patients, 53%, had a favorable treatment response for a high number of treatments.

2.4. Possible Predictors

To evaluate the possible predictors, we compared the characteristics from group A and group B patients. The results are shown in Table 4.

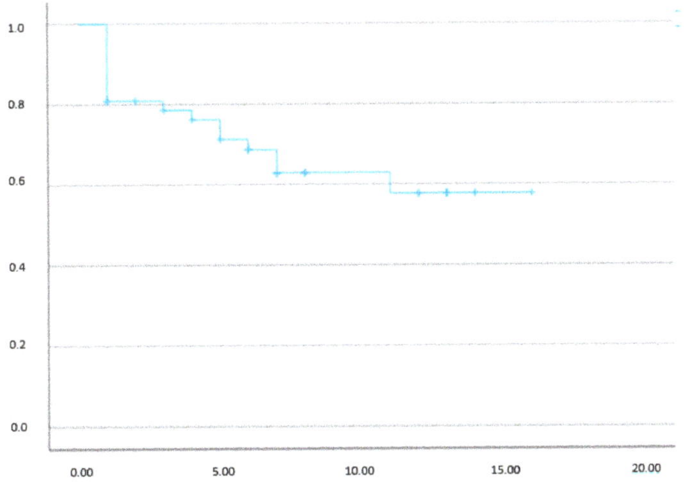

Figure 2. Kaplan-Meier curve of the cohort maintenance in OnaBotA treatment. The *X*-axis represents the number of injections, and the *Y*-axis represents the relative number of patients that were treated (100%). Each drop on the graphic line represents patients that lost treatment efficacy and the vertical dash along the graphic represents the moment patients were lost to follow-up. A total of 53% remained on treatment.

Table 4. Patients' features as possible predictors, per group.

	Groups A and B	Group A	Group B	*p*-Value
N (%)	42 (100%)	25 (59%)	17 (41%)	
Age of 1st treatment	49.7 (±14.0)	51.8 (±11.5)	46.6 (±17.0)	0.29
Initial VAS	6.11 (±1.2)	5.9 (±1.3)	6.8 (±0.5)	0.27
Time between treatments	432.0 (305–645)	337.0 (182–747)	447.5 (310–613)	0.72
Time between 1st and 2nd treatment	350.0 (287–598)	447.5 (310–613)	337.0 (183–392)	0.94
Number of Treatments	4.3 (±3.0)	5.4 (±3.1)	2.6 (±2.1)	0.003
Follow-up (years)	6.9 (4.6)	9.4 (±3.9)	3.3 (±3.0)	0.001

As shown, 25 patients remain in treatment and 17 were non-responders to OnabotA. Notice that only one patient in group A had just one treatment (the patient has no symptoms after an injection carried out 15 months ago, with occasional flares easily managed with simple conservative measures).

The initial VAS score and the duration of the effect of the first treatment were not statistically different between responders (group A) and non-responders (Group B). The overall time between treatment and the subsequent request for reinjection was numerically inferior in the long-term responders in group A when compared to Group B, although the difference was not statistically significant ($p = 0.72$).

2.5. Adverse Events

In terms of adverse events, and after analyzing all of the procedures, three types of complications were reported: lower urinary tract infection, straining during micturition, and acute urinary retention with a high post-voiding residual with the need to initiate clean intermittent catheterization (CIC). The results are presented in Table 5.

In 71 procedures, there was no specific mention of adverse events, and thus the adverse events were classified as omitted. Of those procedures with information available, 58 procedures had no adverse event, simple urinary tract infection UTI was recorded in 36 cases, and UTI with symptoms of straining was reported in 13 post-op procedures. Straining without UTI occurred after 14 procedures and straining with incomplete voiding, with the need for CIC, occurred in only one procedure (0.1%). No upper urinary tract infection was recorded.

Table 5. Total frequency of adverse events.

Adverse Events	Number	% (Total of 193)
Omitted	71	36.8%
None	58	30.1%
Urinary Tract Infection (UTI)	36	18.7%
Straining	14	7.2%
UTI + Straining	13	6.7%
Straining + incomplete voiding with the need for CIC	1	0.1%

3. Discussion

In the present paper, we describe our single-center experience with OnaBotA intratrigonal injection in the treatment of BPS/IC patients. To the best of our knowledge, this is the first long-term evaluation of a BPS/IC cohort with this treatment in real-life conditions. Previously, short and mid-term evaluations done in our and other departments had contributed to the validation of OnaBotA treatment in this disease [14,21].

The great majority, 37 patients, corresponding to 78% of the total cohort, requested more than one treatment. In recent years, we changed our approach and started to re-treat the patients that presented an unsatisfactory duration response to the first treatment at least one more time. This change was based on the perception that even patients with a poor response duration after the first injection could have a good response to posterior treatments. Such subjective opinion was now undoubtedly confirmed by the analysis of the present cohort.

There were no significant differences in age, the time to reinjection request, and pain intensity before the first intervention between responders and non-responders. Caution should be taken when interpreting the variables of time length for treatment requests after the first treatment and overall treatments, since group B includes nine patients that only underwent one treatment and, consequently, fewer patients contributed to this variable.

Contrariwise, patients that maintain a positive response to the OnaBotA treatment and longer time in treatment (5.4 ± 3.1 vs. 2.6 ± 2.1, $p = 0.03$), showed a longer period of follow-up in the urologic clinic (9.3 years vs. 3.4 years, $p < 0.001$). The reason is probably a selection bias because those that are more satisfied with the treatment results are more prone to continue in the program.

Interestingly, the intervals between injections were longer than expected, compared to the duration reported in well-controlled cohorts or randomized clinical trials, in which only OnabotA treatment was allowed [5,21]. On average, the duration of each injection among the responders exceeded one year. This may indicate that OnabotA injections eventually combined with simple conservative measures and eventually oral medication with which patients had previous experience and could be used at their own decision (essentially non-opioid analgesic drugs, amitriptyline, the leukotriene receptor antagonist montelukast and antihistaminics [2,24]) may eventually substantially reduce the necessity of toxin injections, decreasing the burden that repeated injections cause to patients and health facilities. The median time between injection and a new request seems independent of the number of total injections and independent of the duration of the previous treatment, with the possible exception of the interval between the first injection and the request for a second treatment.

The sustained duration of the effect, despite the increase in the number of procedures, suggests that intratrigonal sensory neurons do not develop tolerance to OnaBotA, even during long periods of administration. The use of botulinum toxin in other areas of bladder pathologies has shown the rare possibility of the development of antibodies as a cause of the appearance of resistance to the toxin [25,26]. It may be recalled that in a systematic review evaluating long-term treatment with intravesical OnaBotA in another urinary condition, overactive bladder, the data regarding the time between reinjections was heterogeneous among the analysed studies [27]. In some, the interval between injections was stable, while in others it could become either longer or shorter.

As presented, seven of nine patients with a shorter time of effect after their first injection (lower than percentile 25) become good responders in subsequent treatments. As a matter of fact, they presented, in the following interventions, a time between injections and requests for retreatment similar to that found in the rest of the cohort. This could be justified by a cumulative therapeutic effect of the toxin, an adjustment on the parallel oral therapy, or by the stabilization of the disease. This finding could also be related to the inter-surgeon variation of the surgical technique and the process of reconstitution of OnaBotA. However, these two possibilities seem less probable, as if present they only occurred in the first treatment cycle.

Despite the significant number of patients with positive results that maintained the treatment in our cohort, approximately 53%, as seen in Figure 2, a large number of patients abandoned the long-term OnabotA program. One should remember that despite being effective in the long run, OnabotA injections can be rather unpleasant for BPS/IC patients. This had already been observed in overactive bladder and neurogenic detrusor overactivity cohorts, and reflects the low adherence to long-term reinjection programs [28]. Nevertheless, in our series almost half of the patients remained in the long-term program, exceeding the long-term adherence in OAB which may be as low as 10% [28]. Eventually, as the treatment for BPS/IC should be tailored-made for each patient, and since flares and remissions occur frequently, these different circumstances may introduce large variations in the time for patients to request another injection. [29].

The adverse effects observed in this group of patients are in line with other studies, with the risk of UTI and straining being the main concerns. This point should be fully discussed with the patients, since a UTI may markedly aggravate their symptomatology and the need for CIC will surely demand urethral manipulation.

Limitations

The main limitations of the study are the relatively small number of patients recruited, which were limited by the off-label nature of this treatment and the retrospective analysis of clinical records, and with the inherent risk of bias associated with the quality of the information in the files, including missing data. In addition, we could not provide reliable data on day and night time voiding frequency that we observed to decrease significantly in other studies [5]. However, from our perspective, it can be a more accurate representation of this treatment in real-world clinical practice. In this real-life scenario, the therapeutic effect of each treatment was determined by the time until a treatment request was made by the patients to avoid the bias of treatment delays due to fluctuations in the waiting list.

The readers should also be aware that different from evaluating oral pharmacological treatment effects, the OnaBotA treatment is a surgical procedure and there could be inter-surgeon variations of the surgical technique. We believe that this bias has a low impact as the procedure is well standardized.

Another limitation of this real-life study is relative to the use of other drugs other than OnaBotA by patients in this cohort. While patients could be medicated with a small number of pain-killers during the injections performed in a trial setting, these trial setting injections just represent a minor number of the treatments in the cohort. All of the other patients treated outside of a trial setting, and even trial patients once off the trial, were able to be medicated, or even automedicated, with non-opioid analgesics, anti-depressants and anti-histaminics to better control the symptomatology at their own discretion. Additional medication would probably be taken more often when the OnaBotA's effect begun to decrease. However, this is a real-life setting, and BPS/IC patients rarely achieve symptom control with monotherapy (especially the patients represented in this cohort that are refractory to oral and intravesical treatments). Despite the fact that other medical therapies could have a role in explaining a more prolonged time of symptoms being under control and, consequently, a greater interval between OnaBotA injections, what is most important is that the BPS/IC condition was better controlled after OnaBotA treatments in responders.

The fact that this study reflects a real-life scenario could suggest that the mild adverse effects, being easily treated, could be underreported.

4. Conclusions

Intratrigonal injection of botulinum toxin A in patients with BPS/IC is an effective and safe long-term treatment option. Moreover, the duration of each treatment seems to be sustained along all of the treatments, even when the number of injections is high. Age, basal pain severity and short duration of the first treatment effect do not seem to predict whether a patient will be a long-term responder to OnaBotA. The main adverse effects are mild, simple UTIs and straining, occurring in a minority of procedures. A specific phenotype for OnaBotA responders is lacking, but given the widely positive effect of the treatment, it should be offered as a third line of therapy.

5. Material & Methods

This is a retrospective study, analyzing our cohort of patients diagnosed with BPS/IC and treated with intratrigonal botulinum toxin in a tertiary public university hospital in Porto (Porto, Portugal) between 2009 and 2022. The procedure and the OnaBotA preparation, in our institution, are carried out by different surgeons in the urology department and by different nurses in our surgical center.

BPS/IC is diagnosed in compliance with guidelines, following the exclusion of more common conditions through physical examination, patient history, uroculture, urinalysis, cystoscopy, urinary cytology, neurological examination and in some cases pelvic magnetic resonance. All patients performed bladder hydrodistension and urothelium biopsies, before initiating OnaBotA treatment, as part of the diagnostic workup. A total of 47 patients were identified.

The clinical and surgical records of the participants, available in our hospital database, were utilized for the analysis of data related to the interventions—every medical record such as written appointments, date of surgery and surgery details are available in the hospital database. The process of collecting the electronic records into files was conducted following the Ethics Committee's approval for the study. Patients were assessed for pain intensity using a 10-point visual analogue scale (VAS) (results were from 0 to 10; a higher number corresponded to higher pain). For the evaluation of each patient, the authors accessed the number of treatments and the treatment duration (the duration between an injection and the request for a new one). The overall time of disease follow-up was also accessed. Adverse effects of the procedure, such as urinary tract infection, straining and urinary retention were analyzed when recorded.

Three groups of patients were defined to identify possible predictors of outcome. Group A comprised all patients currently in treatment (with the disease controlled after an injection or patients that already requested a reinjection); group B comprised patients who were non-responders to OnaBotA (they could have already shown treatment response but now are non-responders to OnaBotA and abandoned the treatment but not the clinic); and group C are patients lost to follow-up but for non-therapeutic reasons.

A total of 25 patients met the criteria for group A, 17 met the group B criteria, and five met the criteria for group C. For the evaluation of possible predictors of long-term success, we compared the characteristics of group A with group B patients, such as age, the initial pain intensity evaluated by the VAS score, the overall treatment duration, and also the duration of the first treatment (excluding patients that only received one injection). Moreover, we evaluated whether a rapid loss of effect after the first treatment was predictive of a general treatment failure or the need for more frequent injections. The treatment maintenance was evaluated and displayed as a Kaplan-Meier graphic, providing information on the proportion of drop-outs and patients still in OnaBotA. The number of injections performed before abandoning OnaBotA treatment, as well as the number of injections performed by patients still in treatment, are represented in the graphic.

Most treatments were performed outside of a trial, since from a total of 198 treatments, only 71 (35%) of them were in a clinical trial set EudraCT: 2014-001013-81, "Treatment of Bladder Pain Syndrome with Onabotulinum toxin A" (ProBaBle). This leads us to consider that these data reflect real-world practice.

5.1. Procedure Technique and Follow Up

In all our patients, the procedure, the drug and the dose administered were the same. The botulinum toxin A used was OnaBotA (Allergan, Irvine, CA, USA), and it was injected under light sedation through a 23-gauge needle (Coloplast A/S, Humlebaek, Denmark) inserted 3 mm into the trigonal wall with a 70°-lens cystoscopy control. A total of 100 Units were distributed throughout 10 sites (10 U per 1 mL saline)—Figure 3. A preoperative diagnostic workup was performed to guarantee that the individuals had a negative uriculture and no symptoms of cystitis. Patients were evaluated 2 to 3 weeks after the procedure to access early complications.

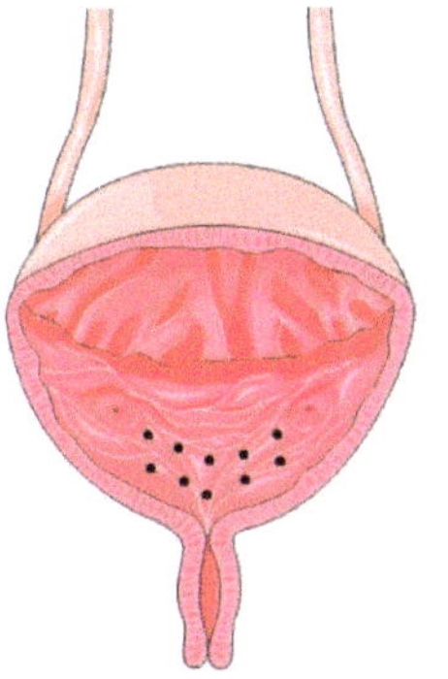

Figure 3. Schematic representation of the 10 bladder sites of OnaBotA injection.

5.2. Statistical Analysis

The statistical program IBM® SPSS® v.28.0 (IBM Corp., Armonk, NY, USA) was used for data analysis. The Kolmogorov-Smirnov test was used to assess the normality of the distribution of continuous variables. Continuous variables with a normal distribution are presented as mean (±standard deviation). Non-normally distributed variables are reported as the median (percentile 25; percentile 75) and a Student's t-test was used to compare the variables with normal distribution.

The authors chose to compare groups A and B for predictor analysis. Group C includes five patients that abandoned OnaBotA treatment early for reasons unrelated to the treatment or their clinical situation.

Clearance from the hospital Ethics Committee (Protocol number 337-21: Effect of intratrigonal botulinum toxin in patients with BPS/IC in a single center) was obtained.

Author Contributions: Conceptualization, R.P. and P.A.-M.; methodology, F.B.; software, P.A.-M.; validation, F.C., R.P. and F.B.; formal analysis, A.F.-M. and F.B.; investigation, A.F.-M. and P.A.-M.; data curation, A.F.-M.; writing—original draft preparation, A.F.-M.; writing—review and editing, P.A.-M., R.P., F.B. and F.C.; visualization, F.B.; supervision, P.A.-M., R.P., F.B. and F.C.; project administration, R.P.; funding acquisition, All authors have read and agreed to the published version of the manuscript.

Funding: This research received no external funding.

Institutional Review Board Statement: The study was conducted according to the guidelines of the Declaration of Helsinki and approved by the Institutional or Ethics Committee of Centro Hospitalar e Universitário de São João, Porto, Portugal (Protocol number 337-21: Effect of intratrigonal botulinum toxin in patients with BPS/IC in a single-centre, on 8 November 2021).

Informed Consent Statement: Patient consent was waived. Since the data is electronically recorded in the hospital system, after the Hospital's Ethics Committee study approval we could use those information without revealing patients' identity (which we did not).

Data Availability Statement: The data presented in this study are available on request from the corresponding author. The data are not publicly available due to Hospitals Ethics Committee policy.

Conflicts of Interest: The author Pedro Abreu-Mendes declares that only Francisco Cruz has the current conflict of interest: he is a consultant for Allergan, Astellas, Bayer, and Recordati; has received lecture fees from Allergan and Astellas; and is a trial investigator for Astellas, Bayer, Ipsen and Recordati.

References

1. Van de Merwe, J.P.; Nordling, J.; Bouchelouche, P.; Bouchelouche, K.; Cervigni, M.; Daha, L.K.; Elneil, S.; Fall, M.; Hohlbrugger, G.; Irwin, P.; et al. Diagnostic Criteria, Classification, and Nomenclature for Painful Bladder Syndrome/Interstitial Cystitis: An ESSIC Proposal. *Eur. Urol.* **2008**, *53*, 60–67. [CrossRef] [PubMed]
2. Engeler, D.; Baranowski, A.P.; Berghmans, B.; Borovicka, J.; Cottrell, A.M.; Dinis-Oliveira, P.; Elneil, S.; Hughes, J.; Messelink, J.M.; Pinto, R.A.; et al. EAU guidelines on chronic pelvic pain 2022. *Eur. Urol.* **2022**. Available online: https://uroweb.org/guidelines/chronic-pelvic-pain (accessed on 4 November 2022).
3. Malde, S.; Palmisani, S.; Al-Kaisy, A.; Sahai, A. Guideline of guidelines: Bladder pain syndrome. *BJU Int.* **2018**, *122*, 729–743. [CrossRef] [PubMed]
4. Engeler, D.; Baranowski, A.P.; Berghmans, B.; Borovicka, J.; Cottrell, A.M.; Dinis-Oliveira, P.; Elneil, S.; Hughes, J.; Messelink, J.M.; Pinto, R.A.; et al. EAU Guidelines on Chronic Pelvic Pain. In *EAU Guidelines, Edn. Presented at the EAU Annual Congress Milan 2021*; Elsevier: Amsterdam, The Netherlands, 2021; pp. 681–689.
5. Pinto, R.A.; Costa, D.; Morgado, A.; Pereira, P.; Charrua, A.; Silva, J.; Cruz, F. Intratrigonal OnabotulinumtoxinA Improves Bladder Symptoms and Quality of Life in Patients with Bladder Pain Syndrome/Interstitial Cystitis: A Pilot, Single Center, Randomized, Double-Blind, Placebo Controlled Trial. *J. Urol.* **2018**, *199*, 998–1003. [CrossRef]
6. Cruz, F. Targets for botulinum toxin in the lower urinary tract. *Neurourol. Urodyn.* **2014**, *33*, 31–38. [CrossRef] [PubMed]
7. Chiu, B.; Tai, H.-C.; Chung, S.-D.; Birder, L. Botulinum Toxin A for Bladder Pain Syndrome/Interstitial Cystitis. *Toxins* **2016**, *8*, 201. [CrossRef]
8. Franciosa, G.; Floridi, F.; Maugliani, A.; Aureli, P. Differentiation of the Gene Clusters Encoding Botulinum Neurotoxin Type A Complexes in Clostridium botulinum Type A, Ab, and A(B) Strains. *Appl. Environ. Microbiol.* **2004**, *70*, 7192–7199. [CrossRef] [PubMed]
9. Jhang, J.F.; Kuo, H.C. Botulinum toxin a and lower urinary tract dysfunction: Pathophysiology and mechanisms of action. *Toxins* **2016**, *8*, 120. [CrossRef]
10. Birder, L.A.; Kullmann, F.A. Role of neurogenic inflammation in local communication in the visceral mucosa. *Semin. Immunopathol.* **2018**, *40*, 261–279. [CrossRef]
11. Ikeda, Y.; Zabbarova, I.V.; Birder, L.A.; De Groat, W.C.; McCarthy, C.J.; Hanna-Mitchell, A.T.; Kanai, A.J. Botulinum neurotoxin serotype a suppresses neurotransmitter release from afferent as well as efferent nerves in the urinary bladder. *Eur. Urol.* **2012**, *62*, 1157–1164. [CrossRef]
12. Jhang, J.F. Using botulinum toxin a for treatment of interstitial cystitis/bladder pain syndrome—Possible pathomechanisms and practical issues. *Toxins* **2019**, *11*, 641. [CrossRef]
13. Coelho, A.; Dinis, P.; Pinto, R.; Gorgal, T.; Silva, C.; Silva, A.; Silva, J.; Cruz, C.D.; Cruz, F.; Avelino, A. Distribution of the High-Affinity Binding Site and Intracellular Target of Botulinum Toxin Type A in the Human Bladder. *Eur. Urol.* **2010**, *57*, 884–890. [CrossRef] [PubMed]
14. Pinto, R.; Lopes, T.; Frias, B.; Silva, A.; Silva, J.A.; Silva, C.M.; Cruz, C.; Cruz, F.; Dinis, P. Trigonal Injection of Botulinum Toxin A in Patients with Refractory Bladder Pain Syndrome/Interstitial Cystitis. *Eur. Urol.* **2010**, *58*, 360–365. [CrossRef] [PubMed]
15. Karsenty, G.; Elzayat, E.; Delapparent, T.; St-Denis, B.; Lemieux, M.; Corcos, J. Botulinum Toxin Type A Injections Into the Trigone to Treat Idiopathic Overactive Bladder do Not Induce Vesicoureteral Reflux. *J. Urol.* **2007**, *177*, 1011–1014. [CrossRef] [PubMed]
16. Yeh, T.-C.; Chen, P.-C.; Su, Y.-R.; Kuo, H.-C. Effect of Botulinum Toxin A on Bladder Pain—Molecular Evidence and Animal Studies. *Toxins* **2020**, *12*, 98. [CrossRef]
17. Smith, C.P.; Radziszewski, P.; Borkowski, A.; Somogyi, G.T.; Boone, T.B.; Chancellor, M.B. Botulinum toxin a has antinociceptive effects in treating interstitial cystitis. *Urology* **2004**, *64*, 871–875. [CrossRef]

18. Kuo, H.-C.; Jiang, Y.-H.; Tsai, Y.-C.; Kuo, Y.-C. Intravesical botulinum toxin-A injections reduce bladder pain of interstitial cystitis/bladder pain syndrome refractory to conventional treatment—A prospective, multicenter, randomized, double-blind, placebo-controlled clinical trial. *Neurourol. Urodyn.* **2016**, *35*, 609–614. [CrossRef]
19. Akiyama, Y.; Nomiya, A.; Niimi, A.; Yamada, Y.; Fujimura, T.; Nakagawa, T.; Fukuhara, H.; Kume, H.; Igawa, Y.; Homma, Y. Botulinum toxin type A injection for refractory interstitial cystitis: A randomized comparative study and predictors of treatment response. *Int. J. Urol.* **2015**, *22*, 835–841. [CrossRef]
20. Giannantoni, A.; Porena, M.; Costantini, E.; Zucchi, A.; Mearini, L.; Mearini, E. Botulinum A Toxin Intravesical Injection in Patients With Painful Bladder Syndrome: 1-Year Followup. *J. Urol.* **2008**, *179*, 1031–1034. [CrossRef]
21. Pinto, R.; Lopes, T.; Silva, J.; Silva, C.; Dinis, P.; Cruz, F. Persistent therapeutic effect of repeated injections of onabotulinum toxin A in refractory bladder pain syndrome/interstitial cystitis. *J. Urol.* **2013**, *189*, 548–553. [CrossRef]
22. Ryul, S.; Young, S.; Cho, J.; Soo, I.; Jae, S.; Kim, H. Efficacy and safety of botulinum toxin injection for interstitial cystitis/bladder pain syndrome: A systematic review and meta-analysis. *Int. Urol. Nephrol.* **2016**, *48*, 1215–1227.
23. Mitcheson, H.D.; Samanta, S.; Muldowney, K.; Pinto, C.A.; Rocha, B.D.A.; Green, S.; Bennett, N.; Mudd, P.N.; Frenkl, T.L. Vibegron (RVT-901/MK-4618/KRP-114V) Administered Once Daily as Monotherapy or Concomitantly with Tolterodine in Patients with an Overactive Bladder: A Multicenter, Phase IIb, Randomized, Double-blind, Controlled Trial. *Eur. Urol.* **2019**, *75*, 274–282. [CrossRef] [PubMed]
24. Hanno, P.M.; Burks, D.A.; Clemens, J.Q.; Dmochowski, R.R.; Fitzgerald, M.P.; Forrest, J.B.; Gordon, B.; Gray, M.; Mayer, R.D.; Moldwin, R.; et al. Diagnosis and Treatment Interstitial Cystitis/Bladder Pain Syndrome Panel Members. *J. Urol.* **2015**, *193*, 1545–1553. [CrossRef] [PubMed]
25. Fabbri, M.; Leodori, G.; Fernandes, R.M.; Bhidayasiri, R.; Marti, M.J.; Colosimo, C.; Ferreira, J.J. Neutralizing Antibody and Botulinum Toxin Therapy: A Systematic Review and Meta-analysis. *Neurotox. Res.* **2016**, *29*, 105–117. [CrossRef] [PubMed]
26. Schulte-Baukloh, H.; Bigalke, H.; Miller, K.; Heine, G.; Pape, D.; Lehmann, J.; Knispel, H.H. Botulinum neurotoxin type A in urology: Antibodies as a cause of therapy failure. *Int. J. Urol.* **2008**, *15*, 407–415. [CrossRef]
27. Eldred-Evans, D.; Sahai, A. Medium- to long-term outcomes of botulinum toxin A for idiopathic overactive bladder. *Ther. Adv. Urol.* **2017**, *9*, 3–10. [CrossRef]
28. Marcelissen, T.A.T.; Rahnama'i, M.S.; Snijkers, A.; Schurch, B.; De Vries, P. Long-term follow-up of intravesical botulinum toxin-A injections in women with idiopathic overactive bladder symptoms. *World J. Urol.* **2017**, *35*, 307–311. [CrossRef]
29. Dellis, A.E.; Papatsoris, A.G. Bridging pharmacotherapy and minimally invasive surgery in interstitial cystitis/bladder pain syndrome treatment. *Expert Opin. Pharmacother.* **2018**, *19*, 1369–1373. [CrossRef]

toxins

MDPI

Article

Treatment Outcomes of Intravesical Botulinum Toxin A Injections on Patients with Interstitial Cystitis/Bladder Pain Syndrome

Wan-Ru Yu [1,2,3], Yuan-Hong Jiang [3], Jia-Fong Jhang [3], Wei-Chuan Chang [4] and Hann-Chorng Kuo [3,*]

1 Department of Nursing, Hualien Tzu Chi Hospital, Buddhist Tzu Chi Medical Foundation, Hualien 970, Taiwan
2 Institute of Medical Sciences, Tzu Chi University, Hualien 970, Taiwan
3 Department of Urology, Hualien Tzu Chi Hospital, Buddhist Tzu Chi Medical Foundation and Tzu Chi University, Hualien 970, Taiwan
4 Department of Medical Research, Buddhist Tzu Chi General Hospital, Hualien 970, Taiwan
* Correspondence: hck@tzuchi.com.tw; Tel.: +886-3-856-1825 (ext. 2117)

Abstract: Botulinum toxin A (BoNT-A) is effective in reducing bladder hypersensitivity and increasing capacity through the effects of anti-inflammation in the bladder urothelium; however, studies on the treatment outcome of interstitial cystitis/bladder pain syndrome (IC/BPS) are lacking. We investigated the treatment outcome in IC/BPS patients receiving intravesical BoNT-A injections. This retrospective study included IC/BPS patients who had 100U BoNT-A intravesical injections in the past 20 years. The treatment outcomes at 6 months following the BoNT-A treatment were evaluated using the global response assessment (GRA) scale. The treatment outcomes according to the GRA scale include clinical symptoms, urodynamic parameters, cystoscopic characteristics, and urinary biomarkers, and it was these predictive factors for achieving satisfactory outcomes which were investigated. Among the 220 enrolled patients (180 women, 40 men) receiving BoNT-A injections, only 87 (40%) had significantly satisfactory treatment outcomes. The satisfactory group showed significantly larger voided volumes, and lower levels of both the urinary inflammatory protein MCP-1 and the oxidative stress biomarker 8-isoprostane in comparison to the unsatisfactory group. The IC severity and detrusor pressure are predictive factors of BoNT-A treatment outcomes. IC/BPS patients with less bladder inflammation showed satisfactory outcomes with intravesical BoNT-A injections. Patients with severe bladder inflammation might require more intravesical BoNT-A injections to achieve a satisfactory outcome.

Keywords: interstitial cystitis/bladder pain syndrome; botulinum toxin A injection; urine biomarkers; bladder inflammation

Key Contribution: Botulinum toxin A injections for interstitial cystitis/Bladder Pain Syndrome (IC/BPS) is effective in 40% of the patients studied. Patients with lesser bladder inflammation as characterized by a larger maximal bladder capacity on hydrodistention, lower urinary biomarker MCP-1 and oxidative stress biomarker 8-isoprostane levels, and fewer IC symptoms might achieve satisfactory treatment outcomes.

Citation: Yu, W.-R.; Jiang, Y.-H.; Jhang, J.-F.; Chang, W.-C.; Kuo, H.-C. Treatment Outcomes of Intravesical Botulinum Toxin A Injections on Patients with Interstitial Cystitis/Bladder Pain Syndrome. *Toxins* **2022**, *14*, 871. https://doi.org/10.3390/toxins14120871

Received: 4 November 2022
Accepted: 9 December 2022
Published: 11 December 2022

Publisher's Note: MDPI stays neutral with regard to jurisdictional claims in published maps and institutional affiliations.

CC BY

Copyright: © 2022 by the authors. Licensee MDPI, Basel, Switzerland. This article is an open access article distributed under the terms and conditions of the Creative Commons Attribution (CC BY) license (https://creativecommons.org/licenses/by/4.0/).

1. Introduction

Interstitial cystitis/bladder pain syndrome (IC/BPS) is a urinary bladder disorder characterized by chronic pelvic pain, pressure, or discomfort, and is accompanied by urinary symptoms, including urinary frequency, nocturia, and urgency [1]. Its prevalence was reported to be 0.04% and 0.26% in Taiwan and Korea, respectively [1]. In other words, there are approximately 100,000 people with IC/BPS in Taiwan. The pathophysiology is still unclear, and patients with this condition have not achieved satisfactory treatment outcomes [2]. IC/BPS can be classified into Hunner's (HIC) or non-Hunner's (NHIC) ulcer types [1]. The most common pathological findings are urothelial denudation and bladder inflammation [2]. Failure to achieve full urothelial regeneration results in potential breaches in barrier function that may increase an individual's susceptibility to infection or increase sensory fiber stimulation [3]. Nevertheless, multimodal therapies may be necessary to improve not only the physiological but also the psychological well-being of patients [4].

Previously, the American Urology Association (AUA) guidelines for IC/BPS recommended six steps of treatment; however, recently most guidelines do not recommend step-by-step treatments. Instead, multiple and simultaneous treatments were suggested [1,4–6]. Overall, the treatments include pain control, lifestyle modification, stress management, pelvic floor muscle therapy, oral therapies, intravesical therapies, and novel treatment for bladder inflammation [2].

As anti-inflammation and pain control is important for IC/BPS patients, the focus on bladder urothelium treatment is indispensable [7]. Botulinum toxin A (BoNT-A) is effective in reducing bladder hypersensitivity and increasing capacity through its anti-inflammatory and antinociceptive effects in the bladder urothelium [8]. BoNT-A not only reduces bladder pain effectively but it also increases bladder capacity in patients with cases of IC/BPS that are refractory to conventional therapy [9,10]. Furthermore, BoNT-A is capable of gradually decreasing bladder inflammation and enhancing urothelial repair, leading to symptomatic relief [11,12].

Due to IC/BPS's refractory nature, further research and investigation is vitally important. In real-world practice, precision medicine can not only assist clinical doctors in identifying suitable treatment options but could also help IC/BPS patients achieve satisfactory treatment outcomes earlier. Recently, the correlations between urinary biomarkers and the pathophysiology of IC/BPS were explored [13]. However, the self-reported outcomes, according to the IC/BPS patients' point of view, have not been investigated. Moreover, data relating to the effects of intravesical BoNT-A injections on improved self-reported treatment outcomes, and the predictive value of urinary biomarkers among IC/BPS patients are still lacking. Therefore, we aimed to investigate the treatment outcomes of intravesical BoNT-A injections in patients with IC/BPS in a real-life setting.

2. Results

In total, 220 patients with IC/BPS (180 women, and 40 men) who had received BoNT-A injections were enrolled. The mean age and IC/BPS duration were 54.1 ± 13.4 and 13.8 ± 10.1 years, respectively. The mean maximal bladder capacity (MBC) under anesthesia was 652 ± 204 mL; with 76 (35%), 114 (51.4%), and 20 (9.1%) patients having grade I glomerulation, grade II–III glomerulation, and HIC, respectively. The mean IC symptom index (ICSI) and mean IC problem index (ICPI) were 12.7 ± 3.7 and 12.0 ± 3.3 points, respectively. The mean numerical rating scale (NRS) score for bladder pain was 5.1 ± 2.7 points. In total, 124 (56%) patients had voiding dysfunction, which included bladder neck dysfunction (n = 8, 4%), dysfunctional voiding (n = 14, 6%), and poor external sphincter relaxation (102, 46%) whilst under videourodynamic study (VUDS), and all patients had storage dysfunction, which included bladder hypersensitivity (n = 198, 90%) and detrusor overactivity (n = 22, 10%); 214 (97%) patients had bladder pain or an intense urge to void during the potassium chloride (KCl) infusion test. In total, 180 (82%) patients reported having bladder, pelvic, or lower abdominal pain or discomfort (Table 1).

Table 1. IC/BPS patients' characteristics and VUDS parameters according to the treatment outcome (n = 220).

Variable		Total (n = 220)	Unsatisfactory Outcome GRA $\leq$ 1 (n = 133)	Satisfactory Outcome GRA $\geq$ 2 (n = 87)	p Value
Characteristics					
Age (years)		54.1 ± 13.4	53.9 ± 14.2	55.2 ± 12.3	0.499
Gender (%)	Men	40 (18%)	25 (19%)	15 (17%)	0.458
	Women	180 (82%)	108 (81%)	72 (83%)	
IC duration (years)		13.8 ± 10.1	14.5 ± 10.9	12.6 ± 8.6	0.176
Numerical rating pain scale		5.1 ± 2.7	4.9 ± 2.7	5.3 ± 2.6	0.332
IC symptoms index (ICSI)		12.7 ± 3.7	12.5 ± 3.7	13.1 ± 3.8	0.307
IC problem index (ICPI)		12.0 ± 3.3	11.6 ± 3.2	12.5 ± 3.4	0.052
O'Leary-Sant IC Symptom Index (OSS)		24.7 ± 6.6	24.1 ± 6.5	25.6 ± 6.8	0.118
VUDS parameters					
First sensation of filling (mL)		117 ± 52.4	116 + 51.9	118 ± 53.4	0.751
Full sensation (mL)		182 ± 73.5	180 ± 74.7	184 ± 71.9	0.719
Cystometric bladder capacity (mL)		276 ± 114	267 ± 105	289 ± 126	0.167
Detrusor pressure ($P_{det}Q_{max}$) (cm H_2O)		20.8 ± 12.8	20.8 ± 12.3	21.0 ± 13.3	0.572
Maximum flow rate (mL/s)		12.3 ± 5.7	11.8 ± 5.5	13.1 ± 6.0	0.572
Voided-volume (mL)		251 ± 121	236 ± 111	273 ± 130	0.026 *
Post-void residual (mL)		25.9 ± 51.6	28.8 ± 53.6	21.5 ± 48.4	0.308
KCl test—Pain (%)		167 (77.3%)	101 (76%)	66 (76%)	0.531
KCl test—Urge (%)		68 (31.5%)	47 (35%)	21 (24%)	0.056
Maximum bladder capacity (mL)		652 ± 204	635 ± 199	680 ± 209	0.113
Glomerulation grade	Grade 1	86 (39.5%)	48 (36%)	38 (44%)	0.173
	Grade 2	83 (37.3%)	55 (41%)	28 (32%)	
	Grade 3	31 (14.1%)	20 (15%)	11 (13%)	
Hunner's lesion IC		20 (9.1%)	11 (8%)	9 (10%)	

* Significant $p < 0.05$.

Among the 220 patients receiving BoNT-A injections, 133 (60%) reported unsatisfactory treatment outcomes which were evaluated using the global response assessment (GRA) at 6 months later, and 87 (40%) reported satisfactory treatment outcomes. The unsatisfactory group had a significantly higher rate of urinary tract symptoms (LUTS), including urinary frequency (88.9% vs. 69.9%), nocturia (87.5% vs. 74.2%), and urinary retention (6.9% vs. 1.1%) than the satisfactory group. However, the unsatisfactory group had lower urge incontinence (8.3% vs. 18.3%) rate. Nine (10%) patients in the satisfactory group underwent electrical coagulation of Hunner's lesion. Moreover, as shown in Table 1, there were no significant differences in the subjective awareness items which included the ICSI and ICPI of the O'Leary–Sant symptom scale (OSS), and the NRS for bladder pain severity between the two groups, regardless of their self-reported treatment outcomes. However, the satisfactory group had a much larger voided volume (273 ± 130 vs. 236 ± 111 mL, p = 0.026) at the baseline. Moreover, there were no significant differences in age, sex, IC duration, pain severity, IC symptoms, problem severity, VUDS parameters, glomerulation grade, MBC, and KCl test results at the baseline between the two groups (Table 1).

In contrast, according to their bladder condition, we referred to a previous study that used statistical analysis of the receiver operating characteristic curve to predict satisfactory outcomes [11] and to further define both the MBCs greater or less than 760 mL and the phenotype divided on bladder capacity combined with the glomerulation grade. The unsatisfactory group was found to have a significantly smaller bladder capacity of <760 mL in comparison to the satisfactory group (n = 103, 77% vs. n = 53, 61%, p = 0.007). Interestingly, among 220 patients, excluding those with HIC, who had their urine collected for urinary biomarker analysis, the levels of the inflammatory biomarker monocyte chemoattractant protein-1 (MCP-1) and the oxidative stress biomarker 8-isoprostane were significantly higher in the unsatisfactory group (379 ± 517 vs. 229 ± 259, $p = 0.031$; 115 ± 245 vs. 44.8 ± 48.1, $p = 0.017$) (Table 2). Among the patients with satisfactory outcomes, 37% ($n = 32$) received intravesical BoNT-A injections more than four times, whereas, in the unsatisfactory group, only 27% ($n = 36$) received the BoNT-A injection more than four times.

Table 2. Bladder condition and urinary biomarkers of the IC/BPS patients stratified according to the treatment outcome ($n = 220$).

Variable	Total ($n = 220$)	Unsatisfactory Outcome GRA ≤ 1 ($n = 133$)	Satisfactory Outcome GRA ≥ 2 ($n = 87$)	p Value
Bladder condition (%)				
Maximal bladder capacity < 760 (mL)	156 (70.9%)	103 (77%)	53 (61%)	0.007 *
Glomerulation grade 2/3	114 (51.8%)	75 (56%)	39 (45%)	0.062
Hunner's lesion IC	20 (9.1%)	11 (8%)	9 (10%)	
Glomerulation 0/1, MBC ≥ 760 mL	45 (20.5%)	20 (15%)	25 (29%)	
Glomerulation 0/1, MBC < 760 mL	38 (17.3%)	26 (20%)	12 (14%)	0.097
Glomerulation 2/3, MBC ≥ 760 mL	18 (8.2%)	10 (8%)	8 (10%)	
Glomerulation 2/3, MBC < 760 mL	99 (45%)	66 (47%)	33 (38%)	
Urine biomarker (exclude HIC)				
IL-8	23.7 ± 71.2	18.2 ± 24.2	31.6 ± 108	0.291
CXCL 10	16.4 ± 13.2	19.7 ± 46.7	11.5 ± 37.2	0.289
MCP-1	318 ± 436	379 ± 517	229 ± 259	0.029 *
BDNF	1.48 ± 9.35	2.04 ± 12.1	0.64 ± 0.29	0.398
Eotaxin	7.05 ± 7.63	7.83 ± 8.04	5.92 ± 6.89	0.157
IL-6	8.54 ± 53.7	11.2 ± 67.5	4.71 ± 19.0	0.496
MIP-1β	1.70 ± 8.88	1.79 ± 2.61	1.56 ± 5.23	0.728
RANTES	10.6 ± 61.1	15.5 ± 79	3.59 ± 5.06	0.273
TNF-α	6.91 ± 35.6	8.77 ± 44.6	4.19 ± 14.7	0.468
PGE2	329 ± 346	370 ± 382	269 ± 278	0.100
8-OHdG	34.3 ± 26.5	36.9 ± 29.6	30.5 ± 20.9	0.168
8-Isoprostane	86.5 ± 194	115 ± 245	44.8 ± 48.1	0.015 *
TAC	1214 ± 1203	1323 ± 1288	1058 ± 1063	0.218

MBC: Maximal bladder capacity, IL-8: interleukin-8, CXCL10: C-X-C motif chemokine ligand 10, MCP-1: monocyte chemoattractant protein-1, BDNF: brain-derived neurotrophic factor, IL-6: Interleukin 6, RANTES: regulated upon activation/normal T cell expressed and secreted, PGE2: prostaglandin E2, TNF-α: tumor necrosis factor-alpha, 8-OHdG: 8-hydroxy-2-deoxyguanosine, TAC: total antioxidant capacity; * significant $p < 0.05$.

Finally, to determine the IC/BPS patients' subjective or objective influencing factors, including age, sex, IC duration, IC symptoms and problem severity, VUDS parameters, and phenotype, a supervised machine learning algorithm was used to predict the probability of an outcome. The results of the logistic regression indicated that IC/BPS symptoms and problem severity (odds ratio: 1.06, 95% CI: 1.01–1.13, $p = 0.031$) and detrusor pressure were significant predictors of treatment outcomes. Patients with grade 2–3 glomerulation and MBC < 760 mL might have poor treatment outcomes compared to those with grade 0 to 1 glomerulation and MBC ≥ 760 mL (odds ratio: 0.04, 95% CI: 0.17–0.97, $p = 0.042$) (Figure 1). However, adverse events including hematuria after injection in 6 (2.7%) patients, 4 (1.8%) urinary tract infections, and 36 (16%) mild dysuria cases were found, but these were without reports of urinary retention from any of the patients treated.

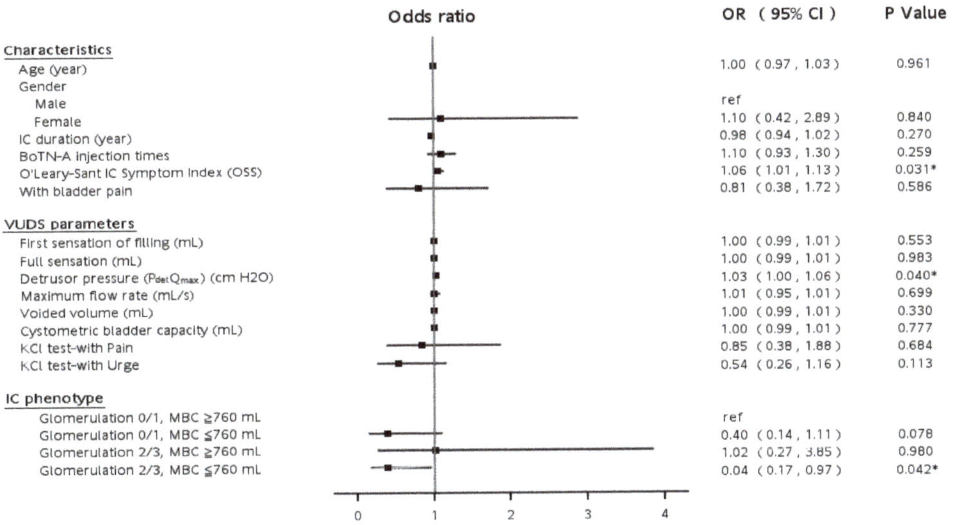

Figure 1. The forest plot results from the logistic regression for predicting satisfactory treatment outcome (GRA $\geq$ 2) effect factors. * significant $p < 0.05$.

3. Discussion

In our study, only 40% of our IC/BPS patients showed symptomatic improvement. IC/BPS patients with less inflammatory bladder conditions would likely have satisfactory outcomes with intravesical BoNT-A treatment. The levels of inflammatory and oxidative stress urinary biomarkers, such as MCP-1 and 8-isoprostane, were higher in IC/BPS patients with unsatisfactory treatment outcomes. Moreover, voided volume and MBC also affect the IC/BPS patients' treatment outcomes. IC/BPS symptom and problem severity and detrusor pressure are significant predictors of treatment outcomes in IC/BPS patients receiving intravesical BoNT-A injections. The IC/BPS patients with severe bladder inflammation might need more intravesical BoNT-A injections to attain a satisfactory outcome.

The urothelium is a stratified epithelium with three cell types (basal, intermediate, and superficial) and its functions include: forming a permeability barrier, acting as a sensory organ, and accommodating large volumes of urine [14]. The bladder urothelium is basically quiescent but regenerates readily upon injury [15]; the turnover rate of quiescent rodent urothelium is approximately once every 200 days [3]. Insufficient urothelial regeneration might decline the defense barrier and impact the barrier function whereby toxic substances or pathogens in the urine further stimulate local tissue inflammation [14], depolarize afferent nerve fibers, raise exposure to urinary toxins, incite chronic bladder inflammation, and aggravate sensory nerve activation, leading to chronic pain and insufficient or overabundant regeneration [3] which further results in higher levels of cytokine biomarkers in the urine.

The first documented therapeutic application of BoNT occurred in 1977. A purified BoNT (Oculinum©) was injected into the extra-ocular muscles to treat strabismus [16]. In 1988, Dykstra et al., first used BoNT in patients with lower urinary tract disorders to treat detrusor external sphincter dyssynergia [17]. Additionally, physicians also attempted to use intravesical BoNT-A injections as treatment for IC/BPS in 2003 [18]. The BoNT-A is one of the most powerful neurotoxins and inhibits the release of neurotransmitters from nerve fibers and urothelium [9]. The therapeutic effects might involve inhibiting the release of acetylcholine into the neuromuscular junctions of the detrusor muscle and anti-inflammatory responses [19]. Intravesical BoNT-A injections are listed in the AUA clinical guidelines as a fourth-line treatment option for IC/BPS [7].

In the present study, we reviewed the data of 220/521 IC/BPS patients receiving intravesical BoNT-A treatment over the past two decades, regardless of the number of BoNT-A injections each received. Only 40% of these patients showed symptomatic improvement, including those with long lasting disease durations and those who were refractory to medical treatments. Additionally, BoNT-A (100 U) is effective and safe as a treatment for IC/BPS [9]. Unfortunately, in the clinical practice, effective treatments for IC/BPS are lacking [1] and the pathophysiology of IC/BPS is also undetermined. However, previous guidelines believe the pathophysiology of NHIC might be multifactorial and include inflammation, post-infection autoimmune process, mast-cell activation, and urothelial dysfunction [1,7,9]. Furthermore, the bladder disorder could be first or secondary, which resulted from another cause [20]. However, bladder treatment combined with multimodal therapy is necessary [21].

Moreover, in the present study, we further explored the inflammatory and oxidative urinary biomarkers in these IC/BPS patients and found that patients without satisfactory treatment outcomes had higher MCP-1 and 8-isoprostane levels. In contrast, the patients reporting satisfactory treatment outcomes had significantly lower levels of inflammatory and oxidative stress urinary biomarkers. This leads us to presume that repeat BoNT-A injections not only reduce pain but also decrease bladder inflammation and improve IC symptoms and problems, resulting in better treatment outcomes. In the previous clinical trial using repeated BoNT-A injections, a higher success rate was found in patients receiving more than two injections over longer therapeutic durations [19]. In practice, when a patient reports no satisfactory outcome after receiving the BoNT-A injection, physicians might not recommend repeat injections and the patient probably would refuse such additional treatment without considering that the anti-inflammatory effect had not been attained during the initial treatment.

In summary, the etiology of IC/BPS might be affected by multiple factors, including a defective/damaged bladder urothelium, activation of C-fibers, neurogenic inflammation with mast cell activation, autoimmunity, occult infection, and pudendal nerve entrapment [1]. However, IC/BPS patients, with or without Hunner's ulcers, had significantly higher levels of urine cytokine biomarkers, including interleukin-8 (IL-8), C-X-C motif chemokine ligand 10 (CXCL-10), brain-derived neurotrophic factor (BDNF), eotaxin, and regulated upon activation/normal T cell expressed and secreted (RANTES) than the general population [13]. This revealed that chronic inflammation might be the fundamental pathophysiology of IC/BPS. Therefore, bladder tissue apoptosis among IC/PBS patients might result from inflammatory signal upregulation [22]. This study, based on the point of view analysis of IC/BPS patients' subjective treatment outcomes in correlation with objective factors, revealed that the unsatisfactory group has higher urine biomarker levels and lesser bladder capacities, indicating that they probably have more severe bladder inflammation and have not yet achieved optimal treatment effects. In these patients, repeat intravesical BoNT-A injections are required to achieve a satisfactory outcome. Regardless of the therapeutic options used by patients with IC/BPS in the past, in the future, precision medicine such as urine biomarkers, are expected to be used during bespoke personal treatment courses irrespective of physiological or psychological treatments, and longer, more complete treatment periods are also essential.

The major limitation of this study is its retrospective study design and single-center. Thus, further research is needed before more definite recommendations can be made, and in addition, longer follow-ups are also needed. Future studies should investigate the correlation between urinary biomarkers before and after BoNT-A treatment. Moreover, a consistent bladder volume must be ensured before collecting a urine sample and any invasive examinations must not be performed on patients for at least 48 h to ensure non-stimulation of the urothelium cell. Furthermore, allocating IC/BPS phenotype to suitable treatment options is another direction for our future efforts.

4. Conclusions

In this study, only 40% of IC/BPS patients had symptomatic improvement after intravesical BoNT-A injections. Patients with less inflammatory bladder conditions characterized by a larger bladder capacity, lower symptom severity, and lower urinary inflammatory and oxidative stress biomarker levels may predict satisfactory outcomes. Patients with severe bladder inflammation might require more intravesical BoNT-A injections to achieve a satisfactory outcome.

5. Materials and Methods

This study involved IC/BPS patients treated with 100 U BoNT-A from February 2000 to December 2021. All patients were diagnosed with IC/BPS in accordance with established IC/BPS characteristic symptoms and cystoscopic findings of glomerulations, petechiae, or mucosal fissures on anesthesia cystoscope hydrodistention [23]. Among the IC/BPS patients, lifestyle and behavioral modification, cystoscopic hydrodistention, intravesical hyaluronic acid instillation, or painkiller medications and treatment modalities were tried in at least two treatment modalities, but the IC symptoms persisted or relapsed. During the study period, some patients were undergoing BoNT-A injection clinical trials. However, we only recorded the outcomes of their first treatments.

All patients were screened thoroughly at the time of enrollment and were not enrolled if they failed the inclusion criteria of the European Society for the Study of Interstitial Cystitis [24]. This is a retrospective analysis of previous clinical trials of BoNT-A injections for patients with IC/BPS. In these clinical trials, the patient inclusion and exclusion criteria were the same (Appendix A).

The treatment outcomes at 6 months after the intravesical BoNT-A injection were evaluated using the GRA scale. Additionally, the IC symptoms were assessed using OSS, including ICSI and ICPI [25]. The ICSI and ICPI are two instruments used to determine the overall level of severity of each symptom and the significance of the problem from the patient's perspective, respectively [26,27]. Both indices included four questions, one each for nocturia, frequency, urgency, and bladder-associated pain. The total ICSI scores range from 0 to 20. Each of the questions in the ICPI has five response options ranging from 0 to 4 with a maximum total ICPI score of 16, with higher scores indicating more severe IC/BPS symptoms and problem severity [26]. Patients were requested to rate their bladder symptoms as compared to that at baseline using a 7-point centered scale, from markedly (−3), moderately (−2), and slightly worse (−1), no change (0), to slightly (+1), moderately (+2), and markedly improved (+3). Patients with moderately and markedly improved results after treatment were considered to have satisfactory treatment outcomes. Otherwise, the treatment outcome was considered unsatisfactory [19].

VUDS was performed before the BoNT-A injection using the multichannel urodynamic system (Life-Tech, Stafford, TX, USA) and a C-arm fluoroscope (Toshiba, Tokyo, Japan). According to International Continence Society recommendations, this study's descriptions and terminologies all follow the compliance criteria [28]. Based on the characteristic VUDS findings, such as the first sensation of filling, first desire to void full bladder sensation, cystometric bladder capacity, detrusor pressure at maximum flow rate, maximum flow rate, voided-volume, and post-void residual (PVR), patients would be diagnosed with hypersensitive bladder, detrusor overactivity, voiding dysfunction, poor pelvic floor muscle relaxation, or intrinsic sphincter deficiency [29]. The KCl test was considered positive if there was bladder pain or an intense urge to void during the KCl infusion after the emptying of the residual urine [30]. was Patients with increased bladder sensation and positive KCl sensitivity tests were encouraged to undergo Cystoscopic hydrodistention. The VUDS was performed to verify the diagnosis of IC/BPS at baseline and recognize other bladder conditions that resemble IC/BPS. A duplicate VUDS was performed 6 months after the primary BoNT-A injection to estimate the bladder condition after treatment and as an action for instigating subsequent treatment.

After cystoscopic hydrodistention, the patients were treated with consecutive bladder-targeting medications for bladder pain, including nonsteroidal-inflammatory drugs, cyclooxygenase-2 inhibitors, antimuscarinics, alpha-blockers, intravesical hyaluronic acid installations, and 4th line of intravesical BoNT-A injections, according to AUA guideline recommendations [20].

BoNT-A medicinal liquid constituted a vial of onabotulinumtoxin A (100 U) diluted with 10 mL 0.9% saline. Twenty injections were performed with this BoNT-A liquid, lead 5-U BoNT-A in each injection site. For the bladder's posterior and lateral walls, an injection needle was inserted approximately 1 mm in the urothelium, sparing the trigone, using a 23-gauge needle and rigid cystoscopic injection instrument (22 Fr, Richard Wolf, and Knittlingen, Germany). After the BoNT-A injections, cystoscopic hydrodistention was performed under slowly dripping 0.9% saline to an intravesical pressure of 80 cm fluid for 15 min. The MBC and glomerulation grade under hydrodistention was also recorded after intravesical pressure release [9]. Based on the appearance of glomerulations for none, less than half, more than half, and more than half and during serious waterfall bleeding of the bladder wall, if patients have Hunner's lesion combined with or without glomerulations were classified as ulcer-type IC/BPS. After that, the glomerulation grade was classified into 0, 1, 2, and 3 [11]. After the BoNT-A treatment, a 14-Fr indwelling urinary catheter was inserted overnight and removed the next day. An antibiotic (cephradine 500 mg every 6 h) was routinely prescribed for a week, and patients visited the outpatient clinic 2 weeks after treatment, followed by monthly visits to the outpatient clinic for outcome assessment. The primary endpoint was 6 months after the BoNT-A injection.

We not only analyzed the patients' subjective and objective characteristics and VUDS parameters but also collected urine specimens to further analyze the urinary biomarkers at baseline. The urinary biomarkers collected included interleukin-8 (IL-8), CXCL10, MCP-1, BDNF, eotaxin, Interleukin 6 (IL-6), RANTES (also known as CCL5), prostaglandin E2, tumor necrosis factor-alpha, 8-hydroxy-2-deoxyguanosine, 8-isoprostane, and total antioxidant capacity [13]. In brief, before cystoscopic hydrodistention, all patients would collect 50 mL urine samples, obtained by self-urination, when patients had a full bladder sensation, and also excluded those with confirmed urinary tract infections. Before transferring to the laboratory, the urine samples were placed on ice. However, HICs would be excluded from further analysis considering the different pathology [13,31].

Statistical Analysis

Statistical analysis was performed using SPSS version 25 (IBM, Armonk, NY, USA); a p value of <0.05 was considered statistically significant. Data were expressed as mean and standard deviations for continuous variables, and categorical variables were presented as counts and proportions. Between-group statistical comparisons were tested for categorical variables using either Pearson's chi-square or Fisher's exact test, and additionally using an independent t-test for continuous variables, excluding outliers of urinary biomarkers.

To examine the association of treatment outcomes, logistic regression models were further estimated for subjective and objective factors in an attempt to predict the factors which influence the expected treatment outcomes. Logistic regression was used to analyze the relationship between IC/BPS patients' characteristics, VUDS parameters, and IC/BPS bladder phenotype and self-reported satisfactory treatment outcomes.

Author Contributions: Conceptualization: W.-R.Y. and H.-C.K.; data curation: W.-R.Y. and W.-C.C.; project administration: W.-R.Y. and H.-C.K.; methodology: W.-R.Y., J.-F.J., Y.-H.J. and H.-C.K.; investigation and formal analysis: W.-R.Y., J.-F.J., Y.-H.J. and H.-C.K.; writing—original draft: W.-R.Y.; writing—review and editing: H.-C.K. All authors have read and agreed to the published version of the manuscript.

Funding: This research was funded by Buddhist Tzu Chi Medical Foundation grants TCMF-SP 108-01 and TCMF-MP 110-03-01.

Institutional Review Board Statement: This study was performed in line with the principles of the Declaration of Helsinki. Approval for convenience sampling at a medical center was granted by the Ethics Committee of Hualien Tzu Chi Hospital, Buddhist Tzu Chi Medical Foundation (Code: IRB: 105-25-B, approved date: 21 June 2017).

Informed Consent Statement: The requirement for obtaining patient informed consent was waived due to the retrospective nature of the study.

Data Availability Statement: Data are available if requested from the corresponding authors.

Acknowledgments: We thank the patients who participated in the trial, their families, and the staff at the Department of Urology, Hualien Tzu Chi Hospital who collected and validated the data. We also thank our colleagues throughout the system who referred cases.

Conflicts of Interest: The authors declare no conflict of interest.

Appendix A. The Inclusion and Exclusion Criteria of Intravesical BoNT-A Injection for IC/BPS

Patient Inclusion Criteria	1. Adults aged 20 years old or above 2. Patients with symptoms of frequency, urgency, nocturia, and/or bladder pain 3. Proven to have glomerulations (at least grade 1) by cystoscopic hydrodistention under anesthesia in recent 1 year 4. Free of active urinary tract infection 5. Free of bladder outlet obstruction on enrolment 6. Free of overt neurogenic bladder dysfunction and limitation of ambulation 7. The patient, or his/her legally acceptable representative, has signed the written informed consent form
Patient Exclusion Criteria	1. Patients with severe cardiopulmonary disease such as congestive heart failure, arrhythmia, poorly controlled hypertension, or those unable to receive regular follow-up treatment 2. Patients with bladder outlet obstruction on enrollment 3. Patients with post-void residual >250mL 4. Patients with an uncontrolled and confirmed diagnosis of acute urinary tract infection 5. Patients with laboratory abnormalities at screening that include: ALT> 3 x upper limit of the normal range, AST> 3 x upper limit of the normal range; Patients with abnormal serum creatinine level > 2 x upper limit of the normal range 6. Patients with any contraindication to urethral catheterization during treatment 7. Female patients who are pregnant, lactating, or with child-bearing potential without contraception. 8. Patients with any other serious disease considered by the investigator not in a condition to enter the trial 9. Patients who had received intravesical onabotulinumtoxinA treatment for IC within the last 6 months 10. Patients who participated in an investigational drug trial within 1 month before entering this study

References

1. Homma, Y.; Akiyama, Y.; Tomoe, H.; Furuta, A.; Ueda, T.; Maeda, D.; Lin, A.T.; Kuo, H.C.; Lee, M.H.; Oh, S.J.; et al. Clinical guidelines for interstitial cystitis/bladder pain syndrome. *Int. J. Urol.* **2020**, *27*, 578–589. [CrossRef] [PubMed]
2. Jhang, J.F.; Jiang, Y.H.; Kuo, H.C. Current understanding of the pathophysiology and novel treatments of interstitial cystitis/bladder pain syndrome. *Biomedicines* **2022**, *10*, 2380. [CrossRef] [PubMed]

3. Balsara, Z.R.; Li, X. Sleeping beauty: Awakening urothelium from its slumber. *Am. J. Physiol. Ren. Physiol.* **2017**, *312*, F732–F743. [CrossRef]
4. Clemens, J.Q.; Erickson, D.R.; Varela, N.P.; Lai, H.H. Diagnosis and treatment of interstitial cystitis/bladder pain syndrome. *J. Urol.* **2022**, *208*, 34–42. [CrossRef] [PubMed]
5. Cox, A.; Golda, N.; Nadeau, G.; Nickel, J.C.; Carr, L.; Corcos, J.; Teichman, J. CUA guideline: Diagnosis and treatment of interstitial cystitis/bladder pain syndrome. *Can. Urol. Assoc. J.* **2016**, *10*, E136–E155. [CrossRef] [PubMed]
6. Malde, S.; Palmisani, S.; Al-Kaisy, A.; Sahai, A. Guideline of guidelines: Bladder pain syndrome. *BJU Int.* **2018**, *122*, 729–743. [CrossRef]
7. Hanno, P.M.; Burks, D.A.; Clemens, J.Q.; Dmochowski, R.R.; Erickson, D.; FitzGerald, M.P.; Forrest, J.B.; Gordon, B.; Gray, M.; Mayer, R.D.; et al. AUA guideline for the diagnosis and treatment of interstitial cystitis/bladder pain syndrome. *J. Urol.* **2011**, *185*, 2162–2170. [CrossRef]
8. Jiang, Y.H.; Yu, W.R.; Kuo, H.C. Therapeutic effect of botulinum toxin A on sensory bladder disorders—from bench to bedside. *Toxins* **2020**, *12*, 166. [CrossRef]
9. Kuo, H.C.; Jiang, Y.H.; Tsai, Y.C.; Kuo, Y.C. Intravesical botulinum toxin-A injections reduce bladder pain of interstitial cystitis/bladder pain syndrome refractory to conventional treatment—a prospective, multicenter, randomized, double-blind, placebo-controlled clinical trial. *Neurourol. Urodyn.* **2016**, *35*, 609–614. [CrossRef]
10. Chiu, B.; Tai, H.C.; Chung, S.D.; Birder, L.A. Botulinum toxin A for bladder pain syndrome/interstitial cystitis. *Toxins* **2016**, *8*, 201. [CrossRef]
11. Wang, H.J.; Yu, W.R.; Ong, H.L.; Kuo, H.C. Predictive factors for a satisfactory treatment outcome with intravesical botulinum toxin A injection in patients with interstitial cystitis/bladder pain syndrome. *Toxins* **2019**, *11*, 676. [CrossRef] [PubMed]
12. Keller, J.J.; Chen, Y.K.; Lin, H.C. Comorbidities of bladder pain syndrome/interstitial cystitis: A population-based study. *BJU Int.* **2012**, *110*, E903–E909. [CrossRef] [PubMed]
13. Yu, W.R.; Jiang, Y.H.; Jhang, J.F.; Kuo, H.C. Use of urinary cytokine and chemokine levels for identifying bladder conditions and predicting treatment outcomes in patients with interstitial cystitis/bladder pain syndrome. *Biomedicines* **2022**, *10*, 1149. [CrossRef] [PubMed]
14. Yamany, T.; Van Batavia, J.; Mendelsohn, C. Formation and regeneration of the urothelium. *Curr. Opin. Organ Transplant* **2014**, *19*, 323–330. [CrossRef] [PubMed]
15. Wiessner, G.B.; Plumber, S.A.; Xiang, T.; Mendelsohn, C.L. Development, regeneration and tumorigenesis of the urothelium. *Development* **2022**, *149*, dev198184. [CrossRef]
16. Choudhury, S.; Baker, M.R.; Chatterjee, S.; Kumar, H. Botulinum toxin: An update on pharmacology and newer products in development. *Toxins* **2021**, *13*, 58. [CrossRef]
17. Moore, D.C.; Cohn, J.A.; Dmochowski, R.R. Use of botulinum toxin A in the treatment of lower urinary tract disorders: A review of the literature. *Toxins* **2016**, *8*, 88. [CrossRef]
18. Kuo, H.C. Preliminary results of suburothelial injection of botulinum a toxin in the treatment of chronic interstitial cystitis. *Urol. Int.* **2005**, *75*, 170–174. [CrossRef]
19. Kuo, H.C. Repeated onabotulinumtoxin-a injections provide better results than single injection in treatment of painful bladder syndrome. *Pain. Phys.* **2013**, *16*, E15–E23. [CrossRef]
20. Hanno, P.M.; Erickson, D.; Moldwin, R.; Faraday, M.M. Diagnosis and treatment of interstitial cystitis/bladder pain syndrome: AUA guideline amendment. *J. Urol.* **2015**, *193*, 1545–1553. [CrossRef]
21. Shatkin-Margolis, A.; White, J.; Jedlicka, A.E.; Tam, T.; Hill, A.; Yeung, J.; Crisp, C.C.; Pauls, R.N. The effect of mindfulness-based stress reduction on the urinary microbiome in interstitial cystitis. *Int. Urogynecol. J.* **2022**, *33*, 665–671. [CrossRef] [PubMed]
22. Shie, J.H.; Liu, H.T.; Kuo, H.C. Increased cell apoptosis of urothelium mediated by inflammation in interstitial cystitis/painful bladder syndrome. *Urology* **2012**, *79*, 484.e7-13. [CrossRef] [PubMed]
23. Hanno, P.M.; Landis, J.R.; Matthews-Cook, Y.; Kusek, J.; Nyberg, L. The diagnosis of interstitial cystitis revisited: Lessons learned from the National Institutes of Health Interstitial Cystitis Database study. *J. Urol.* **1999**, *161*, 553–557. [CrossRef] [PubMed]
24. Van de Merwe, J.P.; Nordling, J.; Bouchelouche, P.; Bouchelouche, K.; Cervigni, M.; Daha, L.K.; Elneil, S.; Fall, M.; Hohlbrugger, G.; Irwin, P.; et al. Diagnostic criteria, classification, and nomenclature for painful bladder syndrome/interstitial cystitis: An ESSIC proposal. *Eur. Urol.* **2008**, *53*, 60–67. [CrossRef] [PubMed]
25. Grinberg, K.; Sela, Y.; Nissanholtz-Gannot, R. New insights about chronic pelvic pain syndrome (CPPS). *Int. J. Environ. Res. Public Health* **2020**, *17*, 3005. [CrossRef]
26. Esen, B.; Obaid, K.; Süer, E.; Gökçe, M.İ.; Gökmen, D.; Bedük, Y.; Gülpınar, Ö. Reliability and validity of Turkish versions of the interstitial cystitis symptom index and interstitial cystitis problem index. *Neurourol. Urodyn.* **2020**, *39*, 2338–2343. [CrossRef]
27. O'Leary, M.P.; Sant, G.R.; Fowler, F.J.; Whitmore, K.E.; Spolarich-Kroll, J. The interstitial cystitis symptom index and problem index. *Urology* **1997**, *49*, 58–63. [CrossRef]
28. Abrams, P.; Cardozo, L.; Fall, M.; Griffiths, D.; Rosier, P.; Ulmsten, U.; Van Kerrebroeck, P.; Victor, A.; Wein, A. The standardisation of terminology of lower urinary tract function: Report from the Standardisation Sub-committee of the International Continence Society. *Am. J. Obstet. Gynecol.* **2002**, *187*, 116–126. [CrossRef]
29. Hsiao, S.M.; Lin, H.H.; Kuo, H.C. Videourodynamic studies of women with voiding dysfunction. *Sci. Rep.* **2017**, *7*, 1–8. [CrossRef]

30. Parsons, C.L.; Stein, P.C.; Bidair, M.; Lebow, D. Abnormal sensitivity to intravesical potassium in interstitial cystitis and radiation cystitis. *Neurourol. Urodyn.* **1994**, *13*, 515–520. [CrossRef]
31. Kuo, H.C. Potential urine and serum biomarkers for patients with bladder pain syndrome/interstitial cystitis. *Int. J. Urol.* **2014**, *21*, 34–41. [CrossRef] [PubMed]

toxins MDPI

Article

Predictive Factors for a Successful Treatment Outcome in Patients with Different Voiding Dysfunction Subtypes Who Received Urethral Sphincter Botulinum Injection

Yao-Lin Kao [1], Yin-Chien Ou [1,2], Kuen-Jer Tsai [2,3] and Hann-Chorng Kuo [4,*]

1 Department of Urology, National Cheng Kung University Hospital, College of Medicine, National Cheng Kung University, Tainan 704, Taiwan
2 Institute of Clinical Medicine, College of Medicine, National Cheng Kung University, Tainan 704, Taiwan
3 Research Center of Clinical Medicine, National Cheng Kung University Hospital, College of Medicine, National Cheng Kung University, Tainan 704, Taiwan
4 Department of Urology, Hualien Tzu Chi Hospital, Buddhist Tzu Chi Medical Foundation and Tzu Chi University, Hualien 970, Taiwan
* Correspondence: hck@tzuchi.com.tw

Abstract: Voiding dysfunction is a common but bothersome problem in both men and women. Urethral sphincter botulinum toxin A (BoNT-A) injections could serve as an option in refractory cases. This study analyzed the efficacy and outcome predictors of the injections in patients with functional, non-neurogenic voiding dysfunction. Patients who received urethral sphincter BoNT-A injection for refractory voiding dysfunction due to detrusor underactivity (DU) or urethral sphincter dysfunction were retrospectively reviewed. A successful outcome was defined as a marked improvement as reported in the global response assessment. The study evaluated the therapeutic efficacy of urethral sphincter BoNT-A injections and measured the changes in urodynamic parameters after the procedure in the patients. A total of 181 patients including 138 women and 43 men were included. The overall success rate was 64%. A lower success rate was noted in patients with DU compared to those with urethral sphincter dysfunction in both genders. In the multivariable analysis, recurrent urinary tract infection (UTI) and bladder voiding efficiency (BVE) were positive predictors for a successful outcome, while DU was a negative predictor. Urethral sphincter BoNT-A injection is an effective treatment for refractory non-neurogenic voiding dysfunction. Baseline BVE and history of recurrent UTI positively predict a successful outcome. DU is a negative outcome predictor.

Keywords: botulinum toxin; urethral; voiding dysfunction; detrusor underactivity; urethral sphincter dysfunction

Key Contribution: Urethral sphincteric BoNT-A injection provides comparative responses in refractory functional, non-neurogenic voiding dysfunction. DU and poor bladder voiding efficiency predict inferior therapeutic outcomes.

Citation: Kao, Y.-L.; Ou, Y.-C.; Tsai, K.-J.; Kuo, H.-C. Predictive Factors for a Successful Treatment Outcome in Patients with Different Voiding Dysfunction Subtypes Who Received Urethral Sphincter Botulinum Injection. *Toxins* **2022**, *14*, 877. https://doi.org/10.3390/toxins14120877

Received: 8 November 2022
Accepted: 13 December 2022
Published: 15 December 2022

Publisher's Note: MDPI stays neutral with regard to jurisdictional claims in published maps and institutional affiliations.

Copyright: © 2022 by the authors. Licensee MDPI, Basel, Switzerland. This article is an open access article distributed under the terms and conditions of the Creative Commons Attribution (CC BY) license (https://creativecommons.org/licenses/by/4.0/).

1. Introduction

Voiding dysfunction is a urological condition characterized by slow or incomplete bladder emptying [1,2]. Being a major component of lower urinary tract symptoms (LUTS) in men, voiding dysfunction is actually not uncommon in women in clinical practice [3]. Detrusor underactivity (DU) and bladder outlet obstruction (BOO) are two fundamental etiologies of voiding dysfunction and both could result from either neurogenic or non-neurogenic origins [4]. The latter could further be subdivided into anatomical obstruction and functional obstruction.

Urodynamic study is often required for the diagnosis of voiding dysfunction. Invasive urodynamic studies such as pressure flow studies or videourodynamic studies (VUDS)

could differentiate DU from BOO as causes of voiding dysfunction [5]. VUDS could further undermine the underlying lower urinary tract dysfunction of BOO including urethral stricture, benign prostate obstruction (BPO), high-grade pelvic organ prolapse as anatomical obstruction, primary bladder neck obstruction, or urethral sphincter dysfunction as functional obstructions [6]. The accurate diagnosis and measurement of urodynamic parameters from VUDS may predict and even improve the outcomes of different voiding dysfunctions [7].

Except for simple anatomical obstruction such as BPO or high-grade pelvic organ prolapse, treating entities of voiding dysfunction may be challenging for urologists. Botulinum toxin A (BoNT-A) has been used to treat the neurogenic voiding dysfunction since the late 1980s [8]. Urethral sphincter injection of BoNT-A could decrease urethral resistance and improve voiding efficiency (VE) via chemical sphincterotomy through the blocking of acetylcholine release from presynaptic efferent nerves at the neuromuscular junctions [9]. Benefits of urethral sphincter BoNT-A injections in non-neurogenic voiding dysfunction were also reported afterwards [10,11]. This article aims to explore the effects of urethral sphincter BoNT-A injections in different types of functional, non-neurogenic voiding dysfunction in both genders and search for the predictive factor for treatment outcome.

2. Results

There were 181 patients including 138 females and 43 males receiving urethral BoNT-A injections in this study. The mean age at injection was 59.7 ± 21.1 years old in women and 67.3 ± 14.1 years old in men, which was significant younger in the former (p = 0.003). Compared to men, women had a higher percentage of recurrent urinary tract infection (43% vs. 5%, p < 0.001) and history of receiving transurethral incision or resection of the bladder neck (TUIBN) (50% vs. 19%, p < 0.001), but a lower percentage of Parkinson's disease (1% vs. 14%, p = 0.003) and dementia (1% vs. 7%, p = 0.042). A total of 56% of men had received transurethral resection of the prostate (TURP). Detailed baseline characteristics and comorbidities stratified by gender are shown in Table 1.

Table 1. Baseline characteristics and comorbidities stratified by gender.

	Female (n = 138) Mean ± SD or No. (%)		Male (n = 43) Mean ± SD or No. (%)		p Value
Age	59.7	±21.1	67.3	±14.0	0.003
Diagnosis					
Detrusor underactivity	61	(44)	17	(40)	
Urethral sphincter dysfunction *	77	(56)	26	(60)	0.589
Diabetes mellitus	36	(26)	11	(26)	0.947
Hypertension	65	(47)	18	(42)	0.547
CAD	13	(9)	1	(2)	0.193
CKD	3	(2)	1	(2)	1.000
COPD			1	(2)	0.238
Parkinson disease	2	(1)	6	(14)	0.003
CVA	19	(14)	7	(16)	0.682
Dementia	1	(1)	3	(7)	0.042
Recurrent UTI	47	(34)	2	(5)	<0.001
History of TURP			24	(56)	<0.001
History of TUI-BN	69	(50)	8	(19)	<0.001

CKD: Chronic kidney disease; COPD: Chronic obstructive pulmonary disease; CVA: Cerebrovascular accident; UTI: Urinary tract infection; TURP: Transurethral Resection of Prostate; TUI-BN: Transurethral Incision or Resection of the Bladder Neck. * Urethral sphincter dysfunction including dysfunctional voiding and poor relaxation of urethral sphincter.

Table 2 shows the baseline and post-injection VUDS parameters and the post-injection GRA in women with different types of voiding dysfunction. There were 61 women with DU and 77 with urethral sphincter dysfunctions in this study. A significantly lower rate of successful outcome was noted in women with DU compared to those with urethral sphincter dysfunction (56% vs. 74%, p = 0.024). Except for mild decrease of US, no obvious change of other VUDS parameters was detected in women diagnosed of DU. Increased

FSF (103.6 ± 60.5 to 125.3 ± 74.6 mL/s, p = 0.034) and decreased Pdet (54.7 ± 36.0 to 45.5 ± 33.9 cmH2O, p = 0.034), as well as BOOI (41.8 ± 37.5 to 31.6 ± 35.9, p = 0.010), were noted in women with urethral sphincter dysfunction. In the male cohort, there were 43 patients receiving urethral sphincter BoNT-A injection. Among them, 17 men were diagnosed with DU and 26 with urethral sphincter dysfunction (Table 3). A significantly lower rate of successful outcome was noted in men with DU compared to those with urethral sphincter dysfunction (36% vs. 73%, p = 0.014). Although there was some dissimilarity in clinical and VUDS parameters, no difference in treatment response rate after urethral sphincter BoNT-A injection was found among different subtypes of urethral sphincter dysfunction (Appendix A Table A1).

Univariable logistic regression analysis for predictors of successful outcome revealed that history of recurrent urinary tract infection (UTI) (OR = 2.37, p = 0.024) and VE (OR = 1.02, p < 0.001) were positively correlated with the outcome; whereas DU (OR = 0.37, p = 0.002), history of hypertension (OR = 0.50, p = 0.026) and FS (OR = 1.00, p = 0.036) in VUDS correlated with the outcome negatively (Table 4). After adjusting for age and gender, history of recurrent UTI and VE were positive predictors for a successful outcome with odds ratios of 3.82 (95% confidence interval: 1.58–9.22, p = 0.003) and 1.02 (95% confidence interval: 1.01–1.03, p = 0.004), respectively. On the other hand, DU was a negative predictor with an odds ratio of 0.46 (95% confidence interval: 0.21–0.99, p = 0.047) in the multivariable logistic regression analysis.

Table 2. Baseline and post-injection urodynamic parameters and the post-injection global response assessment in female patients with different types of voiding dysfunction.

Female (n = 138)	Detrusor Underactivity					Urethral Sphincter Dysfunction *				
	Before Urethral Botox Injection (n = 61) Mean ± SD or No. (%)		After Urethral Botox Injection (n = 61) Mean ± SD or No. (%)		p Value	Before Urethral Botox Injection (n = 77) Mean ± SD or No. (%)		After Urethral Botox Injection (n = 77) Mean ± SD or No. (%)		p Value
VUDS parameters										
FSF (mL)	177.3	±76.6	158.6	78.2	0.152	103.6	±60.5	125.3	±74.6	0.034
FS (mL)	250.1	±86.4	230.0	104.6	0.142	170.3	±78.8	193.2	±98.1	0.059
US (mL)	295.7	±106.5	266.3	109.6	0.042	204.5	±98.3	219.9	±109.5	0.242
Compliance (mL/cm H_2O)	64.3	±80.1	58.0	50.4	0.585	46.3	±62.2	56.3	±64.6	0.258
DO	7	(11)	6	(10)	0.655	51	(66)	42	(55)	0.083
Pdet(cm H_2O)	6.4	±7.9	7.2	±11.1	0.573	54.7	±36.0	45.5	±33.9	0.009
Qmax (mL/s)	4.0	±7.1	4.9	±6.5	0.460	6.5	±4.9	6.9	±5.5	0.430
BOOI	−1.4	±16.4	−2.5	±13.7	0.623	41.8	±37.5	31.6	±35.9	0.010
VV (mL)	89.3	±131.5	101.0	±139.5	0.596	124.2	±102.5	138.8	±124.0	0.337
PVR (mL)	315.4	±210.5	313.3	±220.5	0.952	187.4	±142.8	200.9	±159.0	0.480
BVE (%)	21.5	±30.9	26.1	±35.0	0.402	42.4	±31.9	45.1	±35.8	0.540
Global Response Assessment										
Excellent			5	(8)				20	(26)	
Markedly improved			29	(48)				37	(48)	
Mildly improved			8	(13)				5	(6)	
No change			18	(30)				14	(18)	
Missing			1	(2)				1	(1)	0.024 [b]
Successful outcome [a]			34	(56)				57	(74)	0.024 [b]

BOOI: bladder outlet obstruction index; BVE: bladder voiding efficiency; DO: detrusor overactivity; DU: detrusor underactivity; FS: full sensation; FSF: first sensation of filling; Pdet: maximal detrusor pressure; PVR: post-void residual volume; Qmax: maximal uroflow rate; SD: standard deviation; US: urge sensation; VV: voided volume; VUDS: videourodynamic study. [a] Successful outcome was defined as a global response assessment greater than mildly improved (score ≧ 2). [b] Difference between detrusor underactivity and urethral sphincter dysfunction. * Urethral sphincter dysfunction including dysfunctional voiding and poor relaxation of urethral sphincter.

Table 3. Baseline and post-injection urodynamic parameters and the post-injection global response assessment in male patients with different types of voiding dysfunction.

Male (n = 43)	Detrusor Underactivity					Urethral Sphincter Dysfunction *				
	Before Urethral Botox Injection (n = 17) Mean ± SD or No. (%)		After Urethral Botox Injection (n = 17) Mean ± SD or No. (%)		p Value	Before Urethral Botox Injection (n = 26) Mean ± SD or No. (%)		After Urethral Botox Injection (n = 26) Mean ± SD or No. (%)		p Value
VUDS parameters										
FSF (mL)	181.4	±105.9	172.2	±99.1	0.727	146.2	±89.6	150.8	±68.3	0.818
FS (mL)	265.9	±153.0	275.3	±156.2	0.828	248.8	±116.6	251.6	±134.0	0.919
US (mL)	320.6	±157.3	323.4	±164.4	0.947	283.9	±124.3	281.5	±142.1	0.934
Compliance (mL/cmH_2O)	73.5	±141.5	41.1	±38.0	0.359	44.5	±44.6	56.4	±50.7	0.424
DO	4	(24)	6	(35)	0.157	9	(35)	13	(50)	0.103
Pdet(cm H_2O)	10.5	±11.0	18.0	±24.2	0.285	24.2	±17.5	23.5	±17.3	0.791
Qmax (mL/s)	1.8	±2.6	2.5	±2.6	0.282	5.5	±5.3	6.8	±6.0	0.271
BOOI	6.9	±9.7	12.9	±24.2	0.336	13.3	±16.5	10.0	±15.1	0.405
VV (mL)	24.5	±40.4	38.9	±50.6	0.258	138.5	±137.0	138.6	±150.8	0.997
PVR (mL)	375.3	±162.0	393.8	±185.4	0.712	237.4	±176.5	231.1	±191.8	0.831
BVE (%)	8.2	±12.5	11.4	±13.7	0.348	40.1	±35.2	44.1	±39.0	0.552
Global Response Assessment										
Excellent			3	(18)				7	(27)	
Markedly improved			3	(18)				12	(46)	
Mildly improved			1	(6)				1	(4)	
No change			10	(59)				6	(23)	0.094 [b]
Successful outcome [a]			6	(36)				19	(73)	0.0141 [b]

BOOI: bladder outlet obstruction index; BVE: bladder voiding efficiency; DO: detrusor overactivity; DU: detrusor underactivity; FS: full sensation; FSF: first sensation of filling; Pdet: maximal detrusor pressure; PVR: post-void residual volume; Qmax: maximal uroflow rate; SD: standard deviation; US: urge sensation; VV: voided volume; VUDS: videourodynamic study. [a] Successful outcome was defined as a global response assessment greater than mildly improved (score ≧ 2). [b] Difference between detrusor underactivity and urethral sphincter dysfunction. * Urethral sphincter dysfunction including dysfunctional voiding and poor relaxation of urethral sphincter.

Table 4. Logistic regression analysis for predictors of successful outcomes after urethral sphincteric botulinum toxin A injection.

	Univariate Analysis				Multivariate Analysis			
	OR	95% CI		p Value	OR	95% CI		p Value
Age	0.98	0.97	1.00	0.062	1.00	0.98	1.02	0.728
Gender	0.72	0.36	1.45	0.353	0.88	0.38	2.04	0.769
DU	0.37	0.20	0.70	0.002	0.46	0.21	0.99	0.047
Comorbidities								
DM	0.61	0.31	1.19	0.147				
HTN	0.50	0.27	0.92	0.026	0.53	0.25	1.13	0.099
CAD	2.17	0.58	8.06	0.250				
CKD	1.70	0.17	16.66	0.649				
PD	0.93	0.22	4.02	0.923				
CVA	1.07	0.45	2.56	0.882				
Dementia	0.55	0.08	4.02	0.558				
Recurrent UTI	2.39	1.12	5.09	0.024	3.82	1.58	9.22	0.003
TURP history	0.62	0.26	1.48	0.280				
TUIBN history	0.80	0.43	1.47	0.462				
Baseline VUDS parameters								
FSF (mL)	1.00	0.99	1.00	0.159				
FS (mL)	1.00	0.99	1.00	0.036	1.00	1.00	1.00	0.559
US (mL)	1.00	1.00	1.00	0.164				
Compliance (mL/cm H_2O)	1.00	1.00	1.00	0.500				
DO	1.59	0.84	3.00	0.155				
BVE (%)	1.02	1.01	1.03	<0.001	1.02	1.01	1.03	0.004
BOOI	1.01	1.00	1.02	0.327				

BOOI: bladder outlet obstruction index; BVE: bladder voiding efficiency; CAD: Coronary artery disease; CI: confidence interval; CKD: Chronic kidney disease; COPD: Chronic obstructive pulmonary disease; CVA: Cerebrovascular accident; DM: diabetes mellitus; DO: detrusor overactivity; DU: detrusor underactivity; FS: full sensation; FSF: first sensation of filling; HTN: hypertension; PD: Parkinson's disease; PVR: post-void residual volume; Qmax: maximal uroflow rate; UTI: Urinary tract infection; TURP: Transurethral Resection of Prostate; TUI-BN: Transurethral Incision or Resection of the Bladder Neck; US: urge sensation; VUDS: videourodynamic study.

3. Discussion

This study reveals that urethral sphincter BoNT-A injection is an effective treatment option for refractory non-neurogenic functional voiding dysfunction in both genders. The general success (GRA $\geqq$ 2) rate after injection was 64%. Patients with a history of recurrent UTI and favorable baseline VE had better a subjective response after urethral sphincter BoNT-A injections. DU is a significant predictor for poor outcome. These findings suggest that undertaking urodynamic assessment before the procedure is important for predicting treatment outcomes in patients considering urethral sphincter BoNT-A injection due to voiding dysfunction.

The concept of urethral sphincter BoNT-A injection in treating non-neurogenic voiding dysfunction originated from the positive experience of its usage in treating patients with detrusor sphincter dyssynergia [12]. It was assumed that the improvement of voiding dysfunction is related to lowering of the urethral resistance through chemical sphincterotomy which was induced by blocking the presynaptic release of acetylcholine in the neuromuscular junction of the urethral sphincter after injection [13]. Previous studies have reported about 60–70% overall response rate in non-neurogenic voiding function after the urethral sphincter BoNT-A injections [14,15]. With a greater sample size, our studies demonstrated a similarly successful result in such patients. Notably, high proportion of our patients had history of TUI-BN or TURP. In our practice, we performed TUI-BN in female patients who presented with insufficient bladder neck opening during voiding in the videourodyamic studies prior to urethral sphincteric BoNT-A injection. This treatment sequence could exclude the patients whose voiding dysfunction was attributed to anatomical or functional bladder neck dysfunction. A similar rationale was also applied to the male patients; TURP or TUI-BN were performed first if obstruction in the prostate urethra or bladder neck was suspected. In short, urethral sphincteric BoNT-A was injected in patients with refractory voiding dysfunction due to DU or urethral sphincter dysfunction. In the logistic regression analysis, history of TUI-BN or TURP did not pose significant adverse effects to the outcome of urethral sphincteric BoNT-A injection.

DU and urethral sphincter dysfunction are the two major etiologies of non-neurogenic voiding dysfunction. However, studies comparing the treatment efficacy between the two are lacking and the study subjects were often mixed with those with neurogenic voiding dysfunction [15,16]. DU was reported to be one of the causes of treatment failure after urethral sphincter BoNT-A injections [16]. In this study, both women and men had a significantly lower rate of treatment success in patients diagnosed with DU compared to those with urethral sphincter dysfunction. For DU patients, the major effect of urethral sphincter BoNT-A injection is to release BOO by lowering the urethral resistance while the impaired bladder contractility persisted despite the treatment. This could explain the inferior outcome in these patients. After adjusting for the possible confounding factors including gender difference and age, DU remains a predictive factor for poor treatment response in this study.

It is reasonable that the therapeutic efficacy of urethral BoNT-A might be affected by the severity of baseline pathophysiology of voiding dysfunction. Patients with history of urethral catheterization due to severe emptying failure in idiopathic or neurogenic etiology had been reported to respond poorly to the treatment compared to others [17]. As an index of bladder emptying ability, VE before the treatment might work as an outcome predictor as well. In fact, we found that the baseline VE was positively correlated with the successful outcome in both univariate and multivariate analyses in this study. The best cutoff value for baseline VE were 23% and 4 % for females and males respectively according to the Youden's index in the receiver operating characteristic (ROC) curve. Therefore, patients with DU and poor VE diagnosed in pre-operative urodynamic studies should be adequately informed of the risk of inferior treatment responses.

Aside from the therapeutic effect for voiding function, urethral sphincter BoNT-A injection might also be beneficial for recurrent UTI, a common bothersome nightmare resulting from incomplete urine emptying [18]. Urethral sphincter BoNT-A injection had been reported to achieve a 50% reduction of UTI in spinal cord injury patients with detrusor sphincter dyssynergia [19]. Urethral sphincter BoNT-A injection also decreased UTI in neurologically normal patients with functional voiding dysfunction [20]. The benefit of UTI prevention might explain the finding of higher subjective response rates reported in our patients who had a history of recurrent UTI. As a result, urethral sphincter BoNT-A injection might be considered in those who suffered from refractory voiding dysfunction concomitant with recurrent UTI.

This study provides the treatment response rate of urethral sphincter BoNT-A injection and its predictive factors in patients suffering from functional, non-neurogenic voiding dysfunction with considerable subject numbers as well as complete and detailed urodynamic study before and after the treatment. However, there are still some limitations. First, since the majority of male voiding dysfunction is caused by anatomical obstruction, the number of men in our study is relatively small which makes it difficult to undertake further subgroup analysis. Second, the diagnoses of DU and urethral sphincter dysfunction were based on the image and pressure flow parameters from VUDS which might be somewhat subjective. Nevertheless, it is the most common way to differentiate the cause of voiding dysfunction in clinical practice. Third, the retrospective nature of this study made it difficult to avoid all possible biases during analysis despite our adjusting for the significant variables statistically. A prospective trial with specific inclusion criteria and pre-defined sub-group analysis is required to confirm the results of our study.

4. Conclusions

Urethral sphincter BoNT-A injection is effective in treating refractory functional non-neurogenic voiding dysfunction in both genders. The overall successful rate was 64%. Baseline VE and history of recurrent UTI positively correlate with a successful outcome. DU is a predictive factor for a poor treatment outcome.

5. Materials and Methods

The study was initiated following approval by the Institutional Review Board of the author' hospital (IRB 105-151-B). From January 2010 to November 2019, patients who received urethral sphincter BoNT-A injection due to refractory functional, non-neurogenic voiding dysfunction were retrospectively reviewed. All patients available for baseline and follow-up VUDS data were included. Patients with anatomical urethral conditions including uncorrected BPO and high-grade pelvic organ prolapse, history of lower urinary tract reconstruction, urethral stenosis and urethral tumor were excluded. Patients with uncorrected bladder neck dysfunction, neurogenic abnormality related detrusor sphincter dyssynergia, cauda equina syndrome or peripheral neuropathy were also excluded [21]. The voiding dysfunction among patients with cerebral vascular accident, Parkinson's disease or dementia with subtle neurological clinical manifestation were not considered neurogenic since the lower urinary tract symptoms manifest in these diseases were predominantly detrusor overactivity with or without incontinence [22]. The bladder neck dysfunction was corrected first if the VUDS revealed a narrow bladder neck during the voiding phase in patients with voiding dysfunction. Because the patients still have difficulty in urination after TUI-BN or TUR-P, they were recommended to receive urethral sphincter BoNT-A injection for the urethral sphincter dysfunction.

VUDS performed in accordance with the International Continence Society (ICS) recommendation [23] were utilized for baseline urinary function assessment of every patient with refractory voiding dysfunction before the urethral sphincter BoNT-A injection. The cause of voiding dysfunction was determined by VUDS and electromyography (EMG) as DU or urethral sphincter dysfunction. DU was defined as having a bladder contractility index $\leqq 100$ in men, and maximal detrusor pressure (Pdet) < 10 cm H_2O with maximum flow rate (Qmax) < 10 mL/s and post-void residual (PVR) > 150 mL in women. The external urethral sphincter dysfunction was subclassified into dysfunctional voiding (DV) or poor relaxation of the external sphincter (PRES) according to the features of VUDS and EMG.

DV was diagnosed as the stasis of contrast at the level of urethral sphincter presenting with the typical feature of a "spinning top" urethra during the voiding phase of VUDS with increased external urethral sphincter EMG activity at the same time [24]. PRES was defined as the narrowing of the distal urethra without the presentation of a "spinning top" urethra during the voiding phase of VUDS without the concomitant relaxation of the external urethral sphincter EMG activity [25].

Other parameters of VUDS included first sensation of filling (FSF), full sensation (FS), urge sensation (US), compliance in the storage phase and Pdet, Qmax, BOO index (BOOI), PVR, cystometric bladder capacity (CBC) and VE in the voiding phase. The bladder contractility index was calculated as Pdet + 5× Qmax and BOOI was calculated as Pdet—2 × Qmax [26]. CBC was calculated by voided volume plus PVR in the VUDS. VE was defined as the voided volume divided by the CBC in the VUDS. Major comorbidities including diabetes mellitus, hypertension, chronic kidney disease, chronic obstructive lung disease, coronary artery disease, and neurogenic disease beyond the sacral spinal cord–brainstem pontine micturition center pathways, as well as history of recurrent urinary tract infection, transurethral resection of the prostate (TUR-P) or transurethral incision or resection of the bladder neck (TUI-BN) were collected from medical records.

All patients received 100 units onabotulinumtoxinA (BOTOX, Allergan, Irvine, CA, USA) external urethral sphincter injections in the operation room under light intravenous general anesthesia [27]. The location of the external urethral sphincter was identified by direct visualization under cystoscopy in both men and women. In male patients, urethral sphincter injections were performed transurethrally using a 23-gauge needle (22 Fr, Richard Wolf, Knittlingen, Germany) with 4–8 injections circumferentially distributed in the external urethral sphincter at a depth of 0.5 cm along the longitudinal direction of the urethral lumen. Female patients, on the other hand, received urethral sphincter injections periurethrally using 27-gauge 1 mL syringe needles with 4–8 injections circumferentially into the external urethral sphincter at a depth of 1.5 cm along the longitudinal direction of the urethral lumen. A detailed description of the urethral sphincter injection technique was reported in our previous review [28]. Treatment outcomes of urethral sphincter BoNT-A injections were assessed at around 3 months after the procedure since the average therapeutic duration was reported at around 6 months [9]. Subjective outcomes were measured by global response assessment (GRA) as excellent (+3), markedly improved (+2), mildly improved (+1) or no change (0), according to the patients' perception of the voiding condition after the BoNT-A injections. Patients with an excellent outcome can get rid of the catheter, and patients with marked improvements still need CIC occasionally. A successful outcome was defined as GRA equal to or greater than 2. Objective outcomes were also assessed by VUDS follow-up after the injections.

All analyses were performed through SAS Statistics for Windows, Version 9.4, Cary, NC, USA: SAS Inc. Two-sided p-values less than 0.05 were considered significant. The continuous variables of baseline demographics were expressed as the mean $\pm$ standard deviation whereas the categorical ones were expressed as number (percentage). Differences between gender of the above variables were examined with independent t-test in continuous variables and chi-square test in the categorial ones. We applied Fisher's exact test in circumstances when more than 20% of the expected frequencies were less than five. Changes in post-treatment variables in each gender were examined with the paired samples t-test and McNemar test for continuous and categorical variables, respectively. The distribution of the GRA grades after injections between DU and urethral sphincter dysfunction was examined with the chi-square test. Univariate logistic regression analysis was performed to find out the predictive factors for a successful treatment outcome. Variables demonstrating significant differences in the univariable analysis, including age and gender, were further evaluated in the multivariable model.

Author Contributions: Conceptualization, H.-C.K.; Data curation, Y.-C.O., Y.-L.K. and K.-J.T.; Formal analysis, Y.-L.K.; Investigation, Y.-C.O.; Methodology, Y.-L.K.; Project administration, H.-C.K.; Resources, H.-C.K.; Supervision, H.-C.K. and K.-J.T.; Visualization, Y.-C.O. and Y.-L.K.; Writing—original draft, Y.-L.K.; Writing—review and editing, H.-C.K. All authors have read and agreed to the published version of the manuscript.

Funding: The work was supported by grants from the National Cheng Kung University Hospital NCKUH-11103038 and Buddhist Tzu Chi Medical Foundation TCMF-MP-110-03-01 and TCMF-SP-108-01.

Institutional Review Board Statement: The study was conducted according to the guidelines of the Declaration of Helsinki and approved by the Institutional Review Board of the Buddhist Tzu Chi General Hospital (IRB 105-151-B).

Informed Consent Statement: Patient consent was waived due to the retrospective study design.

Data Availability Statement: Data are available on request to the corresponding author.

Acknowledgments: The work was greatly enhanced by the assistance of Chia-Min Liu.

Conflicts of Interest: The authors declare no conflict of interest.

Appendix A

Table A1. Comparison of baseline characteristics and treatment response between different subtypes of urethral sphincter dysfunction including dysfunctional voiding and poor relaxation of external sphincter.

		Female (n = 77)					Male (n = 26)				
		DV (n = 70)		PRES (n = 7)		p [a]	DV (n = 13)		PRES (n = 13)		p [a]
Age		54.7	±22.7	70.6	±8.2 *		63.1	±12.9	74.4	±12.9*	
VUDS parameters											
FSF (mL)	B	104.6	±62.4	93.9	±39.5		119.5	±52.7	172.8	±111.4	
	P	123.6	±75.2	142.7	±70.4	0.518	123.0	±66.4	178.5	±60.3 *	0.038
FS (mL)	B	171.6	±80.8	156.9	±57.8		208.6	±103.9	289.0	±118.4	
	P	193.2	±99.4	192.7	±90.8	0.990	203.2	±140.1	300.0	±112.7	0.059
US (mL)	B	205.9	±100.2	190.4	±80.8		234.4	±119.2	333.4	±112.5 *	
	P	219.0	±111.0	229.6	±101.2	0.794	203.8	±132.3	359.3	±107.1 *	0.003
Compliance	B	41.6	±56.6	92.5	±96.8		45.5	±60.5	43.5	±22.0	
(mL/cm H_2O)	P	57.3	±67.4	46.8	±23.4	0.675	67.3	±68.6	45.6	±19.8	0.281
DO	B	48	(69)	3	(43)		8	(62)	1	(8) *	
	P	41	(59)	1	(14) *	0.081	11	(85)	2	(15) *	0.016
Pdet	B	56.0	±33.0	41.3	±60.7		34.7	±14.5	13.8	±13.7 *	
(cm H_2O)	P	48.2	±34.3	18.1	±9.6 *	0.001	31.8	±17.5	15.2	±12.9 *	0.003
Qmax (mL/s)	B	6.0	±4.4	10.9	±7.0 *		6.5	±6.1	4.4	±4.4	
	P	6.4	±5.1	12.3	±6.5 *	0.003	9.0	±6.2	4.5	±5.0	0.040
BOOI	B	44.0	±33.3	19.6	±66.4		21.6	±16.0	5.0	±12.7 *	
	P	35.4	±35.3	−6.4	±13.4 *	<0.001	13.8	±15.9	6.2	±13.7	0.208
VV (mL)	B	119.7	±103.0	168.9	±91.8		148.3	±132.0	128.6	±146.6	
	P	122.9	±112.6	298.4	±127.1 *	<0.001	163.2	±136.0	113.9	±166.0	0.345
PVR (mL)	B	188.6	±142.8	175.7	±153.2		207.8	±184.5	266.9	±170.2	
	P	211.1	±156.9	100.0	±155.5	0.070	181.2	±206.7	281.1	±168.9	0.090
BVE (%)	B	41.2	±31.8	54.1	±33.6		46.3	±31.00	33.8	±39.2	
	P	41.4	±34.5	82.4	±26.5 *	0.002	59.2	±39.0	29.1	±34.2	0.022
Global Response Assessment											
Excellent		19	(27)	1	(14)		3	(23)	4	(31)	
Markedly improve		33	(47)	4	(57)		7	(54)	5	(38)	
Mildly improve		5	(7)	0	(0)		1	(8)	0	(0)	
No change		12	(17)	2	(29)		2	(15)	4	(31)	
Missing		1	(1)	0	(0)		0	(0)	0	(0)	
Successful outcome [b]		52	(74)	5	(71)	1.000	10	(77)	9	(69)	1.000

B: before urethra botox injection, BOOI: bladder outlet obstruction index, BVE: bladder voiding efficiency, DO: detrusor overactivity, DV: dysfunctional voiding, FS: full sensation, FSF: first sensation of filling, P: post urethra botulinum toxin injection, PVR: post-void residual volume, PRES: poor relaxation of external sphincter, Qmax: maximal uroflow rate, US: urge sensation, VUDS: videourodynamic study. [a] Between-group differences after urethra botulinum toxin injection adjusting by the pre-treatment condition with Analysis of Covariance (ANCOVA). [b] Successful outcome was defined as global response assessment greater than mildly improve (score ≥ 2). * $p < 0.05$

References

1. Haylen, B.T.; Maher, C.F.; Barber, M.D.; Camargo, S.; Dandolu, V.; Digesu, A.; Goldman, H.B.; Huser, M.; Milani, A.L.; Moran, P.A.; et al. An International Urogynecological Association (IUGA)/International Continence Society (ICS) joint report on the terminology for female pelvic organ prolapse (POP). *Int. Urogynecol. J.* **2016**, *27*, 165–194. [CrossRef] [PubMed]
2. D'Ancona, C.; Haylen, B.; Oelke, M.; Abranches-Monteiro, L.; Arnold, E.; Goldman, H.; Hamid, R.; Homma, Y.; Marcelissen, T.; Rademakers, K.; et al. The International Continence Society (ICS) report on the terminology for adult male lower urinary tract and pelvic floor symptoms and dysfunction. *Neurourol. Urodyn.* **2019**, *38*, 433–477. [CrossRef] [PubMed]
3. Choi, Y.S.; Kim, J.C.; Lee, K.S.; Seo, J.T.; Kim, H.J.; Yoo, T.K.; Lee, J.B.; Choo, M.S.; Lee, J.G.; Lee, J.Y. Analysis of female voiding dysfunction: A prospective, multi-center study. *Int. Urol. Nephrol.* **2013**, *45*, 989–994. [CrossRef] [PubMed]
4. Kuo, H.C. Botulinun A toxin urethral sphincter injection for neurogenic or nonneurogenic voiding dysfunction. *Ci Ji Yi Xue Za Zhi* **2016**, *28*, 89–93. [CrossRef]
5. Winters, J.C.; Dmochowski, R.R.; Goldman, H.B.; Herndon, C.D.; Kobashi, K.C.; Kraus, S.R.; Lemack, G.E.; Nitti, V.W.; Rovner, E.S.; Wein, A.J. Urodynamic studies in adults: AUA/SUFU guideline. *J. Urol.* **2012**, *188*, 2464–2472. [CrossRef]
6. Kuo, H.C. Videourodynamic characteristics and lower urinary tract symptoms of female bladder outlet obstruction. *Urology* **2005**, *66*, 1005–1009. [CrossRef]
7. Jiang, Y.H.; Chen, S.F.; Kuo, H.C. Role of videourodynamic study in precision diagnosis and treatment for lower urinary tract dysfunction. *Ci Ji Yi Xue Za Zhi* **2020**, *32*, 121–130. [CrossRef]
8. Dykstra, D.D.; Sidi, A.A.; Scott, A.B.; Pagel, J.M.; Goldish, G.D. Effects of botulinum A toxin on detrusor-sphincter dyssynergia in spinal cord injury patients. *J. Urol.* **1988**, *139*, 919–922. [CrossRef]
9. Kao, Y.L.; Huang, K.H.; Kuo, H.C.; Ou, Y.C. The Therapeutic Effects and Pathophysiology of Botulinum Toxin A on Voiding Dysfunction Due to Urethral Sphincter Dysfunction. *Toxins* **2019**, *11*, 728. [CrossRef]
10. Jiang, Y.H.; Wang, C.C.; Kuo, H.C. OnabotulinumtoxinA Urethral Sphincter Injection as Treatment for Non-neurogenic Voiding Dysfunction—A Randomized, Double-Blind, Placebo-Controlled Study. *Sci. Rep.* **2016**, *6*, 38905. [CrossRef]
11. Lee, C.L.; Chen, S.F.; Jiang, Y.H.; Kuo, H.C. Effect of videourodynamic subtypes on treatment outcomes of female dysfunctional voiding. *Int. Urogynecol. J.* **2022**, *33*, 1283–1291. [CrossRef]
12. Dykstra, D.D.; Sidi, A.A. Treatment of detrusor-sphincter dyssynergia with botulinum A toxin: A double-blind study. *Arch. Phys. Med. Rehabil.* **1990**, *71*, 24–26.
13. Moore, D.C.; Cohn, J.A.; Dmochowski, R.R. Use of Botulinum Toxin A in the Treatment of Lower Urinary Tract Disorders: A Review of the Literature. *Toxins* **2016**, *8*, 88. [CrossRef] [PubMed]
14. Nadeem, M.; Lindsay, J.; Pakzad, M.; Hamid, R.; Ockrim, J.; Greenwell, T. Botulinum toxin A injection to the external urethral sphincter for voiding dysfunction in females: A tertiary center experience. *Neurourol. Urodyn.* **2022**, *41*, 1793–1799. [CrossRef] [PubMed]
15. Lee, Y.K.; Kuo, H.C. Therapeutic Effects of Botulinum Toxin A, via Urethral Sphincter Injection on Voiding Dysfunction Due to Different Bladder and Urethral Sphincter Dysfunctions. *Toxins* **2019**, *11*, 487. [CrossRef] [PubMed]
16. Liao, Y.M.; Kuo, H.C. Causes of failed urethral botulinum toxin A treatment for emptying failure. *Urology* **2007**, *70*, 763–766. [CrossRef]
17. Ou, Y.C.; Huang, K.H.; Jan, H.C.; Kuo, H.C.; Kao, Y.L.; Tsai, K.J. Therapeutic Efficacy of Urethral Sphincteric Botulinum Toxin Injections for Female Sphincter Dysfunctions and a Search for Predictive Factors. *Toxins* **2021**, *13*, 398. [CrossRef]
18. Jiang, Y.H.; Chen, S.F.; Kuo, H.C. Frontiers in the Clinical Applications of Botulinum Toxin A as Treatment for Neurogenic Lower Urinary Tract Dysfunction. *Int. Neurourol. J.* **2020**, *24*, 301–312. [CrossRef]
19. Mehta, S.; Hill, D.; Foley, N.; Hsieh, J.; Ethans, K.; Potter, P.; Baverstock, R.; Teasell, R.W.; Wolfe, D. A meta-analysis of botulinum toxin sphincteric injections in the treatment of incomplete voiding after spinal cord injury. *Arch. Phys. Med. Rehabil.* **2012**, *93*, 597–603. [CrossRef]
20. Franco, I.; Landau-Dyer, L.; Isom-Batz, G.; Collett, T.; Reda, E.F. The use of botulinum toxin A injection for the management of external sphincter dyssynergia in neurologically normal children. *J. Urol.* **2007**, *178*, 1775–1779; discussion 1779–1780. [CrossRef]
21. Wein, A.; Rovner, E. Adult voiding dysfunction secondary to neurologic disease or injury. *AUA Update Ser.* **1999**, *18*, 42–48.
22. Panicker, J.N. Neurogenic Bladder: Epidemiology, Diagnosis, and Management. *Semin Neurol* **2020**, *40*, 569–579. [CrossRef] [PubMed]
23. Chapple, C. International Continence Society guidelines on urodynamic equipment performance. *Neurourol. Urodyn.* **2014**, *33*, 369. [CrossRef] [PubMed]
24. Austin, P.F.; Bauer, S.B.; Bower, W.; Chase, J.; Franco, I.; Hoebeke, P.; Rittig, S.; Walle, J.V.; von Gontard, A.; Wright, A.; et al. The standardization of terminology of lower urinary tract function in children and adolescents: Update report from the standardization committee of the International Children's Continence Society. *Neurourol. Urodyn.* **2016**, *35*, 471–481. [CrossRef] [PubMed]
25. Hsiao, S.M.; Lin, H.H.; Kuo, H.C. Videourodynamic Studies of Women with Voiding Dysfunction. *Sci. Rep.* **2017**, *7*, 6845. [CrossRef]
26. Abrams, P. Bladder outlet obstruction index, bladder contractility index and bladder voiding efficiency: Three simple indices to define bladder voiding function. *BJU Int.* **1999**, *84*, 14–15. [CrossRef]
27. Deindl, F.M.; Vodusek, D.B.; Bischoff, C.; Hofmann, R.; Hartung, R. Dysfunctional voiding in women: Which muscles are responsible? *Br. J. Urol.* **1998**, *82*, 814–819. [CrossRef]
28. Kuo, Y.C.; Kuo, H.C. Botulinum toxin injection for lower urinary tract dysfunction. *Int. J. Urol.* **2013**, *20*, 40–55. [CrossRef]

toxins MDPI

Article

Urethral Sphincter Botulinum Toxin A Injection for Non-Spinal Cord Injured Patients with Voiding Dysfunction without Anatomical Obstructions: Which Patients Benefit Most?

Sheng-Fu Chen [1,2] and Hann-Chorng Kuo [1,2,*]

1 Department of Urology, Hualien Tzu Chi Hospital, Buddhist Tzu Chi Medical Foundation, Hualien 970, Taiwan
2 Department of Urology, Buddhist Tzu Chi University, Hualien 970, Taiwan
* Correspondence: hck@tzuchi.com.tw

Abstract: Objective: Treating voiding dysfunction without anatomical obstructions is challenging. Urethral onabotulinum toxin A (BoNT-A) is used in treating voiding dysfunction; however, the success rate varies widely, and patients may not be satisfied with the treatment outcome. This study compared the efficacy of the urethral BoNT-A injection between patients with different non-spinal cord injury (SCI) voiding dysfunctions. Materials and Methods: This study retrospectively analyzed patients with refractory voiding dysfunction, including detrusor underactivity (DU), dysfunctional voiding (DV), and poor relaxation of the external sphincter (PRES) who received the urethral sphincter 100 U BoNT-A injection. The treatment outcomes were assessed via a global response assessment (GRA) one month after treatment. Baseline and follow-up videourodynamic study (VUDS) parameters were also compared. Results: Totally, 161 patients (60 with DU, 77 with DV, and 24 with PRES) with a mean age of 58.8 $\pm$ 20.2 were enrolled, of which 62.1% had a good response (GRA $\geq$ 2) after urethral BoNT-A injection. DV patients had a higher success rate (76.6%) than DU (50%) and PRES (45.8%) patients (p = 0.002). A diagnosis of DV, higher voided volume and recurrent urinary tract infection were predictors of a good treatment response, while the cervical cancer status post-radical surgery predicted a poor response. Receiver operating characteristic (ROC) curve analyses identified PVR > 250 mL as a negative predictor (p = 0.008) in DU patients. Conclusions: The urethral BoNT-A injection provides a satisfactory success rate for non-SCI voiding dysfunction. Patients with DV benefit most from both subjective and objective parameters. Approximately 50% of patients with DU and PRES also had a fair response. PVR > 250 mL was a negative predictor in DU patients.

Keywords: voiding dysfunction; detrusor underactivity; dysfunctional voiding; poor relaxation of the external sphincter; onabotulinum toxin A

Key Contribution: The urethral BoNT-A injection provides good therapeutic effects for non-SCI voiding dysfunction, especially for dysfunctional voiding.

Citation: Chen, S.-F.; Kuo, H.-C. Urethral Sphincter Botulinum Toxin A Injection for Non-Spinal Cord Injured Patients with Voiding Dysfunction without Anatomical Obstructions: Which Patients Benefit Most? *Toxins* **2023**, *15*, 87. https://doi.org/10.3390/toxins15020087

Received: 28 November 2022
Revised: 25 December 2022
Accepted: 11 January 2023
Published: 17 January 2023

Copyright: © 2023 by the authors. Licensee MDPI, Basel, Switzerland. This article is an open access article distributed under the terms and conditions of the Creative Commons Attribution (CC BY) license (https://creativecommons.org/licenses/by/4.0/).

1. Introduction

Neurogenic or non-neurogenic voiding dysfunction, with symptoms of difficulty voiding and large post-void residual (PVR) volumes, which may result in upper urinary tract deterioration if not well managed. Voiding dysfunction without neurogenic insult may be due to detrusor underactivity (DU) and bladder outlet obstruction (BOO, such as benign prostate hyperplasia, bladder neck dysfunction, or urethral sphincter hyperactivity, like dysfunctional voiding (DV) [1] or poor relaxation of the external urethral sphincter (PRES) during micturition [2].

DU is a common urological condition whose treatment has remained challenging. In a recent study, detrusor contractility may be reversed by the medical or surgical treatment [3]. Surgical techniques such as transurethral incision of the bladder neck (TUI-BN) or transurethral resection of the prostate (TUR-P) and urethral onabulinumtoxinA (BoNT-A) injection aim to decrease bladder outlet resistance [3]. Urethral injections of BoNT-A were first used for patients with detrusor sphincter dyssynergia or patients with spinal cord injury (SCI), and it effectively decreased the urethral pressure profile and PVR volume [4]. Phelan et al. confirmed the therapeutic efficacy of sphincteric BoNT-A injections in SCI patients with various etiologies of DSD in both men and women. BoNT-A decreases urethral resistance in pharmacology by paralyzing the striated sphincter muscle through the inhibition of acetylcholine release from the neuromuscular junction [5]. In recent years, some studies reported different causes of urethral sphincter dysfunction, be it neurogenic or non-neurogenic, and significant improvements in voiding after sphincteric BoNT-A injections [6].

Although urethral BoNT-A injections have been used in treating non-SCI patients with voiding dysfunction in recent years, the success rate varies widely, and patients could be unsatisfied with the outcome. A previous randomized, double-blind, placebo-controlled trial showed the success rate was not superior to that of normal saline injections [7]. We believe inducing powerful abdominal pressure by straining is necessary for voiding in DU patients; conversely, in patients with DV or PRES, adequate relaxation of the urethral resistance is needed to achieve efficient voiding. Therefore, some patients have benefits in terms of subjective or objective responses. Our previous study reported a 60% success rate in DU and voiding dysfunction after BoNT-A injections [8]. Nowadays, it still is an alternative treatment and not a standard one, and which of them benefits patients with voiding dysfunction most is unclear. We aimed to analyze the efficacy of urethral BoNT-A injections in treating voiding dysfunction in non-SCI patients and compare the therapeutic efficacy between the different etiologies of voiding dysfunction (DU, DV, and PRES).

2. Results

A total of 161 patients with voiding dysfunction refractory to medical therapy with a mean age of 58.8 ± 20.2 years who underwent urethral BoNT-A injection were enrolled. The patients were divided into three subgroups as follows: 60 DU patients (19 males and 41 females), 77 DV patients (10 males and 67 females), and 24 PRES patients (14 males and 10 females). The probable underlying comorbidities and bladder conditions that could be related to voiding dysfunction are listed in Table 1.

Table 1. Baseline characteristics and demographics of non-spinal cord injured patients with voiding dysfunction.

	DU (*n* = 60)	**DV (*n* = 77)**	**PRES (*n* = 24)**	**Total (*n*=161)**	***p*-Value**
Age	60.3 ± 19.4	54.0 ± 22.5	67.0 ± 11.6	58.1 ± 20.6	0.007
Male	*n* = 19	*n* = 10	*n* = 14	*n* = 43	0.000
Female	*n* = 41	*n* = 67	*n* = 10	*n* = 118	
DM	30.0%	19.5%	29.2%	23.1%	0.320
CVA	18.3%	11.7%	8.3%	12.2%	0.379
Parkinsonism	1.7%	3.9%	8.3%	4.1%	0.309
Cervical cancer s/p radical surgery	18.3%	7.8%	4.2%	12.2%	0.013
s/p spine surgery	13.3%	3.9%	8.3%	8.2%	0.123
s/p bladder outlet surgery	78.3%	26.0%	45.8%	44.2%	0.000
Immune disease	10.0%	1.3%	16.7%	7.5%	0.007
Recurrent UTI	33.3%	18.2%	4.2%	23.8%	0.008

DU: detrusor underactivity, DV: dysfunctional voiding, PRES: poor relaxation of the external sphincter, DM: diabetes, CVA: Cerebrovascular accident, UTI: urinary tract infection.

The VUDS characteristics before and after treatment in the three study groups were compared, and the results are listed in Table 2. In female patients with DV, $P_{det}.Q_{max}$ significantly decreased after urethral BoNT-A injection (from 60.1 ± 36.0 to 47.6 ± 32.6, $p = 0.004$), and bladder outlet obstruction indext (BOOI) also significantly decreased in female DV patients (from 48.2 ± 35.8 to 30.0 ± 33.5, $p = 0.000$). The changes in $P_{det}.Q_{max}$ and BOOI in female DV patients were also statistically significant compared with the DU and PRES groups ($p = 0.000$ and $p = 0.002$). Other videourodymamic parameters did not differ significantly after urethral BoNT-A injections.

Table 2. Comparison of videourodynamic parameters before and after the urethral Botox injection in non-spinal cord injured patients with voiding dysfunction.

		DU (n = 60)	DV (n = 77)	PRES (n = 24)	p-Value
FSF (mL)	Baseline	172.8 ± 80.9	105.4 ± 53.2	149.5 ± 59.0	0.068
	Follow-up	165.8 ± 88.9	121.7 ± 64.5	214.3 ± 45.8	
FS (mL)	Baseline	241.5 ± 76.8	173.9 ± 79.7	236.8 ± 89.8	0.163
	Follow-up	245.1 ± 127.4	202.9 ± 100.9	290.3 ± 55.1	
US (mL)	Baseline	303.3 ± 117.1	209.1 ± 100.9	286.0 ± 113.8	0.151
	Follow-up	286.6 ± 133.9	230.5 ± 105.5	336.4 ± 64.2	
CBC (mL)	Baseline	402.9 ± 174.3	317.9 ± 135.8	432.0 ± 115.4	0.726
	Follow-up	399.5 ± 168.5	296.7 ± 153.3	412.4 ± 173.3	
Compliance (mL/cmH_2O)	Baseline	63.9 ± 96.5	40.4 ± 62.5	53.8 ± 25.8	0.186
	Follow-up	47.4 ± 36.7	59.6 ± 71.5	52.3 ± 19.5	
$P_{det}.Q_{max}$ (cmH_2O)	Male (BL)	10.3 ± 11.6	34.00 ± 15.4	32.0 ± 13.1	0.584
	Follow-up	19.3 ± 25.6	31.1 ± 17.6	27.6 ± 14.6	
	Female (BL)	5.69 ± 8.09	60.1 ± 36.0	74.3 ± 90.0	0.000
	Follow-up	4.89 ± 8.76	47.6 ± 32.6 *	13.3 ± 7.37	
Qmax (mL/s)	Baseline	2.70 ± 4.41	6.54 ± 5.06	8.29 ± 5.96	0.987
	Follow-up	3.44 ± 5.31	7.11 ± 5.58	8.71 ± 6.13	
Volume (mL)	Baseline	60.5 ± 115.7	131.1 ± 117.3	219.1 ± 142.5	0.961
	Follow-up	73.1 ± 130.6	139.3 ± 131.4	214.4 ± 163.7	
PVR (mL)	Baseline	344.4 ± 206.8	183.1 ± 143.8	198.3 ± 160.3	0.680
	Follow-up	326.5 ± 197.1	195.3 ± 147.8	231.0 ± 176.8	
VE	Baseline	0.16 ± 0.29	0.41 ± 0.34	0.52 ± 0.38	0.811
	Follow-up	0.18 ± 0.32	0.38 ± 0.36	0.58 ± 0.41	
BOOI	Male (BL)	8.07 ± 9.21	16.0 ± 13.6	13.5 ± 19.2	0.580
	Follow-up	15.0 ± 24.9	10.1 ± 14.8	9.75 ± 21.6	
	Female (BL)	−1.51 ± 12.4	48.2 ± 35.8	53.6 ± 99.4	0.002
	Follow-up	−2.83 ± 14.2	30.0 ± 33.5 *	−12.6 ± 19.0	

FSF: first sensation of filling; FS: full sensation; US: urge sensation; P_{det}: detrusor pressure; Q_{max}: maximum flow rate; Vol: voided volume; PVR: post-void residual; CBC: cystometric bladder capacity; VE: voiding efficiency; BOOI: bladder outlet obstruction index. P, comparison of the changes in variables from baseline and after treatment among each group. * p value < 0.05 comparison between baseline and after treatment.

Treatment outcomes, per the scaled GRA as described in the methodology, are listed in Table 3. The GRA was recorded a month after treatment. Per the postoperative GRA, we divided patients into three groups (0–1, 2, and 3). GRA ≥ 2 was considered a successful outcome. Overall, 100 of 161 (62.1%) non-SCI patients with voiding dysfunction were successfully treated using urethral BoNT-A injections. As shown in Table 3, younger patients responded better to treatment ($p = 0.016$). On the other hand, sex was not significantly associated with treatment outcomes ($p = 0.127$). Finally, among patients with different voiding dysfunctions, we found that DV patients had better treatment outcomes than those with DU and PRES ($p = 0.002$). Approximately 76.6% of DV patients reported GRA ≥ 2, while 50% of DU patients and 45.8% of PRES patients reported GRA ≥ 2. 64 patients were under CIC and baseline and 30 patients voided well without CIC.

Table 3. Treatment outcome per the scaled Global Response Assessment (GRA) after urethral Botulinum toxin A injections.

		GRA = 0–1 (n = 61)	GRA = 2 (n = 69)	GRA = 3 (n = 31)	p-Value
Age (years)		64.3 ± 17.1	54.2 ± 22.5	58.2 ± 18.2	0.016
Gender	Male	21 (48.8%)	13 (30.2%)	9 (20.1%)	0.127
	Female	40 (33.9%)	56 (47.5%)	22 (18.6%)	
Voiding dysfunction	DU	30 (50.0%)	25 (41.7%)	5 (8.3%)	0.002
	DV	18 (23.4%)	38 (49.4%)	21 (27.8%)	
	PRES	13 (54.2%)	6 (25%)	5 (20.8%)	

DU: detrusor underactivity, DV: dysfunctional voiding, PRES: poor relaxation of the external sphincter.

We searched the predictive factors related to the treatment outcome of the baseline characteristics, including the underlying disease, lower urinary tract condition, and VUDS parameters. During multivariate analyses of factors associated with GRA ≥ 2 in the treatment outcome of patients with non-SCI voiding dysfunction, a diagnosis of DV (OR = 3.630, $p = 0.002$), more voided volume (OR = 1.004, $p = 0.014$) at baseline, and a history of recurrent urinary tract infection (UTI) (OR = 3.949, $p = 0.007$) were predictors of good treatment response. On the other hand, cervical cancer was a predictor of a poor treatment outcome (OR = 0.214, $p = 0.008$) (Table 4). Because only approximately 50% of DU patients had satisfactory outcomes, we further analyzed which factors could be better indicators of a good response. We found that a large PVR was a negative predictive factor for DU patients (OR = 0.995, $p = 0.011$). Because PVR is a predictor of a poor outcome in DU patients, a ROC curve analysis was performed. Figure 1 shows that PVR > 250 mL is a negative predictive factor for urethral BoNT-A injection in DU patients (Sensitivity = 0.567, specificity = 0.767, $p = 0.008$).

Table 4. Multivariate analysis of factors associated with a global response assessment ≥2 in non-spinal cord injured voiding dysfunction.

Variables	Odd Ratio (95% CI)	p-Value
DV	3.630 (1.617–8.152)	0.002
Voided volume	1.004 (1.001–1.008)	0.014
Cervical Cancer s/p radical surgery	0.290 (0.092–0.909)	0.034
Recurrent UTI	3.949 (1.453–10.732)	0.007

DV: dysfunctional voiding, s/p: status post operation, UTI: urinary tract infection.

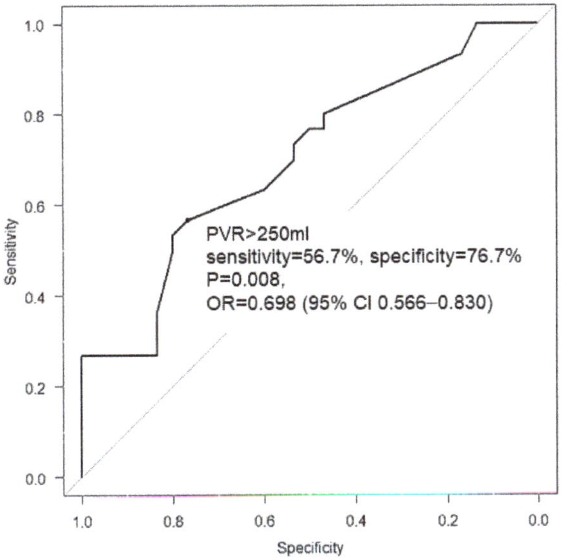

Figure 1. Receiver operating characteristic analysis of the baseline post-void residual (PVR) volume in patients with detrusor underactivity.

3. Discussion

Per our findings, the BoNT-A urethral sphincter injection in non-SCI patients with voiding dysfunction produced a good response in 62.1% of patients after the urethral BoNT-A injection. In different types of voiding dysfunction, patients with DV had better treatment outcomes than those with DU and PRES. In multivariate analyses, DV, more voided volume, and recurrent UTI, were predictors of a good response to treatment, while the cervical cancer status post-radical surgery predicted a poor response. Although VUDS parameters did not differ significantly before and after treatment, they allow physicians to clearly observe the bladder outlet appearance during the voiding phase, which may provide insights into the pathophysiology of the voiding dysfunction [8]. We found that DV is a good predictor of the treatment response; so VUDS is considered to play an important role in making a precise diagnosis before treatment.

BoNT-A is believed to block the presynaptic release of acetylcholine in the neuromuscular junction in striated muscles, which achieves medical sphincterotomy effects. This could reduce the urethral sphincter resistance and improve voiding dysfunction [9]. The application of BoNT-A in urology was first used with urethral sphincter injections for the treatment of detrusor sphincter dyssynergia in patients with SCI and multiple sclerosis [10]. Double-blind placebo-controlled study then confirmed the validity and durability of the therapeutic efficacy of the BoNT-A urethral sphincter injection for patients with SCI and DSD [10]. Therefore, this treatment has been further used in treating non-SCI voiding dysfunction patients nowadays due to urethral sphincter hyperactivity, PRES, and DV or DU [5].

Voiding dysfunction is a frequently encountered clinical problem. In addition to anatomical obstruction-related voiding dysfunctions like benign prostatic hyperplasia and urethral stricture, functional problems like DU, DV, or PRES are more challenging for urologists. The current urodynamic study reported DU would possess in 12.4% of men [11] and 23.1% of women [12] with voiding dysfunction. Urethral sphincter hyperactivity was found in 17.0% of women, and PRES was noted in 39.5% of men and 17.6% of women with voiding dysfunction [11,13].

Treatment of DV is usually challenged because the actual pathophysiology has not been well explained currently and is thought to be a dysregulated urethral function with a spastic or non-relaxing external urethral sphincter during voiding [14]. DV results in difficult voiding and leads to a weak stream of urination and a large PVR. Therefore, attempts to reduce the hypertonicity or hyperactivity of the urethral sphincter via oral medication and resume smooth voiding are often futile. It is also postulated that voiding dysfunction due to psychological origins such as anxiety or depression might cause low detrusor contractility and urethral sphincter non-relaxation by inhibiting detrusor contraction [15]. Liao et al. previously reported an overall success rate of 86.7% for DV patients with sphincteric injections (50–100 units of Botox) [14]. Lee et al. also reported a 62.2% success rate in non-neurogenic DV [16]. In our study, approximately 76.6% of DV patients treated using BoNT-A urethral sphincter injections had a GRA of ≥2. VUDS also showed significantly decreased $P_{det}.Q_{max}$ and BOOI in female patients. On the other hand, our result showed no significant difference in male DV after treatment in VUDS data. It may be due to the case number being small (n = 10), and we also found that male DV baseline detrusor contractility is relatively not strong enough.

The etiology of DU is known to be neurogenic, myogenic, obstructive, or idiopathic. Sustained abdominal pressure is necessary to facilitate emptying the bladder [17]. Urethral BoNT-A sphincter injections help to decrease bladder outlet resistance and achieve successful outcomes. We need to be sure that the bladder neck should open during voiding. Otherwise, BoNT-A injections to the urethral sphincter may not be successful [14]. Therefore, if bladder neck dysfunction was confirmed by VUDS, patients with DU and voiding dysfunction should receive transurethral incision of the bladder neck (TUIBN) rather than urethral BoNT-A injection. In this study, we carefully excluded patients with bladder neck dysfunction and those previously treated for TUIBN (73.9%). In this study, approximately 50% of DU patients had GRA ≥ 2. This means the recovery of detrusor function combined with a hyperactive sphincter also suggested the potential neuromodulatory effect of the sphincteric BoNT-A injection. Sufficient abdominal pressure is necessary for triggering spontaneous voiding after urethral BoNT-A injections in patients with DU. In our previous study, female DU patients exhibited VE improvement after active treatment, and intact bladder sensations and smaller PVR had better treatment outcomes [18]. In this study, we also found that a large PVR is a negative predictor, and the receiver operating characteristic curve showed that PVR > 250 mL at baseline indicates a poor outcome. We supposed that a large PVR indicates a lower abdominal pressure or decreased bladder sensation. Another important factor for efficient urination is acceptable bladder sensation. The sensory afferents from the bladder urothelium and detrusor play important roles in the voiding reflex circuit. Decreased bladder sensation will render the initiation of voiding difficult [19]. Overall, DU patients treated using BoNT-A urethral sphincter injections in our study showed a 50% success rate. We also found that female patients with cervical cancer status post-radical hysterectomy had poor outcomes. We believe radical surgery causes nerve injury and, thus, irreversible DU; so, we could predict that patients with poor sensations and large PVRs were usually not satisfied with the treatment.

PRES, as a diagnosis, was determined based on the voiding phase in the VUDS, which shows non-relaxed surface EMG activity combined with a narrow membranous urethra [2]. The etiology of PRES was considered multifactorial, such as potential neuropathy, learned habituation, pelvic floor hypertonicity, and bladder hypersensitivity [20]. PRES is characterized by relatively small but stable bladders and low-pressure/low-flow during the voiding phase [21], which is different from the typical high-pressure/low-flow presentation in DV. Urethral BoNT-A injections may provide benefits by inhibiting acetylcholine release in the neuromuscular junction to reduce urethral resistance. Because the typical PRES is low-pressure during the voiding phase, we supposed that there was also inadequate detrusor contractility. Therefore, the success rate of urethral BoNT-A injections is not as high as that of DV. On the other hand, a previous study showed that detrusor contractility might be restored after BoNT-A injections in DU patients with PRES [22]. This result supports the hypothesis that the low-pressure/low-flow dysfunction present in PRES might be the result of the detrusor suppression induced by non-relaxed urethral sphincter activity [7].

The primary limitation of this study is its retrospective design, different group sizes, and single-center scope of evaluation. Second, the 1–6-month follow-up VUDS was not consistent, which may have influenced the results of objective parameters. However, we believe the efficacy of BoNT-A durability continued for at least 6 months [23]. Moreover, patients without follow-up VUDS were not enrolled in this study, which might have caused selection bias. In this study, no obvious side was reported. However, we supposed mild side effects might exist in some patients, such as urinary incontinence. Finally, the patient groups were heterogeneous, with varying causes of voiding dysfunction. The identification of the underlying causes of failure may improve the success rate of the urethral sphincter BoNT-A injection.

4. Conclusions

The urethral sphincter BoNT-A injection is effective in treating voiding dysfunction in non-SCI patients. The results of this study showed that patients with DV may benefit the most in terms of subjective and objective parameters, whereas those with DU and PRES also have a fair response in approximately half of the patients. PVR > 250 mL may indicate a poor treatment outcome in patients with DU.

5. Materials and Methods

This study retrospectively analyzed patients with voiding dysfunction who were refractory to medical treatment. They received 100 U of BoNT-A injection (onabotulinumtoxinA, Allergan, Irvine, CA, USA) via urethral sphincter by cystourethroscope. All patients underwent videourodynamic study (VUDS) assessments to identify the underlying etiology of the lower urinary tract dysfunction before administering BoNT-A injections. Patients with anatomical BOO of various etiologies, such as urethral stricture, bladder neck obstruction, or benign prostatic hyperplasia, were excluded from the study. SCI patients with DSD were also excluded. Finally, patients with DU who required abdominal straining for spontaneous voiding and those who required urethral sphincter non-relaxation while voiding were included in the final analysis. The study was conducted in accordance with the Declaration of Helsinki, and the protocol was approved by the Ethics Committee of Hualien Tzu Chi Hospital, Buddhist Tzu Chi Medical Foundation (IRB 111-247-B), and waived informed consent due to its retrospective nature.

The urethral BoNT-A injection treatment was performed under light intravenous general anesthesia. A total of 100 U BoNT-A was given via transurethral sphincter injections per our previous report [24]. One vial of 100 U botulinum toxin A was reconstituted with normal saline to 5 mL. Every one mL of BoNT-A solution was injected into the urethral sphincter at the 2, 4, 6, 8, and 10 o'clock positions transurethrally in men. Transcutaneous injections were administered to the urethral sphincter along the urethral lumen at the 2, 4, 6, 8, and 10 o'clock positions of the sides of the urethral meatus in women. A Foley catheter was placed overnight after BoNT-A injections and removed the next morning. Self-voiding status was recorded at the outpatient clinic. In our previous experiences, the effect of BoNT-A on the urethral sphincter's function appeared approximately three days after injection and the maximum therapeutic effect was attained 2 weeks after treatment [24]. Three days of antibiotics were given to prevent UTIs. After BoNT-A injections, we discontinued other medication for reducing urethral resistance.

Baseline VUDS parameters, including the cystometric bladder capacity (CBC), voided volume (VV), PVR, Q_{max}, first sensation of bladder filling (FSF), first desire (FS), urge sensation (US), bladder compliance, and detrusor pressure at the maximal flow rate ($P_{det}.Q_{max}$), were recorded. VE was calculated as follows: voided volume/total bladder capacity $\times$ 100 [25]. The maximum filling volume was defined if patients consistently had no urge to void at 600mL. Bladder compliance was measured at CBC. The terminology used in this study was based on the recommendations of the International Continence

Society [1]. All patients were regularly followed up at a single center, and repeated VUDS was performed within 6 months. For analysis of the treatment outcome, the urethral sphincter dysfunctions were categorized as DV and PRES, according to the electromyographic reports and pictures during voiding cystourethrography on VUDS. DV was diagnosed when high detrusor pressure, intermittent or increased external sphincter EMG activity, and a "spinning top" urethral appearance on cinefluoroscopy during voiding occurred together. On the other hand, PRES was diagnosed based on low voiding $P_{det}.Q_{max}$, with non-relaxation of urethral sphincter EMG and narrow urethral during urination.

The primary outcome of this study is the VE after treatment which was assessed after the urethral BoNT-A injection to report their global response assessment (GRA) by reviewing the patient's chart over 1 month and graded from 0 to 3. Patients who needed indwelling urethral catheters or suprapubic cystostomy (IDC) and clean intermittent catheterization (CIC) and those with a VE of less than 33% were classified as those with treatment failure (grade 0). When patients who were able to urinate (either abdominal straining or spontaneously) with a VE of 33.3–66.7% were considered to have mild improvement (grade 1). Those who could urinate with a VE of 66.7–90% were considered to have experienced moderate improvement (grade 2). If patients could urinate with VE of 90–100% were considered to have experienced marked improvement (grade 3). Patients who could achieve grade 2 or 3 improvements after treatment were considered to have satisfactory outcomes. For recording the VE, patients were asked to urinate at a strong/urgent desire to the uroflowmetry. If voided volume plus PVR was less than 250 mL, patients were requested to urinate again. The secondary endpoint is the VUDS parameters before and 6 months after treatment. Adverse effects after BoNT-A injections were also recorded.

Statistical Analysis

Categorical variables were presented as frequencies (proportions), while continuous variables were expressed as the mean ± standard deviation. Urodynamic parameters at baseline and after treatment were compared using the paired *t*-test, which was also used to determine differences in symptom scores and objective parameters between groups. On the other hand, the analysis of variance was used to determine differences between subgroups. The Chi-square test was used to analyze categorical variables.

To identify the predictive factors of a good treatment outcome, we used a forward selection method to perform multivariate analyses. Receiver operating characteristic (ROC) curve analyses were performed to identify the optimum cutoff value for predicting better outcomes for DU patients. Accordingly, the optimal cutoff value was indicated by the point on the ROC curve that was closest to the upper left-hand corner. All statistical analyses were performed using SPSS for Windows (Version 16.0; SPSS, Chicago, IL, USA). A *p*-value of <0.05 was considered statistically significant.

Author Contributions: Conceptualization, H.-C.K.; Methodology, S.-F.C.; Writing—original draft, S.-F.C.; Writing—review and editing, H.-C.K. All authors have read and agreed to the published version of the manuscript.

Funding: This research was funded by the Buddhist Tzu Chi Medical Foundation grants TCMF-SP-108-01 and TCMF-MP-110-03-01.

Institutional Review Board Statement: The study was conducted in accordance with the Declaration of Helsinki, and approved by the Hualien Tzu Chi Hospital, Buddhist Tzu Chi Medical Foundation (protocol code IRB 111-247-B and date of approval: 13 December 2022).

Informed Consent Statement: Patient consent was waived due to retrospective chart review study.

Conflicts of Interest: The authors have no conflict of interest relevant to this article.

References

1. Abrams, P.; Cardozo, L.; Fall, M.; Griffiths, D.; Rosier, P.; Ulmsten, U.; Van Kerrebroeck, P.; Victor, A.; Wein, A.; Standardisation Sub-Committee of the International Continence Society. The standardisation of terminology of lower urinary tract function: Report from the Standardisation Sub-committee of the International Continence Society. *Neurourol. Urodyn.* **2002**, *21*, 167–178. [CrossRef] [PubMed]
2. Kuo, H.-C. Pathophysiology of Lower Urinary Tract Symptoms in Aged Men without Bladder Outlet Obstruction. *Urol. Int.* **2000**, *64*, 86–92. [CrossRef] [PubMed]
3. Chen, S.; Peng, C.; Kuo, H. Will detrusor acontractility recover after medical or surgical treatment? A longitudinal long-term urodynamic follow-up. *Neurourol. Urodyn.* **2021**, *40*, 228–236. [CrossRef] [PubMed]
4. Dykstra, D.D.; Sidi, A.A.; Scott, A.B.; Pagel, J.M.; Goldish, G.D. Effects of Botulinum a Toxin on Detrusor-Sphincter Dyssynergia in Spinal Cord Injury Patients. *J. Urol.* **1988**, *139*, 919–922. [CrossRef] [PubMed]
5. Phelan, M.W.; Franks, M.; Somogyi, G.T.; Yokoyama, T.; Fraser, M.O.; Lavelle, J.P.; Yoshimura, N.; Chancellor, M.B. Botulinum toxin urethral sphincter injection to restore bladder emptying in men and women with voiding dysfunction. *J. Urol.* **2001**, *165*, 1107–1110. [CrossRef] [PubMed]
6. Dong, M.; Yeh, F.; Tepp, W.H.; Dean, C.; Johnson, E.A.; Janz, R.; Chapman, E.R. SV2 Is the Protein Receptor for Botulinum Neurotoxin A. *Science* **2006**, *312*, 592–596. [CrossRef]
7. Kao, Y.-L.; Huang, K.-H.; Kuo, H.-C.; Ou, Y.-C. The Therapeutic Effects and Pathophysiology of Botulinum Toxin A on Voiding Dysfunction Due to Urethral Sphincter Dysfunction. *Toxins* **2019**, *11*, 728. [CrossRef]
8. Jiang, Y.-H.; Jhang, J.-F.; Chen, S.-F.; Kuo, H.-C. Videourodynamic factors predictive of successful onabotulinumtoxinA urethral sphincter injection for neurogenic or non-neurogenic detrusor underactivity. *LUTS Low. Urin. Tract Symptoms* **2019**, *11*, 66–71. [CrossRef] [PubMed]
9. Jhang, J.-F.; Kuo, H.-C. Botulinum Toxin A and Lower Urinary Tract Dysfunction: Pathophysiology and Mechanisms of Action. *Toxins* **2016**, *8*, 120. [CrossRef]
10. Dykstra, D.D.; Sidi, A.A. Treatment of detrusor-sphincter dyssynergia with botulinum A toxin: A double-blind study. *Arch. Phys. Med. Rehabil.* **1990**, *71*, 24–26.
11. Jiang, Y.H.; Kuo, H.C. Video-urodynamic characteristics of non-neurogenic, idiopathic underactive bladder in men—A comparison of men with normal tracing and bladder outlet obstruction. *PLoS ONE* **2017**, *12*, e0174593. [CrossRef] [PubMed]
12. Yang, T.-H.; Chuang, F.-C.; Kuo, H.-C. Urodynamic characteristics of detrusor underactivity in women with voiding dysfunction. *PLoS ONE* **2018**, *13*, e0198764. [CrossRef] [PubMed]
13. Hsiao, S.-M.; Lin, H.-H.; Kuo, H.-C. Videourodynamic Studies of Women with Voiding Dysfunction. *Sci. Rep.* **2017**, *7*, 6845. [CrossRef] [PubMed]
14. Liao, Y.-M.; Kuo, H.-C. Causes of Failed Urethral Botulinum Toxin A Treatment for Emptying Failure. *Urology* **2007**, *70*, 763–766. [CrossRef]
15. Chen, Y.-C.; Kuo, H.-C. Clinical and video urodynamic characteristics of adult women with dysfunctional voiding. *J. Formos. Med. Assoc. = Taiwan Yi Zhi* **2014**, *113*, 161–165. [CrossRef] [PubMed]
16. Lee, Y.-K.; Kuo, H.-C. Therapeutic Effects of Botulinum Toxin A, via Urethral Sphincter Injection on Voiding Dysfunction Due to Different Bladder and Urethral Sphincter Dysfunctions. *Toxins* **2019**, *11*, 487. [CrossRef]
17. Hoeritzauer, I.; Phé, V.; Panicker, J. Urologic symptoms and functional neurologic disorders. *Handb. Clin. Neurol.* **2016**, *139*, 469–481. [CrossRef]
18. Chen, S.-F.; Jhang, J.-F.; Jiang, Y.-H.; Kuo, H.-C. Treatment outcomes of detrusor underactivity in women based on clinical and videourodynamic characteristics. *Int. Urol. Nephrol.* **2022**, *54*, 1215–1223. [CrossRef] [PubMed]
19. Jiang, Y.-H.; Kuo, H.-C. Urothelial Barrier Deficits, Suburothelial Inflammation and Altered Sensory Protein Expression in Detrusor Underactivity. *J. Urol.* **2017**, *197*, 197–203. [CrossRef]
20. Shao, I.-H.; Kuo, H.-C. Role of poor urethral sphincter relaxation in men with voiding dysfunction refractory to α-blocker therapy: Clinical characteristics and predictive factors. *LUTS Low. Urin. Tract Symptoms* **2019**, *11*, 8–13. [CrossRef]
21. Kuo, H.-C. Videourodynamic Analysis of Pathophysiology of Men with Both Storage and Voiding Lower Urinary Tract Symptoms. *Urology* **2007**, *70*, 272–276. [CrossRef] [PubMed]
22. Kuo, H.-C. Recovery of Detrusor Function After Urethral Botulinum A Toxin Injection in Patients with Idiopathic Low Detrusor Contractility and Voiding Dysfunction. *Urology* **2007**, *69*, 57–61. [CrossRef] [PubMed]
23. Apostolidis, A.; Fowler, C.J. The use of botulinum neurotoxin type A (BoNTA) in urology. *J. Neural Transm.* **2008**, *115*, 593–605. [CrossRef] [PubMed]
24. Kuo, H.-C. Botulinum A Toxin Urethral Injection for the Treatment of Lower Urinary Tract Dysfunction. *J. Urol.* **2003**, *170*, 1908–1912. [CrossRef] [PubMed]
25. Abrams, P. Bladder outlet obstruction index, bladder contractility index and bladder voiding efficiency: Three simple indices to define bladder voiding function. *BJU Int.* **1999**, *84*, 14–15. [CrossRef] [PubMed]

Disclaimer/Publisher's Note: The statements, opinions and data contained in all publications are solely those of the individual author(s) and contributor(s) and not of MDPI and/or the editor(s). MDPI and/or the editor(s) disclaim responsibility for any injury to people or property resulting from any ideas, methods, instructions or products referred to in the content.

toxins

MDPI

Article

Intravesical Injection of Botulinum Toxin Type A in Patients with Refractory Overactive Bladder—Results between Young and Elderly Populations, and Factors Associated with Unfavorable Outcomes

Yin-Chien Ou [1], Yao-Lin Kao [1], Yi-Hui Ho [2], Kuan-Yu Wu [1] and Hann-Chorng Kuo [3,*]

1 Department of Urology, National Cheng Kung University Hospital, College of Medicine, National Cheng Kung University, Tainan 704, Taiwan
2 Department of Anesthesiology, National Cheng Kung University Hospital, College of Medicine, National Cheng Kung University, Tainan 704, Taiwan
3 Department of Urology, Hualien Tzu Chi Hospital, Buddhist Tzu Chi Medical Foundation and Tzu Chi University, Hualien 970, Taiwan
* Correspondence: hck@tzuchi.com.tw

Abstract: Intravesical botulinum toxin type A (BoNT-A) injection has been recognized as the standard treatment for refractory overactive bladder (OAB). However, its therapeutic efficacy and safety have not been thoroughly reviewed in elderly patients. This study aims to provide treatment outcomes for patients aged ≥75 years, and to identify factors associated with unfavorable outcomes. Patients receiving intradetrusor injections of 100 U onabotulinumtoxinA for refractory OAB between 2011 and 2021 were retrospectively reviewed. Urodynamic parameters, underlying comorbidities, subjective success, and unfavorable outcomes were assessed. A total of 192 patients were included, and 65 of them were classified into the elderly group. For the elderly group, 60.0% experienced subjective dryness, and 84.6% remained subjective success at 6 months after the injections. The prevalence rates of common unfavorable outcomes, including urinary tract infections, large post-void residual urine volume, and urinary retention, were 9.2%, 27.7%, and 12.3%, respectively. Multivariate analysis revealed that female, baseline urodynamic parameters, and diabetes mellitus were associated with unfavorable outcomes in the elderly group. Intravesical BoNT-A injections provide comparable therapeutic efficacy and safety concerns in elderly patients with refractory OAB. A thorough consultation for treatment benefits and possible adverse events is mandatory before the procedure.

Keywords: botulinum toxins; type A; urinary bladder; overactive; aged; postoperative complications

Key Contribution: This study highlights the treatment outcomes of intravesical botulinum toxin type A injections for refractory overactive bladder syndrome in an extremely old population (≥75 years). Factors associated with unfavorable outcomes will provide more prudent and precise patient selection in this fragile population.

Citation: Ou, Y.-C.; Kao, Y.-L.; Ho, Y.-H.; Wu, K.-Y.; Kuo, H.-C. Intravesical Injection of Botulinum Toxin Type A in Patients with Refractory Overactive Bladder—Results between Young and Elderly Populations, and Factors Associated with Unfavorable Outcomes. *Toxins* **2023**, *15*, 95. https://doi.org/10.3390/toxins15020095

Received: 14 December 2022
Revised: 16 January 2023
Accepted: 16 January 2023
Published: 19 January 2023

Copyright: © 2023 by the authors. Licensee MDPI, Basel, Switzerland. This article is an open access article distributed under the terms and conditions of the Creative Commons Attribution (CC BY) license (https://creativecommons.org/licenses/by/4.0/).

1. Introduction

Overactive bladder (OAB) is a syndrome defined by the International Continence Society and is characterized by urinary urgency, with or without urgency urinary incontinence, and usually accompanied by frequency and nocturia [1,2]. Large population-based surveys revealed that the prevalence of OAB increases with age, and is slightly higher for elderly males over females [3,4]. Many studies have described the negative influence of OAB on health-related quality of life, including anxiety, depression, sleep disorder, social withdrawal, and sexual life impairment [5–10]. Likewise, urinary incontinence is known to negatively affect the quality of life in the elderly population [11] and is also responsible for low self-esteem and depression [12]. To treat the bothersome storage symptoms of

OAB, antimuscarinic agents have been developed to inhibit spontaneous detrusor smooth muscle contractions and reduce afferent signals during bladder filling [13]. The therapeutic effect of antimuscarinic agents has been proven; however, insufficient symptom relief and concomitant adverse events cause poor medication persistence and adherence [14]. Solifenacin and fesoterodine have been shown to have limited impact on cognitive function and few central nervous system adverse events for patients ≥65 years after short-term exposure [15–17]. Even though, uncertainty regarding cognitive decline after long-term cumulative anticholinergic exposure still limits their use in the elderly population [18,19]. On the other hand, β3-adrenoceptor agonists facilitate relaxation of the detrusor muscle during bladder filling. Both mirabegron and vibegron have been confirmed to be effective and well-tolerated in the elderly population [20–25]. However, most participants in the clinical trials were relatively healthy and did not have uncontrolled cardiovascular diseases. The long-term application of these pharmacological agents in the elderly population remains questionable.

The efficacy of intravesical injection of botulinum toxin type A (BoNT-A) has been established for patients with OAB who have an insufficient response to first-line pharmacological agents [26,27]. However, most of these published data did not focus on the elderly population, and only a handful of studies included a population with a mean age of ≥65 years old [28–35]. In addition, 75 years of age has been proposed as a new cutoff value to redefine the elderly because of the global extension of life expectancy [36]. Exploring the therapeutic outcomes and adverse events associated with BoNT-A injections in this vulnerable population is urgently necessary [37]. The commonly reported adverse events after BoNT-A injection include large post-void residual urine volume (PVR), urinary retention, and urinary tract infection (UTI) [38]. However, factors that can help identify patients at risk of these unfavorable outcomes are still limited, especially in the elderly population. Therefore, the primary aim of our study is to retrospectively evaluate the therapeutic efficacy of intravesical BoNT-A injection for refractory OAB, and the secondary aim is to investigate the factors associated with unfavorable outcomes in an elderly population aged ≥75 years.

2. Results

In total, 192 patients received intravesical BoNT-A injections for refractory OAB symptoms during the study period. During the administration of injections, 65 (33.9%) patients were classified into the elderly group (≥75 years old), and the remaining 127 (66.1%) patients were classified into the young group. For the young and elderly groups, the mean age was 58.8 ± 11.9 and 82.0 ± 4.6 years old, respectively. A higher percentage of males was found in the elderly group compared to the young group (75.5% and 34.6%, respectively). More comorbidities were found in the elderly group, including hypertension, diabetes mellitus (DM), dementia, coronary artery disease, and chronic kidney disease. The multichannel urodynamic parameters for baseline bladder function prior to BoNT-A injection are listed in Table 1. For the filling phase parameters, the elderly bladders are more sensitive to filling, and have a smaller cystometric bladder capacity (CBC) compared to those of the young. For the voiding phase parameters, a higher detrusor pressure at the maximal flow rate (PdetQmax), a slower maximum flow rate (Qmax), and a smaller voided volume (VV) were found for the elderly group compared to the young group.

Primary outcomes after intravesical BoNT-A injections are shown in Table 2. At 6 months after the injection, 77.2% and 84.6% of patients in the young and elderly group remained subjective success, respectively. The subjective success rate was comparable in both groups at 3, 6, and 12 months after the injections. Additionally, more than 60% of patients in both groups experienced a certain period of subjective dryness without any urge incontinence. Compared to the baseline uroflowmetry parameters, the CBC and PVR were significantly increased, and the voiding efficiency was significantly decreased in both groups three months postoperatively. In addition, the postoperative CBC and VV were smaller, and Qmax was slower (265.8 ± 126.0 vs. 332.5 ± 158.1 mL, $p = 0.010$; 156.9 ± 106.1

vs. 220.4 ± 139.6 mL, p = 0.007; and 11.0 ± 7.3 vs. 15.5 ± 10.7 mL/s, p = 0.007, respectively) in the elderly group than in the young group. The prevalence of unfavorable outcomes such as a large PVR, urinary retention, and UTI did not vary between groups. For the young and elderly group, 29 (22.8%) and 18 (27.7%) patients were found to have large PVR, and 11 (8.7%) and 8 (12.3%) patients eventually experienced urinary retention and required catheterization to empty the bladder, respectively. Indwelling Foley catheters were used for all the 11 patients in the elderly group and 4 patients in the young group. Clean intermittent catheterization was used by the other 4 patients in the young group. The catheterization period persisted within one week for 7 patients, between one week to one month for 5 patients, and up to two months for 7 patients. Additionally, 18 (14.2%) and 6 (9.2%) patients in the young and elderly group experienced UTI, respectively.

Table 1. Patient demographics and baseline multichannel urodynamic parameters.

	Young Group (<75) Years Mean ± SD or No. (%)	**Elderly Group (≥75 Years) Mean ± SD or No. (%)**	***p*-Value**
Number of patients	127	65	
Age (years)	58.8 ± 11.9	82.0 ± 4.6	
Gender (male)	44 (34.6)	51 (75.5)	<0.001
Baseline multichannel urodynamic parameters			
FSF (mL)	110.4 ± 64.4	96.3 ± 66.4	0.051
FS (mL)	171.5 ± 102.1	135.6 ± 87.3	0.010
US (mL)	201.7 ± 117.1	152.4 ± 100.8	0.003
CBC (mL)	272.6 ± 161.1	184.7 ± 109.7	<0.001
Compliance (mL/cmH_2O)	66.4 ± 76.8	57.2 ± 65.3	0.437
PdetQmax (cmH_2O)	23.7 ± 16.6	31.5 ± 20.6	0.003
Qmax (mL/s)	12.7 ± 7.8	7.8 ± 4.5	<0.001
VV (mL)	230.3 ± 142.4	155.7 ± 103.4	<0.001
PVR (mL)	42.2 ± 100.8	29.3 ± 50.6	0.109
Comorbidities			
Hypertension	66 (52.0)	46 (70.8)	0.012
DM	24 (18.9)	25 (38.5)	0.003
CVA	16 (12.6)	13 (20.0)	0.175
Dementia	5 (3.9)	10 (15.4)	0.005
CAD	5 (3.9)	13 (20.0)	<0.001
CHF	3 (2.4)	2 (3.1)	1.000
CKD	2 (1.6)	5 (7.7)	0.045

CAD: coronary artery disease; CBC: cystometric bladder capacity; CHF: congestive heart failure; CKD: chronic kidney disease; CVA: cerebrovascular accident; DM: diabetes mellitus; FS: full sensation; FSF: first sensation of filling; No.: number; PdetQmax: detrusor pressure at the maximal flow rate; PVR: post-void residual urine volume; Qmax: maximum flow rate; SD: standard deviation; US: urge sensation; VV: voided volume.

Table 2. Primary outcomes and unfavorable outcomes after intravesical BoNT-A injection.

	Young Group (<75 Years) (*n* = 127) Mean ± SD or No. (%)	**Elderly Group (≥75 Years) (*n* = 65) Mean ± SD or No. (%)**	***p*-Value**
Subjective success (No.)			
At 3 months	124 (97.6%)	63 (96.9%)	1.000
At 6 months	98 (77.2%)	55 (84.6%)	0.225
At 12 months	31 (24.4%)	31 (32.3%)	0.244
Subjective dryness (No.)	85 (66.9%)	39 (60.0%)	0.342

Table 2. *Cont.*

	Young Group (<75 Years) (n = 127) Mean ± SD or No. (%)	Elderly Group (≥75 Years) (n = 65) Mean ± SD or No. (%)	p-Value
Uroflowmetry			
Qmax (mL/s)			
Baseline	17.0 ± 13.3	11.3 ± 7.4	0.001
3 months	15.5 ± 10.7	11.0 ± 7.3	0.004
VV (mL)			
Baseline	211.8 ± 149.6	138.6 ± 84.7	0.002
3 months	220.4 ± 139.6	156.9 ± 106.1	0.007
PVR (mL)			
Baseline	48.7 ± 85.0	38.5 ± 48.7	0.876
3 months	144.4 ± 114.9 *	149.3 ± 117.3 *	0.757
CBC (mL)			
Baseline	260.6 ± 164.8	177.1 ± 99.1	0.001
3 months	332.5 ± 158.1 *	265.8 ± 126.0 *	0.010
VE (%)			
Baseline	81.8 ± 21.6	79.8 ± 21.0	0.292
3 months	65.2 ± 71.8 *	57.4 ± 27.3 *	0.106
Unfavorable outcomes			
Large PVR (> 200 mL) (No.)	29 (22.8%)	18 (27.7%)	0.459
Urinary retention (No.)	11 (8.7%)	8 (12.3%)	0.423
UTI (No.)	18 (14.2%)	6 (9.2%)	0.327

CBC: cystometric bladder capacity; No.: number; PVR: post-void residual urine volume; Qmax: maximum flow rate; SD: standard deviation; UTI: urinary tract infection; VE: voiding efficiency; VV: voided volume. * Wilcoxon signed-rank test $p < 0.001$ at 3 months compared to baseline.

Table 3 shows the baseline clinical characteristics and multichannel urodynamic parameters of elderly patients with or without postoperative unfavorable outcomes: 6 (9.2%), 18 (27.7%), and 8 (12.3%) patients in the elderly group had postoperative UTI, large PVR, and urinary retention, respectively. For baseline multichannel urodynamic parameters, patients with postoperative UTI tended to have lower bladder compliance (19.7 ± 12.5 vs. 61.0 ± 67.3 mL/cmH_2O, p = 0.014) and a higher PdetQmax (56.2 ± 33.2 vs. 29.0 ± 17.4 cmH_2O, p = 0.013) compared to those without UTI, whereas patients with post-operative large PVR or with urinary retention tended to have higher PdetQmax (40.1 ± 23.4 vs. 28.3 ± 18.6 cmH_2O, p = 0.029; 55.5 ± 27.1 vs. 28.2 ± 17.3 cmH_2O, p = 0.001, respectively) compared to those with normal PVR or without urinary retention. Regarding underlying comorbidities, patients with postoperative UTI had a higher prevalence of dementia, while patients suffering postoperative urinary retention had a greater prevalence of DM and cerebrovascular accidents.

For the elderly population, multivariate analysis revealed that female, lower baseline bladder compliance, and higher PdetQmax were significantly associated with postoperative UTI. In addition, a higher baseline PdetQmax and a history of DM were associated with urinary retention. However, the association between higher baseline PdetQmax and postoperative large PVR failed to achieve significance (OR: 1.027, p = 0.075) after adjusting for age and gender (Table 4).

Forty-three (33.9%) patients in the young group and 14 (21.5%) patients in the elderly group received subsequent injection cycles after the initial BoNT-A effect vanished, whereas the other 135 (70.4%) patients received only one episode of BoNT-A injection. The injection cycles between young and old patient groups are shown in Table 5.

Table 3. Baseline clinical characteristics and multichannel urodynamic parameters in elderly population with or without each unfavorable outcome.

Unfavorable Outcomes	UTI			Large PVR			Urinary Retention		
	No	Yes	*p*-Value	≤200 mL	>200 mL	*p*-Value	No	Yes	*p* Value
Number of patients	59	6		47	18		57	8	
Age (years)	81.9 ± 4.6	82.8 ± 5.5	0.650	81.4 ± 4.5	83.4 ± 4.8	0.106	81.7 ± 4.6	84.1 ± 4.5	0.176
Gender (male)	48 (81.4)	3 (50.0)	0.108	36 (76.6)	15 (83.3)	0.740	44 (77.2)	7 (87.5)	0.675
Baseline multichannel urodynamic parameters									
FSF (mL)	98.1 ± 68.9	78.8 ± 29.5	0.903	94.6 ± 66.6	100.8 ± 67.6	0.747	95.7 ± 67.8	100.4 ± 59.6	0.660
FS (mL)	137.1 ± 89.7	120.8 ± 62.1	0.903	133.7 ± 86.2	140.3 ± 92.6	0.889	135.1 ± 86.5	138.6 ± 98.9	0.944
US (mL)	154.5 ± 103.9	131.8 ± 66.8	0.834	150.0 ± 97.4	158.7 ± 112.1	1.000	152.4 ± 100.5	152.8 ± 110.2	0.992
CBC (mL)	189.8 ± 111.1	135.0 ± 88.2	0.223	179.7 ± 96.7	197.7 ± 140.6	0.953	188.3 ± 109.7	159.3 ± 113.5	0.442
Compliance (mL/cmH_2O)	61.0 ± 67.3	19.7 ± 12.5	0.014	53.9 ± 63.1	65.7 ± 71.8	0.639	59.0 ± 68.2	43.9 ± 39.5	0.472
PdetQmax (cmH_2O)	29.0 ± 17.4	56.2 ± 33.2	0.013	28.3 ± 18.6	40.1 ± 23.4	0.029	28.2 ± 17.3	55.5 ± 27.1	0.001
Qmax (mL/s)	7.9 ± 4.4	6.5 ± 5.7	0.485	7.8 ± 4.5	7.6 ± 4.6	0.860	7.9 ± 4.5	6.6 ± 4.5	0.496
VV (mL)	162.5 ± 102.4	85.0 ± 92.7	0.048	154.7 ± 93.6	157.2 ± 128.5	0.671	159.6 ± 99.8	125.5 ± 130.0	0.235
PVR (mL)	27.2 ± 47.9	50.0 ± 75.4	0.214	25.0 ± 47.0	40.6 ± 59.1	0.332	28.7 ± 48.2	33.8 ± 69.5	0.550
Comorbidities									
Hypertension	42 (71.2%)	4 (66.7%)	1.000	33 (70.2)	13 (72.2)	0.873	39 (68.4)	7 (87.5)	0.420
DM	24 (40.7%)	1 (16.7%)	0.393	15 (31.9)	10 (55.6)	0.080	19 (33.3)	6 (75.0)	0.047
CVA	11 (18.6%)	2 (33.3%)	0.591	7 (14.9)	6 (33.3)	0.162	9 (15.8)	4 (50.0)	0.044
Dementia	7 (11.9%)	3 (50.0%)	0.042	7 (14.9)	3 (16.7)	1.000	7 (12.3)	3 (37.5)	0.098
CAD	11 (18.6%)	2 (33.3%)	0.591	9 (19.1)	4 (22.2)	0.743	12 (21.1)	1 (12.5)	1.000
CHF	2 (3.4%)	0 (0.0%)	1.000	2 (4.3)	0 (0.0)	1.000	2 (3.5)	0 (0.0)	1.000
CKD	4 (6.8%)	1 (16.7%)	0.394	4 (8.5)	1 (5.6)	1.000	4 (7.0)	1 (12.5)	0.493

CAD: coronary artery disease; CBC: cystometric bladder capacity; CHF: congestive heart failure; CKD: chronic kidney disease; CVA: cerebrovascular accident; DM: diabetes mellitus; FS: full sensation; FSF: first sensation of filling; No.: number; PdetQmax: detrusor pressure at the maximal flow rate; PVR: post-void residual urine volume; Qmax: maximum flow rate; SD: standard deviation; US: urge sensation; UTI: urinary tract infection; VV: voided volume. Data expressed by mean ± standard deviation or number (%).

Table 4. Univariate and multivariate logistic regression to identify factors associated with each unfavorable outcome in elderly population.

	Postoperative UTI ($n = 6$)			Large PVR > 200 mL ($n = 18$)			Urinary Retention ($n = 8$)		
	OR (95% CI)	**Adjusted OR (95% CI)**	***p*-Value ****	**OR (95% CI)**	**Adjusted OR (95% CI)**	***p*-Value ****	**OR (95% CI)**	**Adjusted OR (95% CI)**	***p*-Value ****
Age	1.044 (0.873–1.249)	1.344 (0.892–2.026)	0.157	1.101 (0.975–1.242)	1.099 (0.960–1.257)	0.170	1.120 (0.953–1.315)	1.245 (0.942–1.646)	0.124
Gender (male)	0.229 (0.041–1.292)	0.000 (0.000–0.400)	0.029	1.528 (0.372–6.268)	0.803 (0.167–3.866)	0.785	2.068 (0.233–18.382)	0.309 (0.018–5.255)	0.416
Compliance	0.951 (0.904–1.000)	0.903 (0.820–0.995)	0.040	1.003 (0.995–1.010)			0.994 (0.976–1.013)		
PdetQmax	1.048 (1.009–1.089) *	1.214 (1.007–1.464)	0.042	1.028 (0.999–1.057)	1.027 (0.997–1.058)	0.075	1.058 (1.013–1.104) *	1.077 (1.012–1.145)	0.019
DM	0.292 (0.032–2.656)			2.667 (0.876–8.122)			6.000 (1.104–32.595) *	29.042 (1.114–756.870)	0.043
CVA	2.182 (0.354–13.458)			2.857 (0.805–10.143)			5.333 (1.123–25.331) *	4.683 (0.587–37.359)	0.145
Dementia	7.429 (1.247–44.239) *	0.026 (0.000–3.144)	0.136	1.143 (0.261–5.005)			4.286 (0.835–21.991)		

CI: Confidence interval; CVA: cerebrovascular accident; DM: diabetes mellitus; OR: odds ratio; PdetQmax: detrusor pressure at the maximal flow rate; PVR: post-void residual urine; UTI: urinary tract infection. * Univariate logistic regression $p < 0.05$. ** Multivariate Binary logistic regression.

Table 5. The subsequent BoNT-A injection cycles during the follow-up period after the first time BoNT-A injection for young and elderly patients with refractory overactive bladder.

Subsequent Injection Cycle(s)	0	1	2	3	4	5	6	7
Young patients (n)	84	22	10	4	2	2	2	1
Elderly patients (n)	51	10	3	1	0	0	0	0

3. Discussion

The role of BoNT-A in treating refractory OAB is well established in both sexes [26,27]. However, studies focusing on efficacy and adverse events in the elderly population are limited [38]. In addition, with the extension of life expectancy, "75 years of age and over" is increasingly being used to define the elderly population [36]. Hence, our study defined the elderly population as patients aged 75 years or older. We aimed to determine the therapeutic outcome of intravesical BoNT-A in this population and identify valuable factors associated with adverse events. Our results revealed that although elderly bladders were more sensitive at baseline compared to young bladders, BoNT-A intravesical injection was equally effective for OAB symptom control. In addition, the prevalence of adverse events was equal in both age groups. Female sex, lower bladder compliance, and higher PdetQmax were associated with postoperative UTI, while DM and higher PdetQmax were associated with postoperative urinary retention in the elderly population.

Several possible pathophysiologies have been proposed to explain refractory OAB [39], including urothelial dysfunction with aging [40], undetected bladder outlet obstruction (BOO), chronic bladder ischemia or inflammation [41,42], and central sensitization [43,44]. These conditions are commonly found in the elderly population owing to aging-induced changes from the brain to the bladder itself [45–47]. In our study, more than 75% of patients in the elderly group were men, a proportion much higher than that in the young group. This may further emphasize the importance of chronic undetected BOO in bladder remodeling [48]. It is well-documented that the presence of BOO will result in large PVR and could be a risk of urinary retention after the intravesical BoNT-A injection, especially in the elderly [29,30]. Therefore, in our clinical practice, we will investigate patients with refractory OAB by video-urodynamic study to find if there is BOO, and the BoNT-A injection can only be performed in patients without BOO, or if their BOO has been well-treated. In addition, our findings of the preoperative multichannel urodynamic study in these elderly bladders, including increased bladder sensation and reduction in bladder capacity, were consistent with the known changes in the aging bladder [46]. Intravesical BoNT-A injection provides sensory blockade in addition to chemo-denervation of the bladder detrusor muscle [49,50]. This may explain why patients who are refractory to conventional OAB medications can be successfully treated with BoNT-A.

To the best of our knowledge, no case-control study has compared the therapeutic efficacy of BoNT-A between patients aged ≥75 years and those aged <75 years. White et al. [34] reported a case series of 21 refractory OAB patients aged 75 years and older and concluded that BoNT-A injection is efficacious, durable, and has a low incidence of adverse events in the short term. Frailty has been proposed as a negative factor for long-term treatment success, but this study used "age greater than 65 years" as the definition of elderly [29]. Our study demonstrated that the elderly population (≥75 years old) had similar subjective success rates at 3, 6, and 12 months postoperatively compared with the young population. Furthermore, with no between-group differences, >60% of patients in both groups eventually experienced a certain period of subjective dryness without urge incontinence. This highlights that age itself is not a direct factor that affects the bladder response to BoNT-A. Instead, the underlying pathophysiologies that develop during the aging process to induce refractory OAB are key factors in determining therapeutic outcomes.

Considering the direct chemo-denervation effect on the bladder detrusor muscle, PVR elevation and urinary retention are common concerns after intravesical BoNT-A injections [51]. A large PVR is commonly defined as a PVR greater than 150 or 200 mL, and approximately 6–61% of patients with a mean age > 65 years have been reported to experience a large PVR after receiving injections [28–30,35]. Miotla et al. reported that female patients with PVR > 200 mL or retention after injections were older than those with PVR < 200 mL [52]. Liao and Kuo proposed that instead of age, frailty was associated with post-injection PVR > 150 mL [29]. In our elderly population (≥75 years old), 18 (27.7%) patients were found to have a large PVR > 200 ml after BoNT-A intravesical injection, and eight (12.3%) patients eventually experienced urinary retention and needed temporary Foley catheter indwelling. There was no difference in the prevalence of a large PVR and urinary retention between the elderly and young populations. Although no valuable factor could be found to be associated with large postoperative PVR in our elderly population, a higher baseline PdetQmax and a history of DM were identified as factors associated with postoperative urinary retention. DM is a well-known factor that induces overactive bladder and affects detrusor contractility during the voiding phase [53]. Wang et al. reported that intravesical BoNT-A successfully managed detrusor overactivity and achieved a similar treatment success rate in both DM and non-DM patients but with a higher risk of large PVR and general weakness in DM patients [54]. In elderly patients with DM, detailed consultation and close follow-up for postoperative PVR are necessary.

UTI is another common but frustrating unfavorable outcome after intravesical BoNT-A injections [55]. A recent systemic review revealed that the prevalence rate of UTI after intravesical BoNT-A injection for treating OAB is approximately 29.8% [56]. Both storage and emptying dysfunction have been proposed to impact UTI recurrence [57,58]. In our study, we found that female sex, lower bladder compliance, and a higher PdetQmax were associated with postoperative UTI in the elderly population. Lower bladder compliance and higher PdetQmax are common bladder dysfunctions that increase intravesical pressure during both the storage and emptying phases. Increased intravesical pressure is known to cause bladder ischemia, which may predispose the bladder to infection because of a delayed or insufficient immune response [59,60].

Although the present study successfully demonstrated the therapeutic outcomes and adverse events of intravesical BoNT-A injections in a population older than most of the published data, some limitations still exist. First, its retrospective design made it possible to involve biases during patient selection, data collection, and statistical analysis. Moreover, we could not further define 'frailty' by retrospectively reviewing the medical records. Instead, we believe that using 75 years as the cutoff value would be indeed a reasonable choice. Second, the small sample size in the elderly group limited the statistical power in multivariate logistic regression analyses, and also hindered the subgroup analysis for different sexes. Third, no postoperative multichannel urodynamic data were available to provide detailed bladder storage function after BoNT-A injection. Considering the invasiveness of the test, a simple uroflowmetry with PVR is commonly used to represent postoperative bladder function. Finally, in the long-term follow-up, we found only 29.7% of refractory OAB patients received subsequent BoNT-A injection in our hospital. This result indicates that the patients might not be satisfied with the unfavorable treatment outcome after the first BoNT-A injection and would choose medical therapy for their bothersome OAB symptoms. However, understanding the treatment effect of BoNT-A on the sensory blockade in the elderly population remains limited. Prospective case-control studies are necessary to evaluate treatment outcomes and outcome predictors in this population in detail.

4. Conclusions

Intravesical BoNT-A injections provided equally effective and durable therapeutic outcomes in both young and elderly patients (≥75 years old) with refractory OAB. The prevalence rates of common unfavorable outcomes were equal between the two age groups. For elderly patients receiving intravesical BoNT-A injection, female, lower bladder compliance, and higher PdetQmax were associated with postoperative UTI, whereas a history of DM and higher PdetQmax were associated with urinary retention postoperatively. A thorough consultation for possible benefits and adverse events is mandatory, especially in elderly patients with certain risk factors.

5. Materials and Methods

We retrospectively reviewed patients with idiopathic OAB symptoms refractory to conventional medications who received intravesical injections of BoNT-A for the first time at a tertiary medical center in eastern Taiwan. All patients had persistent urgency urinary incontinence even with antimuscarinics, β3-adrenoceptor agonists, or a combination of both for more than three months. A multichannel urodynamic study, including cystometry and a pressure flow study, was performed preoperatively in accordance with the International Continence Society's good urodynamic practice recommendations [61] to confirm the presence of detrusor overactivity. All patients have been proven to be non-BOO by the video-urodynamic study before receiving the intravesical BoNT-A injections. Patients with underlying neurological factors that may cause neurogenic detrusor overactivity, or intrinsic sphincter deficiency were excluded from this study. Patients who were ≥75 years old while receiving the injections were classified into the elderly group, whereas the others belonged to the young group.

Baseline lower urinary tract function was assessed for each patient using uroflowmetry, PVR, and a multichannel urodynamic study before BoNT-A injection. Parameters including the VV, Qmax, CBC, and voiding efficiency were collected from the uroflowmetry. CBC was defined as the sum of VV and PVR, and voiding efficiency was defined as VV divided by CBC. For the multichannel urodynamic study, bladder sensations, compliance, and the presence of detrusor overactivity were recorded as the filling phase parameters, whereas PdetQmax, Qmax, VV, CBC, and PVR were recorded as the voiding phase parameters. BOO was defined as BOO index >40 for men [62], and as PdetQmax > 35 cmH_2O for women [63]. Bladder sensations were further classified as the first sensation of filling, full sensation, and urge sensation, according to the patients' reports.

All patients were hospitalized and received intravesical injections of 100 units of Botox® (Allergan, Irvine, CA, USA), which is the standard dosage used to treat refractory OAB [26], under general anesthesia in the operating room. The injection method has been described previously [26]. Briefly, 10 mL normal saline was used to dilute each Botox vial. The injection needle was inserted into the posterior and lateral bladder walls under the guidance of rigid cystoscopy, and a total of 20 evenly distributed intradetrusor injections (0.5 mL for each injection) were performed while sparing the trigone area. A 14 Fr. urethral Foley catheter was placed and remained in place for one day after the Botox injection. Objective outcomes were assessed three months after the injections using uroflowmetry and PVR. Subjective treatment success and improvement of urge incontinence were reviewed according to the medical records at the out-patient department during serial follow-ups. As improvement of urinary incontinence and difficult urination might coexist after intravesical BoNT-A injection, patients might consider that they had unsuccessful treatment if they had severe difficulty in urination even though urinary incontinence had improved. Therefore, a subjective success was defined by having a Global Response Assessment (scoring from −3 to +3, indicating markedly worse to markedly improved after the treatment [64]) of +2 or +3. Underlying comorbidities and postoperative unfavorable outcomes, including a large PVR (defined as PVR >200 mL during the follow-up period), urinary retention, and UTI, were also collected from the patients' medical records. All patients were followed up regularly at the out-patient clinic with or without OAB medication, and repeat BoNT-A injections were performed if patients had recurrence of OAB symptoms and requested for injection, otherwise they were continuously treated with oral medications.

Statistical analyses were performed using SPSS Statistics for Windows, Version 17.0. Chicago: SPSS Inc. Continuous and categorical variables are expressed as mean ± standard deviation and as numbers and percentages, respectively. Statistical comparisons between groups were performed using the Mann–Whitney U test for continuous variables and the chi-square test for categorical variables. Fisher's exact test was applied when > 20% of the expected frequencies were less than five. Comparisons between baseline and follow-up within-group differences were performed using the Wilcoxon signed-rank test. Age, gender, and variables demonstrating significant differences between patients with or without each unfavorable outcome were further analyzed with multivariate logistic regression analyses to identify factors associated with postoperative unfavorable outcomes in the elderly group. All statistical assessments were considered significant when the two-sided p-value was <0.05.

Author Contributions: Conceptualization, H.-C.K.; Data Curation, Y.-C.O. and H.-C.K.; Formal Analysis, Y.-C.O., Y.-L.K. and H.-C.K.; Investigation, Y.-C.O. and Y.-L.K.; Methodology, Y.-C.O., Y.-L.K., Y.-H.H. and K.-Y.W.; Project Administration, H.-C.K.; Resources, H.-C.K.; Supervision, H.-C.K.; Visualization, Y.-C.O., Y.-L.K., Y.-H.H. and K.-Y.W.; Writing—Original Draft, Y.-C.O.; Writing—Review and Editing, Y.-C.O., Y.-L.K. and H.-C.K. All authors have read and agreed to the published version of the manuscript.

Funding: The work was supported by grants from the National Cheng Kung University Hospital NCKUH-11206016 and Buddhist Tzu Chi Medical Foundation TCMF-SP-108-01 and TCMF-MP-110-03-01.

Institutional Review Board Statement: The study was conducted according to the guidelines of the Declaration of Helsinki and approved by the Institutional Review Board of the Buddhist Tzu Chi General Hospital (IRB 104-23-A).

Informed Consent Statement: Patient informed consent was waived due to the retrospective study design.

Data Availability Statement: Data are available on request to the corresponding author.

Conflicts of Interest: The authors declare no conflict of interest.

References

1. Haylen, B.T.; de Ridder, D.; Freeman, R.M.; Swift, S.E.; Berghmans, B.; Lee, J.; Monga, A.; Petri, E.; Rizk, D.E.; Sand, P.K.; et al. An International Urogynecological Association (IUGA)/International Continence Society (ICS) joint report on the terminology for female pelvic floor dysfunction. *Int. Urogynecol. J.* **2010**, *21*, 5–26. [CrossRef] [PubMed]
2. Abrams, P.; Cardozo, L.; Fall, M.; Griffiths, D.; Rosier, P.; Ulmsten, U.; van Kerrebroeck, P.; Victor, A.; Wein, A. The standardisation of terminology of lower urinary tract function: Report from the Standardisation Sub-committee of the International Continence Society. *Neurourol. Urodyn.* **2002**, *21*, 167–178. [CrossRef] [PubMed]
3. Irwin, D.E.; Milsom, I.; Hunskaar, S.; Reilly, K.; Kopp, Z.; Herschorn, S.; Coyne, K.; Kelleher, C.; Hampel, C.; Artibani, W.; et al. Population-based survey of urinary incontinence, overactive bladder, and other lower urinary tract symptoms in five countries: Results of the EPIC study. *Eur. Urol.* **2006**, *50*, 1306–1314; discussion 1305–1314. [CrossRef] [PubMed]
4. Milsom, I.; Abrams, P.; Cardozo, L.; Roberts, R.G.; Thüroff, J.; Wein, A.J. How widespread are the symptoms of an overactive bladder and how are they managed? A population-based prevalence study. *BJU Int.* **2001**, *87*, 760–766. [CrossRef] [PubMed]
5. Teloken, C.; Caraver, F.; Weber, F.A.; Teloken, P.E.; Moraes, J.F.; Sogari, P.R.; Graziottin, T.M. Overactive bladder: Prevalence and implications in Brazil. *Eur. Urol.* **2006**, *49*, 1087–1092. [CrossRef] [PubMed]
6. Gomes, C.M.; Averbeck, M.A.; Koyama, M.; Soler, R. Impact of OAB symptoms on work, quality of life and treatment-seeking behavior in Brazil. *Curr. Med. Res. Opin.* **2020**, *36*, 1403–1415. [CrossRef]
7. Patrick, D.L.; Khalaf, K.M.; Dmochowski, R.; Kowalski, J.W.; Globe, D.R. Psychometric performance of the incontinence quality-of-life questionnaire among patients with overactive bladder and urinary incontinence. *Clin. Ther.* **2013**, *35*, 836–845. [CrossRef] [PubMed]
8. Bartoli, S.; Aguzzi, G.; Tarricone, R. Impact on quality of life of urinary incontinence and overactive bladder: A systematic literature review. *Urology* **2010**, *75*, 491–500. [CrossRef] [PubMed]
9. Amarenco, G.; Arnould, B.; Carita, P.; Haab, F.; Labat, J.J.; Richard, F. European psychometric validation of the CONTILIFE: A Quality of Life questionnaire for urinary incontinence. *Eur. Urol.* **2003**, *43*, 391–404. [CrossRef]
10. Kosilov, K.; Loparev, S.; Kuzina, I.; Kosilova, L.; Prokofyeva, A. Socioeconomic status and health-related quality of life among adults and older with overactive bladder. *Int. J. Qual. Health Care J. Int. Soc. Qual. Health Care* **2019**, *31*, 289–297. [CrossRef]
11. El-Gharib, A.K.; Manzour, A.F.; El-Mallah, R.; El Said, S.M.S. Impact of urinary incontinence on physical performance and quality of life (QOL) amongst a group of elderly in Cairo. *Int. J. Clin. Pract.* **2021**, *75*, e14947. [CrossRef] [PubMed]
12. Dugan, E.; Cohen, S.J.; Bland, D.R.; Preisser, J.S.; Davis, C.C.; Suggs, P.K.; McGann, P. The association of depressive symptoms and urinary incontinence among older adults. *J. Am. Geriatr. Soc.* **2000**, *48*, 413–416. [CrossRef] [PubMed]
13. Abrams, P.; Andersson, K.E. Muscarinic receptor antagonists for overactive bladder. *BJU Int.* **2007**, *100*, 987–1006. [CrossRef] [PubMed]

14. Chapple, C.R.; Nazir, J.; Hakimi, Z.; Bowditch, S.; Fatoye, F.; Guelfucci, F.; Khemiri, A.; Siddiqui, E.; Wagg, A. Persistence and Adherence with Mirabegron versus Antimuscarinic Agents in Patients with Overactive Bladder: A Retrospective Observational Study in UK Clinical Practice. *Eur. Urol.* **2017**, *72*, 389–399. [CrossRef]
15. Hampel, C.; Betz, D.; Burger, M.; Nowak, C.; Vogel, M. Solifenacin in the Elderly: Results of an Observational Study Measuring Efficacy, Tolerability and Cognitive Effects. *Urol. Int.* **2017**, *98*, 350–357. [CrossRef] [PubMed]
16. Wagg, A.; Arumi, D.; Herschorn, S.; Angulo Cuesta, J.; Haab, F.; Ntanios, F.; Carlsson, M.; Oelke, M. A pooled analysis of the efficacy of fesoterodine for the treatment of overactive bladder, and the relationship between safety, co-morbidity and polypharmacy in patients aged 65 years or older. *Age Ageing* **2017**, *46*, 620–626. [CrossRef]
17. Wagg, A.; Khullar, V.; Michel, M.C.; Oelke, M.; Darekar, A.; Bitoun, C.E. Long-term safety, tolerability and efficacy of flexible-dose fesoterodine in elderly patients with overactive bladder: Open-label extension of the SOFIA trial. *Neurourol. Urodyn.* **2014**, *33*, 106–114. [CrossRef]
18. Cai, X.; Campbell, N.; Khan, B.; Callahan, C.; Boustani, M. Long-term anticholinergic use and the aging brain. *Alzheimers Dement. J. Alzheimers Assoc.* **2013**, *9*, 377–385. [CrossRef]
19. Gray, S.L.; Anderson, M.L.; Dublin, S.; Hanlon, J.T.; Hubbard, R.; Walker, R.; Yu, O.; Crane, P.K.; Larson, E.B. Cumulative use of strong anticholinergics and incident dementia: A prospective cohort study. *JAMA Intern. Med.* **2015**, *175*, 401–407. [CrossRef]
20. Nitti, V.W.; Rosenberg, S.; Mitcheson, D.H.; He, W.; Fakhoury, A.; Martin, N.E. Urodynamics and safety of the β_3-adrenoceptor agonist mirabegron in males with lower urinary tract symptoms and bladder outlet obstruction. *J. Urol.* **2013**, *190*, 1320–1327. [CrossRef]
21. Herschorn, S.; Staskin, D.; Schermer, C.R.; Kristy, R.M.; Wagg, A. Safety and Tolerability Results from the PILLAR Study: A Phase IV, Double-Blind, Randomized, Placebo-Controlled Study of Mirabegron in Patients $\geq$ 65 years with Overactive Bladder-Wet. *Drugs Aging* **2020**, *37*, 665–676. [CrossRef] [PubMed]
22. Wagg, A.; Staskin, D.; Engel, E.; Herschorn, S.; Kristy, R.M.; Schermer, C.R. Efficacy, safety, and tolerability of mirabegron in patients aged $\geq$65yr with overactive bladder wet: A phase IV, double-blind, randomised, placebo-controlled study (PILLAR). *Eur. Urol.* **2020**, *77*, 211–220. [CrossRef] [PubMed]
23. Staskin, D.; Frankel, J.; Varano, S.; Shortino, D.; Jankowich, R.; Mudd, P.N., Jr. International Phase III, Randomized, Double-Blind, Placebo and Active Controlled Study to Evaluate the Safety and Efficacy of Vibegron in Patients with Symptoms of Overactive Bladder: EMPOWUR. *J. Urol.* **2020**, *204*, 316–324. [CrossRef] [PubMed]
24. Staskin, D.; Frankel, J.; Varano, S.; Shortino, D.; Jankowich, R.; Mudd, P.N., Jr. Once-Daily Vibegron 75 mg for Overactive Bladder: Long-Term Safety and Efficacy from a Double-Blind Extension Study of the International Phase 3 Trial (EMPOWUR). *J. Urol.* **2021**, *205*, 1421–1429. [CrossRef]
25. Varano, S.; Staskin, D.; Frankel, J.; Shortino, D.; Jankowich, R.; Mudd, P.N., Jr. Efficacy and Safety of Once-Daily Vibegron for Treatment of Overactive Bladder in Patients Aged $\geq$65 and $\geq$75 Years: Subpopulation Analysis from the EMPOWUR Randomized, International, Phase III Study. *Drugs Aging* **2021**, *38*, 137–146. [CrossRef]
26. Nitti, V.W.; Dmochowski, R.; Herschorn, S.; Sand, P.; Thompson, C.; Nardo, C.; Yan, X.; Haag-Molkenteller, C. OnabotulinumtoxinA for the treatment of patients with overactive bladder and urinary incontinence: Results of a phase 3, randomized, placebo controlled trial. *J. Urol.* **2013**, *189*, 2186–2193. [CrossRef]
27. Chapple, C.; Sievert, K.D.; MacDiarmid, S.; Khullar, V.; Radziszewski, P.; Nardo, C.; Thompson, C.; Zhou, J.; Haag-Molkenteller, C. OnabotulinumtoxinA 100 U significantly improves all idiopathic overactive bladder symptoms and quality of life in patients with overactive bladder and urinary incontinence: A randomised, double-blind, placebo-controlled trial. *Eur. Urol.* **2013**, *64*, 249–256. [CrossRef] [PubMed]
28. Liao, C.H.; Chen, S.F.; Kuo, H.C. Different number of intravesical onabotulinumtoxinA injections for patients with refractory detrusor overactivity do not affect treatment outcome: A prospective randomized comparative study. *Neurourol. Urodyn.* **2016**, *35*, 717–723. [CrossRef] [PubMed]
29. Liao, C.H.; Kuo, H.C. Increased risk of large post-void residual urine and decreased long-term success rate after intravesical onabotulinumtoxinA injection for refractory idiopathic detrusor overactivity. *J. Urol.* **2013**, *189*, 1804–1810. [CrossRef]
30. Kuo, H.C.; Liao, C.H.; Chung, S.D. Adverse events of intravesical botulinum toxin a injections for idiopathic detrusor overactivity: Risk factors and influence on treatment outcome. *Eur. Urol.* **2010**, *58*, 919–926. [CrossRef]
31. Mateu Arrom, L.; Mayordomo Ferrer, O.; Sabiote Rubio, L.; Gutierrez Ruiz, C.; Martínez Barea, V.; Palou Redorta, J.; Errando Smet, C. Treatment Response and Complications after Intradetrusor OnabotulinumtoxinA Injection in Male Patients with Idiopathic Overactive Bladder Syndrome. *J. Urol.* **2020**, *203*, 392–397. [CrossRef] [PubMed]
32. Habashy, D.; Losco, G.; Tse, V.; Collins, R.; Chan, L. Botulinum toxin (OnabotulinumtoxinA) in the male non-neurogenic overactive bladder: Clinical and quality of life outcomes. *BJU Int.* **2015**, *116* (Suppl. S3), 61–65. [CrossRef] [PubMed]
33. Kim, S.H.; Habashy, D.; Pathan, S.; Tse, V.; Collins, R.; Chan, L. Eight-Year Experience With Botulinum Toxin Type-A Injections for the Treatment of Nonneurogenic Overactive Bladder: Are Repeated Injections Worthwhile? *Int. Neurourol. J.* **2016**, *20*, 40–46. [CrossRef]
34. White, W.M.; Pickens, R.B.; Doggweiler, R.; Klein, F.A. Short-term efficacy of botulinum toxin a for refractory overactive bladder in the elderly population. *J. Urol.* **2008**, *180*, 2522–2526. [CrossRef] [PubMed]

35. Yokoyama, O.; Honda, M.; Yamanishi, T.; Sekiguchi, Y.; Fujii, K.; Nakayama, T.; Mogi, T. OnabotulinumtoxinA (botulinum toxin type A) for the treatment of Japanese patients with overactive bladder and urinary incontinence: Results of single-dose treatment from a phase III, randomized, double-blind, placebo-controlled trial (interim analysis). *Int. J. Urol. Off. J. Jpn. Urol. Assoc.* **2020**, *27*, 227–234. [CrossRef] [PubMed]
36. Ouchi, Y.; Rakugi, H.; Arai, H.; Akishita, M.; Ito, H.; Toba, K.; Kai, I. Redefining the elderly as aged 75 years and older: Proposal from the Joint Committee of Japan Gerontological Society and the Japan Geriatrics Society. *Geriatr. Gerontol. Int.* **2017**, *17*, 1045–1047. [CrossRef]
37. Manns, K.; Khan, A.; Carlson, K.V.; Wagg, A.; Baverstock, R.J.; Trafford Crump, R. The use of onabotulinumtoxinA to treat idiopathic overactive bladder in elderly patients is in need of study. *Neurourol. Urodyn.* **2022**, *41*, 42–47. [CrossRef]
38. Kao, Y.L.; Ou, Y.C.; Kuo, H.C. Bladder Dysfunction in Older Adults: The Botulinum Toxin Option. *Drugs Aging* **2022**, *39*, 401–416. [CrossRef]
39. Chen, L.C.; Kuo, H.C. Pathophysiology of refractory overactive bladder. *Low. Urin. Tract Symptoms* **2019**, *11*, 177–181. [CrossRef]
40. Mansfield, K.J.; Liu, L.; Mitchelson, F.J.; Moore, K.H.; Millard, R.J.; Burcher, E. Muscarinic receptor subtypes in human bladder detrusor and mucosa, studied by radioligand binding and quantitative competitive RT-PCR: Changes in ageing. *Br. J. Pharmacol.* **2005**, *144*, 1089–1099. [CrossRef]
41. Azadzoi, K.M.; Shinde, V.M.; Tarcan, T.; Kozlowski, R.; Siroky, M.B. Increased leukotriene and prostaglandin release, and overactivity in the chronically ischemic bladder. *J. Urol.* **2003**, *169*, 1885–1891. [CrossRef] [PubMed]
42. Lowe, E.M.; Anand, P.; Terenghi, G.; Williams-Chestnut, R.E.; Sinicropi, D.V.; Osborne, J.L. Increased nerve growth factor levels in the urinary bladder of women with idiopathic sensory urgency and interstitial cystitis. *Br. J. Urol.* **1997**, *79*, 572–577. [CrossRef] [PubMed]
43. Avelino, A.; Cruz, C.; Nagy, I.; Cruz, F. Vanilloid receptor 1 expression in the rat urinary tract. *Neuroscience* **2002**, *109*, 787–798. [CrossRef] [PubMed]
44. Baron, R.; Hans, G.; Dickenson, A.H. Peripheral input and its importance for central sensitization. *Ann. Neurol.* **2013**, *74*, 630–636. [CrossRef] [PubMed]
45. Birder, L.A.; Kullmann, A.F.; Chapple, C.R. The aging bladder insights from animal models. *Asian J. Urol.* **2018**, *5*, 135–140. [CrossRef]
46. Suskind, A.M. The Aging Overactive Bladder: A Review of Aging-Related Changes from the Brain to the Bladder. *Curr. Bladder Dysfunct. Rep.* **2017**, *12*, 42–47. [CrossRef]
47. de Rijk, M.M.; Wolf-Johnston, A.; Kullmann, A.F.; Taiclet, S.; Kanai, A.J.; Shiva, S.; Birder, L.A. Aging-Associated Changes in Oxidative Stress Negatively Impacts the Urinary Bladder Urothelium. *Int. Neurourol. J.* **2022**, *26*, 111–118. [CrossRef]
48. Fusco, F.; Creta, M.; De Nunzio, C.; Iacovelli, V.; Mangiapia, F.; Li Marzi, V.; Finazzi Agrò, E. Progressive bladder remodeling due to bladder outlet obstruction: A systematic review of morphological and molecular evidences in humans. *BMC Urol.* **2018**, *18*, 15. [CrossRef]
49. Lin, Y.H.; Chiang, B.J.; Liao, C.H. Mechanism of Action of Botulinum Toxin A in Treatment of Functional Urological Disorders. *Toxins* **2020**, *12*, 129. [CrossRef]
50. Chen, J.L.; Kuo, H.C. Clinical application of intravesical botulinum toxin type A for overactive bladder and interstitial cystitis. *Investig. Clin. Urol.* **2020**, *61*, S33–S42. [CrossRef]
51. Anger, J.T.; Weinberg, A.; Suttorp, M.J.; Litwin, M.S.; Shekelle, P.G. Outcomes of intravesical botulinum toxin for idiopathic overactive bladder symptoms: A systematic review of the literature. *J. Urol.* **2010**, *183*, 2258–2264. [CrossRef] [PubMed]
52. Miotla, P.; Cartwright, R.; Skorupska, K.; Bogusiewicz, M.; Markut-Miotla, E.; Futyma, K.; Rechberger, T. Urinary retention in female OAB after intravesical Botox injection: Who is really at risk? *Int. Urogynecol. J.* **2017**, *28*, 845–850. [CrossRef] [PubMed]
53. Wang, C.C.; Jiang, Y.H.; Kuo, H.C. The Pharmacological Mechanism of Diabetes Mellitus-Associated Overactive Bladder and Its Treatment with Botulinum Toxin A. *Toxins* **2020**, *12*, 186. [CrossRef] [PubMed]
54. Wang, C.C.; Liao, C.H.; Kuo, H.C. Diabetes mellitus does not affect the efficacy and safety of intravesical onabotulinumtoxinA injection in patients with refractory detrusor overactivity. *Neurourol. Urodyn.* **2014**, *33*, 1235–1239. [CrossRef]
55. Kuo, H.C. Clinical Application of Botulinum Neurotoxin in Lower-Urinary-Tract Diseases and Dysfunctions: Where Are We Now and What More Can We Do? *Toxins* **2022**, *14*, 498. [CrossRef]
56. Truzzi, J.C.; Lapitan, M.C.; Truzzi, N.C.; Iacovelli, V.; Averbeck, M.A. Botulinum toxin for treating overactive bladder in men: A systematic review. *Neurourol. Urodyn.* **2022**, *41*, 710–723. [CrossRef]
57. Lee, P.J.; Kuo, H.C. High incidence of lower urinary tract dysfunction in women with recurrent urinary tract infections. *Low. Urin. Tract Symptoms* **2020**, *12*, 33–40. [CrossRef]
58. Seki, N.; Masuda, K.; Kinukawa, N.; Senoh, K.; Naito, S. Risk factors for febrile urinary tract infection in children with myelodysplasia treated by clean intermittent catheterization. *Int. J. Urol. Off. J. Jpn. Urol. Assoc.* **2004**, *11*, 973–977. [CrossRef]
59. Vasudeva, P.; Madersbacher, H. Factors implicated in pathogenesis of urinary tract infections in neurogenic bladders: Some revered, few forgotten, others ignored. *Neurourol. Urodyn.* **2014**, *33*, 95–100. [CrossRef]
60. McKibben, M.J.; Seed, P.; Ross, S.S.; Borawski, K.M. Urinary Tract Infection and Neurogenic Bladder. *Urol. Clin. N. Am.* **2015**, *42*, 527–536. [CrossRef]
61. Drake, M.J.; Doumouchtsis, S.K.; Hashim, H.; Gammie, A. Fundamentals of urodynamic practice, based on International Continence Society good urodynamic practices recommendations. *Neurourol. Urodyn.* **2018**, *37*, S50–S60. [CrossRef] [PubMed]

62. Nitti, V.W. Pressure flow urodynamic studies: The gold standard for diagnosing bladder outlet obstruction. *Rev. Urol.* **2005**, *7* (Suppl. 6), S14–S21. [PubMed]
63. Hsiao, S.M.; Lin, H.H.; Kuo, H.C. Videourodynamic Studies of Women with Voiding Dysfunction. *Sci. Rep.* **2017**, *7*, 6845. [CrossRef]
64. Lee, E.S.; Lee, S.W.; Lee, K.W.; Kim, J.M.; Kim, Y.H.; Kim, M.E. Effect of transurethral resection with hydrodistention for the treatment of ulcerative interstitial cystitis. *Korean J. Urol.* **2013**, *54*, 682–688. [CrossRef] [PubMed]

Disclaimer/Publisher's Note: The statements, opinions and data contained in all publications are solely those of the individual author(s) and contributor(s) and not of MDPI and/or the editor(s). MDPI and/or the editor(s) disclaim responsibility for any injury to people or property resulting from any ideas, methods, instructions or products referred to in the content.

toxins

Article

Botulinum Toxin A Injection for Autonomic Dysreflexia—Detrusor Injection or Urethral Sphincter Injection?

Po-Ming Chow [1,2] and Hann-Chorng Kuo [3,*]

1 Department of Urology, National Taiwan University Hospital and College of Medicine, No. 7, Chung-Shan South Road, Taipei 100225, Taiwan
2 Glickman Urologic and Kidney Institute, Cleveland Clinic, 9500 Euclid Avenue, Cleveland, OH 44195, USA
3 Department of Urology, Hualien Tzu Chi Hospital, Buddhist Tzu Chi Medical Foundation and Tzu Chi University, 707, Sec. 3, Chung-Yang Rd., Hualien 970, Taiwan
* Correspondence: hck@tzuchi.com.tw; Tel.: +886-3-856-1825

Abstract: Spinal cord injuries (SCI) have a profound impact on autonomic systems, sometimes resulting in multi-organ dysfunction, including of the neurogenic bladder. Autonomic dysreflexia (AD) is commonly seen in patients with SCI above T6 when the injured cord develops a deregulated sympathetic reflex, which can be induced by bladder sensation and can cause hypertensive crisis. While intravesical injection of botulinum toxin A (Botox) is a standard therapy for neurogenic detrusor overactivity, the role of Botox for AD has rarely been described. This study reviewed the medical records of SCI patients who reported AD and received either detrusor or urethral sphincter injection with Botox. The primary endpoint is the subjective improvement of AD. The secondary endpoint is a change in videourodynamic parameters before and after Botox injection. A total of 200 patients were enrolled for analysis. There were 125 (62.5%) patients in the detrusor injection group, and 75 (37.5%) in the urethral sphincter injection group. There were 79 (63.2%) patients in the detrusor injection group and 43 (57.3%) in the urethral sphincter injection group reporting moderate or marked improvement. Detrusor injection leads to a greater improvement in AD, probably because of decreased detrusor pressure and increased compliance after Botox injection. Urethral sphincter injection appears to have a modest effect on AD, despite general improvements in the voiding parameters of videourodynamic study.

Keywords: spinal cord injury; neurogenic bladder; onabotulinumtoxinA

Key Contribution: We report the largest cohort describing the effect of botulinum toxin A injection on the improvement of autonomic dysreflexia in patients with spinal cord injuries.

Citation: Chow, P.-M.; Kuo, H.-C. Botulinum Toxin A Injection for Autonomic Dysreflexia—Detrusor Injection or Urethral Sphincter Injection? *Toxins* **2023**, *15*, 108. https://doi.org/10.3390/toxins15020108

Received: 14 December 2022
Revised: 19 January 2023
Accepted: 24 January 2023
Published: 26 January 2023

Copyright: © 2023 by the authors. Licensee MDPI, Basel, Switzerland. This article is an open access article distributed under the terms and conditions of the Creative Commons Attribution (CC BY) license (https://creativecommons.org/licenses/by/4.0/).

1. Introduction

The spinal cord can be affected by various disorders, which may be classified into traumatic or non-traumatic. Traumatic injuries are often marked by distinct events, whereas non-traumatic injuries are caused by medical conditions, including degenerative, autoimmune, vascular, infectious, or neoplastic diseases. The leading etiology for non-traumatic disease is cervical spondylosis, followed by multiple sclerosis and tumors [1]. The most common causes of traumatic injuries are vehicular accidents and falls. According to the National Spinal Cord Injury Statistical Center (Birmingham, AL, USA), the annual incidence of traumatic spinal cord injury (SCI) is approximately 54 cases per one million people in the United States [2]. The average age is 43, and 78% of the affected patients are male. The cervical spine is the most common site of injury, comprising more than 50% of the cases [3].

The high prevalence of C-spine SCI results in multi-organ dysfunction. Cardiac risks are elevated due to a more prevalent adverse lipid profile, insulin resistance, and abnormal glucose metabolism in SCI patients. Pneumonia is frequent due to an impairment of the respiratory muscles and poor clearance of lung secretions. Constipation is common in patients who have injuries above the conus medullaris, resulting in hypertonic pelvic muscles. Pressure ulcers are directly related to immobility, and are difficult to manage in SCI patients [4]. The immobility resulting from either tetraplegia or paraplegia further aggravates cardiac, respiratory, metabolic, wound, and urinary complications through deprivation of exercises, muscle power reduction, sensation impairment, and fluid and nutritional imbalance. Higher mortality from the above conditions is observed in these patients due to their atypical presentations and delayed diagnosis. Multi-organ dysfunction also shortens the life expectancy of SCI patients to approximately 90 percent that of the normal population [5].

Bladder function is altered in SCI patients regardless of the level of the lesion [6]. In higher-level injuries, uninhibited contraction of the detrusor muscle results in detrusor hyperreflexia, with or without bladder sensation, leading to urinary incontinence, poor bladder compliance, and vesicoureteral reflux. These disorders can be worsened by the un-relaxation or dyssynergic contraction of the external sphincter during the voiding phase, which further increases intravesical pressure. In lower-level injuries, acontractile detrusors result in urinary retention, and insufficient sphincters result in urinary incontinence [7]. Both storage and voiding function require assistance to maintain a low-pressure, compliant, contractile bladder, as well as a continent sphincter. The wellness of the bladder directly reflects the quality of life in terms of the reduction in infection, stone formation, ureteral reflux, and renal function impairment [8].

Autonomic dysreflexia (AD) is a distinct cardiovascular complication commonly seen in SCI above T6. The injury separates the sympathetic neurons from the supraspinal regulation, resulting in a decentralized cord. An episode of AD presents with hypertension and concomitant baroreflex-mediated bradycardia, initiated by unmodulated sympathetic reflexes [9]. The reflex is often triggered by a stimulation below the injury level, such as constipation, bladder distention, pressure sores, or even tight clothing in SCI patients. During an episode of AD, the systolic pressure can reach as high as 325 mmHg [10]. Hypertensive crisis can result in cardiac arrest, seizure, stroke, or sudden death. In patients with SCI and neurogenic bladder, episodes of AD can be discerned by their symptoms, including headache, sweating, and flushing above the injured level.

Intravesical injection of botulinum toxin A (Botox) is a standard therapy for neurogenic detrusor overactivity (NDO). The toxin works on the neuro-muscular junction and relaxes the detrusor muscle, thus improving bladder compliance and reducing urinary incontinence [11]. Another application of Botox is urethral sphincter injection for the purpose of lowering bladder outlet resistance [12]. Both detrusor and urethral sphincter injections of Botox can theoretically improve AD by reducing intravesical pressure during storage and reducing bladder outlet resistance during voiding. However, few studies have investigated the clinical effect of Botox on AD. Schurch et al. first reported the disappearance of AD in 3 of 31 SCI patients who received botulinum-A toxin injections [13]. Fougere et al. found that AD was reduced and blood pressure was stabilized after botulinum-A toxin injections in 17 patients [14]. Herein, we report our experience with Botox injection in either the detrusor or the urethral sphincter, and its effect on AD in patients with SCI.

2. Results

A total of 200 patients were enrolled for analysis. There were 125 (62.5%) patients in the detrusor injection group, and 75 (37.5%) in the urethral sphincter injection group. The average age was 40.8 years, and 131 (65.5%) were men. The levels of injuries were 52 (26%) at the C-spine and 148 (74%) at the T-spine. Symptoms included 2 (1%) with normal voiding, 71 (35.5%) with difficult voiding, 107 (53.5%) with urgency incontinence, and 32 (16%) with urinary retention. Types of bladder management among the participants included 38 (19%) self-voiding, 45 (22.5%) using diapers, 20 (10%) using abdominal pressure, 102 (51%) using percussion voiding, 41 (20.5%) using reflex voiding, 31 (15.5%) using intermittent catheterization, 11 (5.5%) using indwelling catheters, and 7 (3.5%) using cystostomy. The baseline characteristics of each group are summarized in Table 1.

Table 1. Baseline characteristics in detrusor injection and urethral sphincter injection groups.

	Detrusor (n = 125)	Sphincter (n = 75)	p-Value *
Age	37.75 (12.67)	45.90 (15.78)	**<0.001**
Sex			0.071
Men	76 (60.8%)	55 (73.3%)	
Women	49 (39.2%)	20 (26.7%)	
SCI level			0.067
Cervical	27 (21.6%)	25 (33.3%)	
Thoracic	98 (78.4%)	50 (66.7%)	
Symptom			
Normal voiding	2 (1.6%)	0 (0.0%)	0.529
Difficult voiding	23 (18.4%)	48 (64.0%)	**<0.001**
Urge incontinence	92 (73.6%)	15 (20.0%)	**<0.001**
Retention	17 (13.6%)	15 (20.0%)	0.232
Bladder management			
Spontaneous voiding	28 (22.4%)	10 (13.3%)	0.114
On diaper	27 (21.6%)	18 (24.0%)	0.694
Abdominal pressure	10 (8.0)	10 (13.3%)	0.224
Percussion voiding	63 (50.4%)	39 (52.0%)	0.827
Reflex voiding	29 (23.2%)	12 (16.0%)	0.222
CIC/CISC	21 (16.8%)	10 (13.3%)	0.512
Urethral Foley	6 (4.8%)	5 (6.7%)	0.575
Cystostomy	2 (1.6%)	5 (6.7%)	0.105

* p-value by Student's t test and Chi-square test.

The patient-reported improvements in AD are presented as GRA. Of the 200 patients, 28 (14%) reported no improvement, 50 (25%) reported mild improvement, 75 (32.5%) reported moderate improvement, and 47 (23.5%) reported marked improvement. There were more patients in the detrusor group reporting moderate or marked improvement in AD (Table 2). AD was found to increase immediately after intradetrusor injection in two patients, but in none after urethral sphincter injection. However, there were no patients who reported having a worsened GRA of AD after treatment at the follow-up time-point in this study.

Table 2. Subjective improvement after treatment.

	Detrusor (n = 125)	Sphincter (n = 75)	p-Value *
Satisfaction with treatment			**0.019**
No improvement	20 (16.0%)	8 (10.7%)	
Mild improvement	26 (20.8%)	24 (32.0%)	
Moderate improvement	42 (33.6%)	33 (44.0%)	
Marked improvement	37 (29.6%)	10 (13.3%)	

*p-value by Chi-square test.

At baseline, the patients in the detrusor groups had more sensitive bladders, evidenced by a smaller filling volume at first sensation (171 mL vs. 210 mL, p = 0.019), urge sensation (189 mL vs. 235 mL, p = 0.015), as well as maximal bladder capacity (254 mL vs. 293 mL, p = 0.038). After Botox injection, the urethral group showed significant increases in Qmax, voided volume, and VE (Table 3).

Table 3. Baseline and post-treatment videourodynamic parameters in the detrusor and urethral Botox injection groups.

VUDS Parameters		Detrusor (n = 125)	Urethra (n = 75)	p-Value *
PVR	Baseline	184.75 (173.29)	210.16 (156.01)	0.106
	Post-BTX	279.77 (195.26)	223.41 (227.62)	0.032
	Change	97.27 (247.97)	26.82 (271.63)	0.033
FSF	Baseline	131.29 (86.16)	152.08 (97.10)	0.116
	Post-BTX	152.17 (92.55)	155.11 (97.28)	0.854
	Change	26.87 (103.29)	14.86 (114.71)	0.534
FS	Baseline	171.71 (106.12)	210.79 (121.92)	0.019
	Post-BTX	207.53 (115.40)	215.95 (129.10)	0.904
	Change	41.12 (135.68)	27.18 (147.79)	0.557
US	Baseline	189.32 (120.83)	235.41 (137.31)	0.015
	Post-BTX	226.30 (127.85)	241.64 (134.91)	0.540
	Change	45.72 (148.35)	32.64 (158.09)	0.699
Compliance	Baseline	45.61 (59.52)	55.47 (69.86)	0.106
	Post-BTX	38.22 (44.80)	44.14 (81.95)	0.857
	Change	−12.12 (76.48)	−12.28 (108.99)	0.434
Pdet	Baseline	37.34 (23.32)	36.31 (24.54)	0.735
	Post-BTX	26.06 (18.63)	27.25 (20.25)	0.838
	Change	−10.60 (24.02)	−11.7 (26.67)	0.943
Qmax	Baseline	5.51 (5.97)	4.69 (5.17)	0.329
	Post-BTX	4.10 (5.60)	6.55 (9.44)	0.128
	Change	−1.73 (6.21)	2.25 (7.88)	0.017
Vol	Baseline	67.98 (81.50)	83.07 (113.29)	0.949
	Post-BTX	61.47 (93.53)	112.23 (137.08)	0.050
	Change	−8.41 (103.13)	44.86 (152.88)	0.029
CBC	Baseline	254.11 (164.37)	293.23 (153.51)	0.038
	Post-BTX	341.23 (177.62)	335.64 (188.11)	0.652
	Change	88.86 (217.34)	71.68 (257.48)	0.290
VE	Baseline	0.33 (0.33)	0.29 (0.31)	0.354
	Post-BTX	0.21 (0.30)	0.38 (0.40)	0.027
	Change	-0.11 (0.37)	0.12 (0.42)	0.004
BCI	Baseline	64.89 (39.83)	59.77 (36.44)	0.411
	Post-BTX	46.58 (36.85)	59.98 (51.83)	0.121
	Change	−19.27 (46.25)	−0.45 (48.25)	0.044
BOOI	Baseline	26.32 (25.00)	26.92 (26.17)	0.995
	Post-BTX	17.85 (19.56)	14.16 (27.33)	0.491
	Change	−7.14 (22.17)	−16.20 (30.57)	0.171

BCI: bladder contractility index, BOOI: bladder outlet obstruction index, CBC: cystometric bladder capacity, FS: full sensation, FSF: first sensation of filling, Pdet: detrusor pressure at maximum flow rate, PVR: post-voiding residual, Qmax: maximal flow rate, US: urge sensation, VE: voiding efficiency, * p-value by Mann–Whitney U test.

In the detrusor group, patients who had moderate or marked improvement in AD had poorer bladder compliance (31.14 vs. 70.47, $p < 0.001$), higher Pdet (45.42 vs. 23.48 cmH2O, $p < 0.001$), and higher BOOI (35.93 vs. 9.83, $p < 0.001$) at baseline compared to patients who had no or mild improvement. The post-treatment changes of the moderate or marked improvement subgroups and those of the no or mild subgroups were significantly different in bladder compliance and BOOI (Table 4). DO was present in 77 (61.6%) patients before Botox treatment and in 69 (55.2%) patients after Botox treatment (p = 0.052). DSD was present in 61 (48.8%) patients before Botox treatment and in 53 (42.4%) patients after Botox treatment (p = 0.268).

Table 4. Baseline and post-treatment videourodynamic parameters in the detrusor Botox injection patients.

VUDS Parameters		No/Mild Improvement (n = 46)	Moderate/Marked Improvement (n = 79)	p-Value *
PVR	Baseline	184.26 (184.33)	185.04 (167.75)	0.678
	Post-BTX	248.55 (185.82)	299.21 (200.17)	0.260
	Change	53.39 (238.40)	124.58 (252.10)	0.164
FSF	Baseline	130.17 (86.27)	131.94 (86.63)	0.959
	Post-BTX	174.30 (106.29)	138.40 (80.89)	0.159
	Change	41.76 (122.45)	17.60 (89.35)	0.657
FS	Baseline	183.33 (110.70)	164.95 (103.48)	0.388
	Post-BTX	224.70 (125.42)	196.85 (108.57)	0.419
	Change	40.67 (150.21)	41.40 (127.30)	0.950
US	Baseline	201.72 (127.17)	182.10 (117.20)	0.414
	Post-BTX	243.09 (134.12)	215.85 (123.92)	0.429
	Change	42.64 (163.30)	47.64 (139.84)	0.972
Compliance	Baseline	70.47 (78.70)	31.14 (38.48)	<0.001
	Post-BTX	27.60 (21.93)	44.83 (53.56)	0.212
	Change	−44.04 (84.90)	7.76 (63.85)	0.003
Pdet	Baseline	23.48 (14.59)	45.42 (23.72)	<0.001
	Post-BTX	22.12 (17.12)	28.51 (19.27)	0.108
	Change	−3.00 (20.01)	−15.34 (25.24)	0.015
Qmax	Baseline	6.83 (7.41)	4.74 (4.83)	0.181
	Post-BTX	5.73 (6.40)	3.09 (4.83)	0.038
	Change	−0.97 (6.66)	−2.21 (5.92)	0.261
Vol	Baseline	83.39 (93.17)	59.00 (73.00)	0.290
	Post-BTX	89.82 (119.91)	43.81 (67.99)	0.043
	Change	14.58 (110.90)	−22.72 (96.29)	0.184
CBC	Baseline	267.65 (166.98)	246.23 (163.37)	0.467
	Post-BTX	338.36 (161.02)	343.02 (188.70)	0.821
	Change	67.97 (212.74)	101.87 (221.17)	0.520
VE	Baseline	0.37 (0.35)	0.31 (0.32)	0.396
	Post-BTX	0.28 (0.33)	0.17 (0.27)	0.050
	Change	−0.05 (0.31)	−0.15 (0.40)	0.091
BCI	Baseline	57.61 (44.93)	69.13 (36.17)	0.032
	Post-BTX	50.76 (40.83)	43.98 (34.28)	0.460
	Change	−7.85 (46.91)	−26.38 (44.82)	0.045
BOOI	Baseline	9.83 (16.08)	35.93 (24.30)	<0.001
	Post-BTX	10.67 (17.81)	22.32 (19.41)	0.004
	Change	−1.06 (17.38)	−10.92 (24.07)	0.044

BCI: bladder contractility index, BOOI: bladder outlet obstruction index, CBC: cystometric bladder capacity, FS: full sensation, FSF: first sensation of filling, Pdet: detrusor pressure at maximum flow rate, PVR: post-voiding residual, Qmax: maximal flow rate, US: urge sensation, VE: voiding efficiency. * p-value by Mann–Whitney U test.

In the urethral sphincter group, patients who had moderate or marked improvement in AD had marginally higher Pdet (41.65 vs. 29.13 cmH2O, p = 0.050) and lower capacity (258.86 vs. 399.41 ml, p = 0.023) compared to patients who had no or mild improvement (Table 5). DO was present in 38 (50.7%) patients before Botox treatment and in 33 (44%) patients after Botox treatment (p = 0.180). DSD was present in 30 (40%) patients before Botox treatment and in 20 (26.7%) patients after Botox treatment (p = 0.031).

Table 5. Baseline and post-treatment VUDS parameters in the urethral sphincter Botox injection patients.

VUDS Parameters		No/Mild Improvement (*n* = 32)	Moderate/Marked Improvement (*n* = 43)	*p*-Value *
PVR	Baseline	235.22 (169.81)	191.51 (144.09)	0.304
	Post-BTX	213.33 (221.92)	230.38 (235.58)	0.905
	Change	−33.61 (262.36)	68.65 (275.05)	0.145
FSF	Baseline	170.88 (107.03)	138.09 (87.67)	0.210
	Post-BTX	182.17 (71.61)	136.38 (109.08)	0.016
	Change	16.61 (107.40)	13.65 (121.59)	0.738
FS	Baseline	228.69 (122.39)	197.47 (121.27)	0.197
	Post-BTX	250.28 (131.10)	192.19 (124.68)	0.061
	Change	35.44 (149.40)	21.46 (149.36)	0.793
US	Baseline	255.91 (139.08)	220.16 (135.60)	0.161
	Post-BTX	278.00 (146.92)	216.46 (122.53)	0.145
	Change	37.33 (158.65)	29.38 (160.76)	0.793
Compliance	Baseline	61.60 (68.64)	50.90 (71.22)	0.197
	Post-BTX	40.05 (61.28)	46.97 (94.76)	0.793
	Change	−25.21 (87.26)	−3.33 (122.68)	0.233
Pdet	Baseline	29.13 (19.86)	41.65 (26.48)	0.050
	Post-BTX	26.39 (22.32)	27.85 (19.12)	0.667
	Change	−3.28 (27.10)	−17.54 (25.24)	0.173
Qmax	Baseline	4.78 (6.08)	4.63 (4.44)	0.621
	Post-BTX	7.22 (11.07)	6.08 (8.33)	0.636
	Change	3.17 (7.64)	1.62 (8.13)	0.381
Vol	Baseline	104.19 (140.18)	67.35 (86.69)	0.768
	Post-BTX	137.67 (155.35)	94.62 (122.97)	0.436
	Change	52.06 (192.16)	39.88 (122.58)	0.624
CBC	Baseline	339.41 (165.07)	258.86 (136.29)	0.023
	Post-BTX	351.00 (182.20)	325.00 (194.93)	0.489
	Change	18.44 (274.19)	108.54 (243.83)	0.252
VE	Baseline	0.31 (0.33)	0.28 (0.29)	0.965
	Post-BTX	0.39 (0.41)	0.38 (0.39)	0.855
	Change	0.13 (0.43)	0.12 (0.41)	0.877
BCI	Baseline	53.03 (36.40)	64.79 (36.08)	0.148
	Post-BTX	62.50 (53.66)	58.23 (51.52)	0.793
	Change	12.56 (41.08)	−9.46 (51.49)	0.079
BOOI	Baseline	19.56 (23.23)	32.40 (27.14)	0.056
	Post-BTX	11.94 (35.52)	15.69 (20.52)	0.821
	Change	−9.61 (34.22)	−20.77 (27.53)	0.283

BCI: bladder contractility index, BOOI: bladder outlet obstruction index, CBC: cystometric bladder capacity, FS: full sensation, FSF: first sensation of filling, Pdet: detrusor pressure at maximum flow rate, PVR: post-voiding residual, Qmax: maximal flow rate, US: urge sensation, VE: voiding efficiency. * *p*-value by Mann–Whitney U test.

3. Discussion

Our study revealed that Botox injection to either the detrusor or the urethral sphincter achieved moderate or marked improvement in AD in 61% of SCI patients. There were more patients with marked improvement in the detrusor group, indicating a better control of AD. The baseline VUDS profile suggested that patients with poorer bladder compliance and higher detrusor pressure showed better responses to detrusor injection, and this response was best reflected by an increase in post-treatment compliance and a decrease in DO. The benefits that these patients might report could be related to their inferior pre-treatment conditions, as these treatments did not help patients with borderline bladder dysfunction. In the urethral sphincter group, there were general improvements in VUDS parameters, including Qmax, VE, and BOOI, regardless of the subjective improvements in

AD after Botox injection. To our knowledge, this is the first study that has correlated VUDS findings and AD symptom improvements in SCI patients who received Botox injection at different sites.

The leading cause of death in SCI patients has shifted from urinary complications to cardiovascular events [15], marking the importance of the management of AD. Since AD is highlighted by episodic hypertension, treatments for AD has been focused on blood pressure control with nitrites [16], calcium channel blockers [17], and alpha-adrenergic blockers [18]. However, the pathophysiology of AD includes a serial remodeling of the autonomic system: loss of supraspinal control over the sympathetic preganglionic neurons [19], synaptic reorganization of the sympathetic preganglionic neurons [20], primary afferent sprouting [21], and propriospinal plasticity [22]. This sensitized bladder proprioception, as well as other stimuli below the level of injury, are amplified to form an unregulated sympathetic reflex, resulting in an episode of AD. Considering the pathophysiology of AD, blood pressure control alone does not provide to-the-target management.

Botox paralyzes smooth or striated muscles through its inhibition of acetylcholine release in neuromuscular junctions. Through this mechanism of action, Botox has demonstrated effectiveness in reducing DO and urethral sphincter spasticity [23]. In addition to motor inhibition, Botox also has effects on the sensory neurons. The application of a sensory blockade has been proven effective in patients with bladder pain syndrome treated with intravesical injections [24]. These mechanisms include a decrease in both the release of neurotransmitters and the expression of nociceptors, as well as the suppression of afferent nerve sprouting and reorganization [25]. The diverse mechanisms of action make Botox an ideal therapy for SCI patients, as it targets both lower urinary tract symptoms and AD.

In our cohort of SCI patients who had AD that required anti-hypertensive management, LUTS-directed Botox injection yielded a 61% moderate or marked improvement in AD symptoms. There were two prior series addressing the role of Botox on AD. In the study by Schurch et al. evaluating the effect of Botox on LUTS, AD associated with bladder emptying that manifested as a hypertensive crisis during voiding disappeared after treatment in the three patients with tetraplegia [13]. Although this was a prospective study, AD was not an end point, but an incidental finding. Another study by Fougere et al. prospectively measured blood pressure during UDS and daily activity. The authors found that the amplitude of UDS-induced hypertension was attenuated in 17 patients after Botox injection; however, there were no significant differences found in 24-h ambulatory blood pressure monitoring [14].

Our results suggest that improvement in AD can be more significant in those who have poorer bladder compliance and higher Pdet at baseline, which are typical UDS indications for Botox injection. This finding implies that additional detrusor injection can be considered in patients symptomatically indicated for urethral injection, in order to further eliminate their AD symptoms. Nonetheless, there were still 14% of patients who reported no improvement in AD, indicating insufficient management for either LUTS or other stimulatory conditions such as constipation or pressure sores.

The strengths of our study are the large number of cases and complete VUDS evaluations. There are some limitations to our study. First, the baseline AD severity was unclear, and was not objectively measured. As there are currently no symptom scores or other objective evaluation tools for AD, we relied on patient-reported general assessments of the outcome to evaluate the treatment responses. Some studies used ambulatory blood pressure monitoring, but this method may not always record the blood pressure during AD episodes. Furthermore, there is no consensus on the criteria for blood pressure elevation. Second, this was not a randomized trial, and the decision for detrusor or urethral sphincter injection was based on the patients' main lower urinary tract symptoms and requirements. Although there has been no data suggesting predisposing factors for AD, significant bias might result from any unbalanced factors, such as age, sex, or the injury level between the two arms.

4. Conclusions

Detrusor or urethral sphincter injection of Botox were both shown to improve AD in the majority of SCI patients. Detrusor injection leads to a greater improvement in AD, probably because of decreased detrusor pressure and increased bladder compliance. Urethral sphincter injection appears to have a modest effect on AD, despite general improvement in the VUDS parameters.

5. Methods

5.1. Ethical Approval

The study was approved by the Institutional Review Board of Hualien Tzu Chi Hospital (IRB 110-033-B). Patients' informed consent was waived due to the retrospective nature of this study.

5.2. Patient Enrollment

We retrospectively reviewed the medical records of SCI patients who reported AD and received either detrusor or urethral sphincter injection with Botox from 1998 to 2022. All patients had either storage symptoms, such as urgency and urgency incontinence; emptying symptoms, such as difficult urination or large postvoid residual volume; or both storage and emptying symptoms. Thus, all were ready for detrusor or urethral Botox injection. All patients also had symptoms of AD, such as headache, hypertension, increased reflexes, profuse sweating, bradycardia, and other systemic symptoms either associated with bladder fullness or occurring during urination. These AD symptoms were considered moderate to severe, causing discomfort to the patients and requiring medication to alleviate them. Patient data included age, sex, level of SCI, bladder management, videourodynamic study (VUDS) profiles, and subjective improvement in AD.

5.3. Botulinum Toxin A Injection

The techniques for Botox injection were described previously [12,26,27]. The treatment was performed in an operating room under light intravenous general anesthesia. For detrusor injection, 200 U of onabotulinumtoxinA (Botox, Allergan, Irvine, CA, USA) was diluted with 20 mL of normal saline and injected into 20 well-distributed sites in the bladder wall, sparing the trigone. All cystoscopic injections were performed using a rigid injection instrument (22-Fr, Richard Wolf, Knittlingen, Germany) and a 23-gauge injection needle. For urethral sphincter injection, a total of 100 U Botox was given. A single vial of 100 U Botox was dissolved in 5 mL of normal saline, resulting in a concentration equivalent to 20 U/mL. Each 1 mL of Botox solution was injected transurethrally under cystoscopy into the urethral sphincter at the 2, 4, 8, 10, and 12 o'clock positions in men, and transcutaneously into the urethral sphincter along the urethral lumen at the sides of the urethral meatus in women. The selection of Botox injection to the detrusor or the urethral sphincter was based on the individual patient's main lower urinary tract symptoms. Detrusor Botox injection was performed for NDO with urinary incontinence and AD. Urethral sphincter Botox injection was performed for detrusor sphincter dyssynergia (DSD) to facilitate spontaneous voiding, ease self-catheterization, and improve AD.

5.4. VUDS Parameters

VUDS was performed under fluoroscopy and pressure flow study [28]. The VUDS parameters were defined as follows. Bladder sensation was evaluated by first sensation of filling (FSF), full sensation (FS), and urge sensation (US). Cystometric bladder capacity (CBC) was calculated by adding post-voiding residual (PVR) and voided volume (Vol). Bladder compliance was calculated by dividing the volume at full sensation (FS) by the detrusor pressure (Pdet). Voiding efficiency (VE) was defined as voided volume divided by bladder capacity. Maximal flow rate (Qmax) and detrusor pressure at the maximum flow rate (Pdet@Qmax) were recorded. The bladder outlet obstruction index (BOOI) was calculated by (Pdet@Qmax -2 × Qmax). Detrusor overactivity (DO) was defined as any involuntary detrusor contraction during the filling phase of the pressure flow study [29].

5.5. Outcome Measurement and Statistics Analysis

The primary endpoint was the subjective improvement in AD, as defined by the global response assessment (GRA). The scale we used was as follows: −3 for markedly worse, −2 for moderately worse, −1 for mildly worse, 0 for no change, 1 for mildlimprovement, 2 for moderate improvement, and 3 for marked improvement [30]. The GRA assessments were taken within 1 month after Botox, and VUDS was carried out within 3 months after Botox. GRA and VUDS were evaluated separately. The secondary endpoint was the change in VUDS parameters before and after Botox injection. Either the Student's *t*-test or Mann–Whitney U test was performed to compare numerical data, and the Chi-square test was performed to compare categorical data. Statistical analyses were performed using free software (R version 4.0.0). All statistical tests were two-tailed, with $p < 0.05$ indicating significance.

Author Contributions: Conceptualization, H.-C.K.; methodology, P.-M.C.; software, P.-M.C.; formal analysis, P.-M.C.; investigation, P.-M.C.; resources, H.-C.K.; data curation, H.-C.K.; writing—original draft preparation, P.-M.C.; writing—review and editing, H.-C.K.; visualization, P.-M.C.; supervision, H.-C.K.; project administration, H.-C.K.; funding acquisition, H.-C.K. All authors have read and agreed to the published version of the manuscript.

Funding: This work was supported by Buddhist Tzu Chi Medical Foundation (TCMF-MP 110-03-01), National Taiwan University Hospital (112-S0151), and National Science and Technology Council (109-2314-B-002-173-MY3).

Institutional Review Board Statement: The study was conducted according to the guidelines of the Declaration of Helsinki, and approved by Hualien Tzu Chi Hospital Institutional Review Board (IRB 110-033-B, 7 March 2021).

Informed Consent Statement: Patient consent was waived due to the retrospective nature of this study.

Data Availability Statement: All data were presented with the manuscript.

Conflicts of Interest: The authors declare no conflict of interest.

References

1. Moore, A.P.; Blumhardt, L.D. A prospective survey of the causes of non-traumatic spastic paraparesis and tetraparesis in 585 patients. *Spinal Cord* **1997**, *35*, 361–367. [CrossRef]
2. Jain, N.B.; Ayers, G.D.; Peterson, E.N.; Harris, M.B.; Morse, L.R.; O'Connor, K.C.; Garshick, E. Traumatic Spinal Cord Injury in the United States, 1993-2012. *JAMA* **2015**, *313*, 2236–2243. [CrossRef] [PubMed]
3. Devivo, M.J. Epidemiology of traumatic spinal cord injury: Trends and future implications. *Spinal Cord* **2012**, *50*, 365–372. [CrossRef]
4. McKinley, W.O.; Jackson, A.B.; Cardenas, D.D.; De Vivo, M.J. Long-term medical complications after traumatic spinal cord injury: A regional model systems analysis. *Arch. Phys. Med. Rehabil.* **1999**, *80*, 1402–1410. [CrossRef] [PubMed]
5. Hagen, E.M.; Lie, S.A.; Rekand, T.; Gilhus, N.E.; Gronning, M. Mortality after traumatic spinal cord injury: 50 years of follow-up. *J. Neurol. Neurosurg. Psychiatry* **2009**, *81*, 368–373. [CrossRef] [PubMed]
6. Bellucci, C.; Wöllner, J.; Gregorini, F.; Birnböck, D.; Kozomara, M.; Mehnert, U.; Schubert, M.; Kessler, T.M. Acute Spinal Cord Injury—Do Ambulatory Patients Need Urodynamic Investigations? *J. Urol.* **2013**, *189*, 1369–1373. [CrossRef] [PubMed]
7. Hamid, R.; Averbeck, M.A.; Chiang, H.; Garcia, A.; Al Mousa, R.T.; Oh, S.-J.; Patel, A.; Plata, M.; Del Popolo, G. Epidemiology and pathophysiology of neurogenic bladder after spinal cord injury. *World J. Urol.* **2018**, *36*, 1517–1527. [CrossRef]
8. Wyndaele, J.-J. The management of neurogenic lower urinary tract dysfunction after spinal cord injury. *Nat. Rev. Urol.* **2016**, *13*, 705–714. [CrossRef]
9. Eldahan, K.C.; Rabchevsky, A.G. Autonomic dysreflexia after spinal cord injury: Systemic pathophysiology and methods of management. *Auton. Neurosci.* **2017**, *209*, 59–70. [CrossRef]
10. McBride, F.; Quah, S.P.; E Scott, M.; Dinsmore, W.W. Tripling of Blood Pressure by Sexual Stimulation in a Man with Spinal Cord Injury. *J. R. Soc. Med.* **2003**, *96*, 349–350. [CrossRef]

11. Rovner, E.; Kohan, A.; Chartier-Kastler, E.; Jünemann, K.-P.; Del Popolo, G.; Herschorn, S.; Joshi, M.; Magyar, A.; Nitti, V. Long-Term Efficacy and Safety of OnabotulinumtoxinA in Patients with Neurogenic Detrusor Overactivity Who Completed 4 Years of Treatment. *J. Urol.* **2016**, *196*, 801–808. [CrossRef]
12. Lee, Y.-K.; Kuo, H.-C. Therapeutic Effects of Botulinum Toxin A, via Urethral Sphincter Injection on Voiding Dysfunction Due to Different Bladder and Urethral Sphincter Dysfunctions. *Toxins* **2019**, *11*, 487. [CrossRef]
13. Schurch, B.; Stohrer, M.; Kramer, G.; Schmid, D.M.; Gaul, G.; Hauri, D. Botulinum-A toxin for treating detrusor hyperreflexia in spinal cord injured patients: A new alternative to anticholinergic drugs? Preliminary results. *J. Urol.* **2000**, *164*, 692–697. [CrossRef] [PubMed]
14. Fougere, R.J.; Currie, K.D.; Nigro, M.K.; Stothers, L.; Rapoport, D.; Krassioukov, A.V. Reduction in Bladder-Related Autonomic Dysreflexia after OnabotulinumtoxinA Treatment in Spinal Cord Injury. *J. Neurotrauma* **2016**, *33*, 1651–1657. [CrossRef]
15. Frankel, H.L.; Coll, J.R.; Charlifue, S.W.; Whiteneck, G.G.; Gardner, B.P.; Jamous, M.A.; Krishnan, K.R.; Nuseibeh, I.; Savic, G.; Sett, P. Long-term survival in spinal cord injury: A fifty year investigation. *Spinal Cord* **1998**, *36*, 266–274. [CrossRef] [PubMed]
16. Caruso, D.; Gater, D.; Harnish, C. Prevention of recurrent autonomic dysreflexia: A survey of current practice. *Clin Auton Res* **2015**, *25*, 293–300. [CrossRef]
17. Krassioukov, A.; Warburton, D.; Teasell, R.; Eng, J. A Systematic Review of the Management of Autonomic Dysreflexia After Spinal Cord Injury. *Arch. Phys. Med. Rehabil.* **2009**, *90*, 682–695. [CrossRef] [PubMed]
18. Phillips, A.A.; Elliott, S.L.; Zheng, M.M.; Krassioukov, A.V. Selective Alpha Adrenergic Antagonist Reduces Severity of Transient Hypertension during Sexual Stimulation after Spinal Cord Injury. *J. Neurotrauma* **2015**, *32*, 392–396. [CrossRef]
19. Rabchevsky, A.G. Segmental organization of spinal reflexes mediating autonomic dysreflexia after spinal cord injury. *Prog. Brain Res.* **2006**, *152*, 265–274. [CrossRef]
20. Schramm, L.P. Spinal sympathetic interneurons: Their identification and roles after spinal cord injury. *Prog. Brain. Res.* **2006**, *152*, 27–37. [CrossRef]
21. Hou, S.; Duale, H.; Rabchevsky, A.G. Intraspinal sprouting of unmyelinated pelvic afferents after complete spinal cord injury is correlated with autonomic dysreflexia induced by visceral pain. *Neuroscience* **2009**, *159*, 369–379. [CrossRef]
22. Krassioukov, A.V.; Johns, D.G.; Schramm, L.P. Sensitivity of Sympathetically Correlated Spinal Interneurons, Renal Sympathetic Nerve Activity, and Arterial Pressure to Somatic and Visceral Stimuli after Chronic Spinal Injury. *J. Neurotrauma* **2002**, *19*, 1521–1529. [CrossRef] [PubMed]
23. Chen, S.-L.; Huang, Y.-H. Concomitant Detrusor and External Urethral Sphincter Botulinum Toxin-A Injections in Male Spinal Cord Injury Patients with Detrusor Overactivity and Detrusor Sphincter Dyssynergia. *J. Rehabil. Med.* **2022**, *54*, jrm00264. [CrossRef]
24. Jhang, J.-F. Using Botulinum Toxin A for Treatment of Interstitial Cystitis/Bladder Pain Syndrome—Possible Pathomechanisms and Practical Issues. *Toxins* **2019**, *11*, 641. [CrossRef] [PubMed]
25. Apostolidis, A.; Popat, R.; Yiangou, Y.; Cockayne, D.; Ford, A.; Davis, J.; Dasgupta, P.; Fowler, C.; Anand, P. Decreased sensory receptors P2X3 and TRPV1 in suburothelial nerve fibers following intradetrusor injections of botulinum toxin for human detrusor overactivity. *J. Urol.* **2005**, *174*, 977–982. [CrossRef] [PubMed]
26. Chow, P.-M.; Hsiao, S.-M.; Kuo, H.-C. Obstructive patterns in videourodynamic studies predict responses of female dysfunctional voiding treated with or without urethral botulinum toxin injection: A long-term follow-up study. *Int. Urogynecol. J.* **2020**, *31*, 2557–2564. [CrossRef] [PubMed]
27. Chen, Y.-C.; Kuo, H.-C. The Therapeutic Effects of Repeated Detrusor Injections Between 200 or 300 Units of OnabotulinumtoxinA in Chronic Spinal Cord Injured Patients. *Neurourol. Urodyn.* **2014**, *33*, 129–134. [CrossRef]
28. Chow, P.-M.; Hsiao, S.-M.; Kuo, H.-C. Identifying occult bladder outlet obstruction in women with detrusor-underactivity-like urodynamic profiles. *Sci. Rep.* **2021**, *11*, 23242. [CrossRef] [PubMed]
29. Chow, P.-M.; Kuo, H.-C. Performance of urinary biomarkers in differentiating dysfunctional voiding in women with overactive bladder syndrome: A prospective pilot study. *Int. Urol. Nephrol.* **2022**, *54*, 2497–2502. [CrossRef] [PubMed]
30. Propert, K.; Mayer, R.; Wang, Y.; Sant, G.; Hanno, P.; Peters, K.; Kusek, J. Responsiveness of symptom scales for interstitial cystitis. *Urology* **2006**, *67*, 55–59. [CrossRef] [PubMed]

Disclaimer/Publisher's Note: The statements, opinions and data contained in all publications are solely those of the individual author(s) and contributor(s) and not of MDPI and/or the editor(s). MDPI and/or the editor(s) disclaim responsibility for any injury to people or property resulting from any ideas, methods, instructions or products referred to in the content.

toxins

MDPI

Article

Comparison of the Clinical Efficacy and Adverse Events between Intravesical Injections of Platelet-Rich Plasma and Botulinum Toxin A for the Treatment of Interstitial Cystitis Refractory to Conventional Treatment

Jia-Fong Jhang, Wan-Ru Yu and Hann-Chorng Kuo *

Department of Urology, Hualien Tzu Chi Hospital, Buddhist Tzu Chi Medical Foundation, Tzu Chi University, Hualien 970, Taiwan
* Correspondence: hck@tzuchi.com.tw

Abstract: Background: Intravesical injection of Botulinum toxin A (BoNT-A) and platelet-rich plasma (PRP) have been reported to alleviate bladder pain and decrease nocturia in patients with refractory interstitial cystitis/bladder pain syndrome (IC/BPS). Both treatments are novel and there has no comparison between them. This study compared the therapeutic effects and adverse events between IC/BPS patients receiving PRP or BoNT-A injections. Materials and Methods: This study retrospectively analyzed female patients with IC/BPS who were refractory to conventional treatment and received BoNT-A (n = 26) or PRP (n = 30) injections within the previous two years. Patients were arbitrarily treated with four monthly injections of PRP or a single injection of 100 U of BoNT-A. All injections were followed by cystoscopic hydrodistention. The primary endpoint was the global response assessment (GRA), and secondary endpoints were changes in the O'Leary-Sant IC symptom score, visual analog score (VAS) of bladder pain, voiding diary, and uroflow measures from baseline to six months after the first injection day. Results: The baseline demographics revealed no significant difference between groups. The GRA at one, three, and six months was similar between groups. A significant improvement in IC symptom scores was noted in both groups. Although VAS was significantly improved in overall patients, no significant difference was noted between the PRP and BoNT-A groups at 6 months. Only half of the study cohort had a GRA $\geq$2 at six months. An increase in the post-void residual was noted one month after the BoNT-A injection, but there was no difference between groups at three and six months. More patients reported dysuria (19.2% vs. 3.3%, p = 0.086) and urinary tract infection (UTI, 15.4% vs. 0%, p = 0.041) after BoNT-A injection than after the PRP injections. The time from the first injection to receiving alternative treatment was similar between groups. Conclusion: Both intravesical PRP and BoNT-A injections have similar efficacy in IC symptom improvement. However, only half of the study cohort had a GRA of $\geq$2 at the six-month follow-up BoNT-A injection carries a potential risk of UTI after treatment.

Keywords: botox; platelet-rich plasma; interstitial cystitis; intravesical injection

Key Contribution: Intravesical injections of either PRP or BoNT-A are safe and effective for improving IC/BPS symptoms without significantly increasing the PVR. However, only half of patients remained effective at 6 months; repeat treatment was necessary for both groups.

Citation: Jhang, J.-F.; Yu, W.-R.; Kuo, H.-C. Comparison of the Clinical Efficacy and Adverse Events between Intravesical Injections of Platelet-Rich Plasma and Botulinum Toxin A for the Treatment of Interstitial Cystitis Refractory to Conventional Treatment. *Toxins* **2023**, *15*, 121. https://doi.org/10.3390/toxins15020121

Received: 26 December 2022
Revised: 19 January 2023
Accepted: 31 January 2023
Published: 2 February 2023

Copyright: © 2023 by the authors. Licensee MDPI, Basel, Switzerland. This article is an open access article distributed under the terms and conditions of the Creative Commons Attribution (CC BY) license (https://creativecommons.org/licenses/by/4.0/).

1. Introduction

Interstitial cystitis/bladder pain syndrome (IC/BPS) is a chronic bladder inflammatory disease characterized by bladder pain and frequency urgency. Current treatments using pain killer or anti-inflammatory medications cannot completely eradicate symptoms and increase bladder capacity [1]. Several intravesical or oral medications, such as pentosan-polysulphate, amitryptynine, and cyclosporin have been tried, but their therapeutic efficacy has been proven ineffective [2–6]. The lack of a reliable effective therapy for IC/BPS may be related to its poorly understood pathophysiology. One of the most common findings in bladder mucosal biopsies from patients with IC/BPS is denudation or thinning of the bladder epithelium, suggesting an altered regulation of urothelial homeostasis [7,8]. Other bladder abnormalities include an increased nerve fiber density, inflammatory cell infiltrations, and noxious sensory receptor immunoreactivity [9]. Although investigations on this topic have been enthusiastically performed, the etiology of IC/BPS remains unknown. Treatment based on a single pathophysiology might not be sufficient to solve the underlying pathology of IC/BPS.

Intravesical botulinum toxin A (BoNT-A) and platelet-rich plasma (PRP) injections are novel treatments for IC/BPS refractory to conventional therapies. BoNT-A can reduce the release of acetylcholine and inflammation-related neuropeptides from nerve terminals [10]. The BoNT-A injection can eliminate noxious stimulation and reduce bladder suburothelial inflammation, thus improving urothelial regeneration and IC/BPS symptoms. PRP can also produce new inflammation and override unresolved inflammation in IC/BPS bladders [11]. Through repeated injections, the bladder inflammation is eliminated and regeneration of the defective urothelium is improved, resulting in a healed bladder urothelium with adequate barrier function and a reduction in bladder pain [12]. Although there is solid evidence that BoNT-A improves the IC/BPS condition, a decrease in detrusor contractility following treatment may contribute to a poor response to the BoNT-A injection [13]. On the other hand, the PRP injection does not have such adverse events. However, the effect of PRP on inflammation might be less remarkable than that of BoNT-A; frequent monthly PRP injections are necessary to achieve a therapeutic efficacy similar to that of BoNT-A on IC/BPS [14].

Patients with chronic IC/BPS usually cannot be successfully treated with conventional medical or intravesical treatments. Although previous clinical trials provided evidence that intravesical BoNT-A or PRP injections were effective [11–13], the true clinical efficacy and patients' satisfaction have not been reported in real life practice. To date, there has been no head-to-head comparison between these two treatment modalities. Therefore, we compared these two novel therapies to establish which treatment provides superior treatment efficacy and safety.

2. Results

Among the 56 female patients included in the study, 30 received four monthly PRP injections and 26 received a single BoNT-A injection. Patients' baseline demographics, including symptom score, voiding diary data, uroflowmetry data, findings of cystoscopic hydrodistention, and duration of IC/BPS symptoms are listed in Table 1. There was no significant difference between the two treatment groups; however, a higher VAS score for bladder pain was perceived at baseline in the BoNT-A group.

Table 1. Baseline demographics of patients with interstitial cystitis who underwent intravesical platelet-rich plasma or botulinum toxin A injection.

	PRP (n = 30)	BoNT-A (n = 26)	p-Value
Age (years)	52.57 ± 11.08	49.19 ± 17.03	0.392
ICSI	12.57 ± 4.43	13.15 ± 4.15	0.613
ICPI	11.63 ± 3.21	12.23 ± 3.23	0.492
VAS	3.57 ± 3.14	5.35 ± 3.02	0.036
Frequency	11.70 ± 6.39	13.95 ± 8.35	0.260
Nocturia	3.28 ± 1.59	3.77 ± 5.33	0.651
FBC (mL)	255.83 ± 126.74	264.16 ± 103.70	0.793
Qmax (mL/s)	13.17 ± 7.01	16.54 ± 9.60	0.136
Volume (mL)	192.43 ± 109.65	238.38 ± 112.70	0.128
PVR (mL)	22.97 ± 45.04	21.73 ± 35.38	0.911
MBC (mL)	768.33 ± 173.94	728.40 ± 219.94	0.455

Table 1. *Cont.*

	PRP (n = 30)	BoNT-A (n = 26)	p-Value
Glomerulation	1.37 ± 0.89	1.42 ± 0.93	0.841
Ulcer	0 (0.0%)	2 (7.7%)	0.211
Duration (years)	10.27 ± 8.85	8.92 ± 10.26	0.601

Abbreviations: PRP: platelet-rich plasma, BoNT-A: botulinum toxin A, ICSI: interstitial cystitis symptom index, ICPI: interstitial cystitis problem index, VAS: visual analog score, FBC: functional bladder capacity, Qmax: maximum flow rate, PVR: post-void residual, MBC: maximal bladder capacity.

Table 2 shows the changes in IC symptom score, VAS scores for bladder pain, and GRA from baseline to all follow-up points between groups. The improvement in ICSI and ICPI from baseline to each time-point was significant in both groups, but no significant difference was noted between groups. The change in the VAS score after treatment was significant only in the BoNT-A group; however, the change in VAS score from baseline to the follow-up time points was not significant between groups. Interestingly, the GRA was significantly improved only in the PRP group.

Table 2. Changes in symptom scores and the global response assessment after intravesical PRP or BoNT-A injection for patients with IC/BPS.

		All (n = 56)	PRP (n = 30)	BoNT-A (n = 26)	p-Value
ICSI	BL	12.84 ± 4.27	12.57 ± 4.43	13.15 ± 4.15	
	1M	9.95 ± 4.35 *	9.43 ± 3.32 *	10.54 ± 5.30 *	0.616
	3M	9.55 ± 4.16 *	9.57 ± 3.66 *	9.54 ± 4.75 *	0.598
	6M	9.00 ± 4.21 *	8.33 ± 4.40 *	9.77 ± 3.92 *	0.410
ICPI	BL	11.91 ± 3.20	11.63 ± 3.21	12.23 ± 3.23	
	1M	9.20 ± 4.26 *	8.93 ± 3.54 *	9.50 ± 5.02 *	0.975
	3M	8.50 ± 3.69 *	8.87 ± 3.21 *	8.08 ± 4.20 *	0.137
	6M	8.73 ± 3.97 *	8.60 ± 4.06 *	8.88 ± 3.94 *	0.781
VAS	BL	4.39 ± 3.18	3.57 ± 3.14	5.35 ± 3.02	
	1M	4.27 ± 3.11	4.00 ± 3.22	4.58 ± 3.02	0.062
	3M	3.38 ± 2.90 *	3.20 ± 3.01	3.58 ± 2.80 *	0.068
	6M	3.66 ± 3.06 *	3.17 ± 3.18	4.23 ± 2.87 *	0.239
GRA	1M	0.84 ± 1.16	0.73 ± 1.08	0.96 ± 1.25	
	3M	0.89 ± 1.65	0.83 ± 1.58	0.96 ± 1.75	0.840
	6M	1.36 ± 1.55 *	1.53 ± 1.20 *	1.15 ± 1.89	0.227

* $p < 0.05$ compared with baseline data, Abbreviations: GRA: global response assessment, PRP: platelet-rich plasma, BoNT-A: botulinum toxin A, ICSI: interstitial cystitis symptom index, ICPI: interstitial cystitis problem index, VAS: visual analog score.

Table 3 shows the differences in voiding and uroflowmetry parameters between the PRP and BoNT-A groups. Although nocturia and FBC were improved in the PRP group and frequency was improved at the one-month follow-up in the BoNT-A group, there was no significant difference all follow-up time points in the BoNT-A group; however, the change in post-void residual (PVR) was only significantly higher in the BoNT-A group at one month. We found the GRA increased with repeated monthly injections of PRP, whereas the GRA was mildly improved immediately after BoNT-A injection but improved to a level similar to that of PRP at six months. Nevertheless, more patients in the BoNT-A group complained of dysuria after treatment, and a significantly higher rate of urinary tract infection (UTI) (15.4% vs. none) developed after the BoNT-A injection compared with that of patients receiving the PRP injection (Table 4).

Table 3. Changes in voiding and uroflow measurements after intravesical PRP or BoNT-A injection for patients with IC/BPS.

		All (n= 56)	PRP (n= 30)	BoNT-A (n = 26)	p-Value
Frequency	BL	12.74 ± 7.38	11.70 ± 6.39	13.95 ± 8.35	
	1M	11.40 ± 5.83	10.88 ± 4.98	11.99 ± 6.73 *	0.475
	3M	12.09 ± 6.48	10.77 ± 4.18	13.62 ± 8.21	0.729
	6M	11.72 ± 5.63	10.95 ± 4.08	12.60 ± 6.99	0.694
Nocturia	BL	3.51 ± 3.78	3.28 ± 1.59	3.77 ± 5.33	
	1M	2.74 ± 3.00	2.55 ± 1.50 *	2.97 ± 4.13	0.936
	3M	2.63 ± 3.19 *	2.22 ± 1.42 *	309 ± 4.43	0.484
	6M	2.57 ± 3.06 *	2.35 ± 1.80 *	2.83 ± 4.08	0.977
FBC	BL	259 ± 116	256 ± 127	264 ± 104	
	1M	283 ± 123 *	276 ± 124	292 ± 125	0.783
	3M	299 ± 126 *	303 ± 135 *	295 ± 118	0.935
	6M	314 ± 138 *	305 ± 136 *	325 ± 142	0.465
Qmax	BL	14.73 ± 8.41	13.17 ± 7.01	16.54 ± 9.60	
	1M	14.74 ± 9.61	13.76 ± 8.02	15.88 ± 11.23	0.548
	3M	16.04 ± 9.49	16.87 ± 10.48	15.10 ± 8.29	0.043
	6M	15.98 ± 10.08	15.93 ± 10.80	16.03 ± 9.40	0.188
Volume	BL	214 ± 112	192 ± 110	238 ± 113	
	1M	207 ± 132	196 ± 123	218 ± 143	0.425
	3M	212 ± 106	199 ± 93.9	227 ± 118	0.512
	6M	232 ± 114	218 ± 114	248 ± 115	0.608
PVR	BL	22.39 ± 40.49	22.97 ± 45.04	21.73 ± 35.38	
	1M	39.88 ± 56.78 *	25.97 ± 37.95	55.92 ± 70.16 *	0.045
	3M	34.46 ± 50.64	21.70 ± 27.06	49.19 ± 66.11 *	0.070
	6M	43.79 ± 78.38 *	40.97 ± 88.59	47.04 ± 66.26 *	0.735

* $p < 0.05$ compared with baseline data, Abbreviations: PRP: platelet-rich plasma, BoNT-A: botulinum toxin A, FBC: functional bladder capacity, Qmax: maximum flow rate, PVR: post-void residual.

Table 4. Changes in the global response assessment and adverse events after intravesical PRP or BoNT-A injection for patients with IC/BPS.

	PRP (n = 30)	BoNT-A (n = 26)	p-Value
1M GRA $\geq$ 2	5 (16.7%)	9 (34.6%)	0.122
3M GRA $\geq$ 2	12 (40.0%)	10 (38.5%)	0.906
6M GRA $\geq$ 2	14 (46.7%)	13 (50.0%)	0.803
AE-Dysuria	1 (3.3%)	5 (19.2%)	0.086
AE-UTI	0 (0.0%)	4 (15.4%)	0.041

Abbreviations: GRA: global response assessment, PRP: platelet-rich plasma, BoNT-A: botulinum toxin A, AE: adverse event, UTI: urinary tract infection.

Figure 1 shows the cumulative success rate curve after intravesical PRP or BoNT-A injection. Approximately 50% of patients in each group received an additional bladder therapy for bothersome symptoms after six months. There was no significant difference in the successful curves with time between groups.

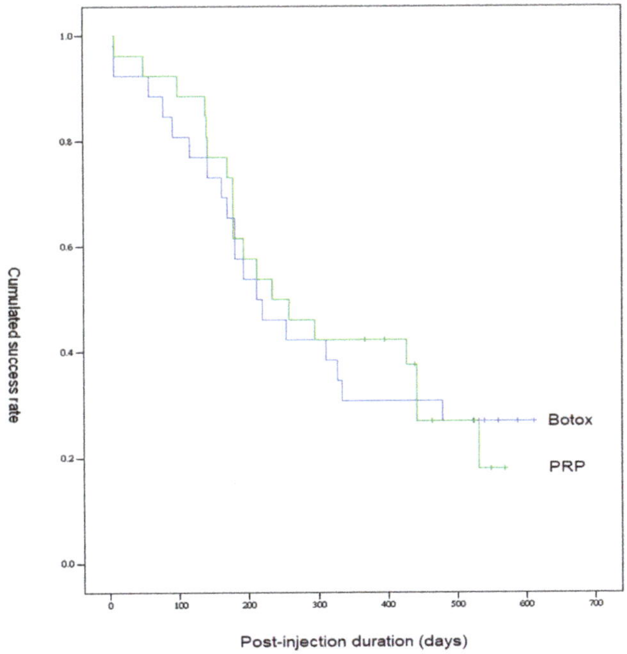

Figure 1. Survival curves of patients with IC/BPS who received either intravesical PRP or BoNT-A injections. Curves from the initial treatment day to the time in which they received additional treatment.

3. Discussion

This study demonstrated that intravesical injections of either PRP or BoNT-A are safe and effective in IC/BPS symptoms improvement without significantly increasing the PVR. Bladder pain reduction was not significant between groups at 6 months. Patients who received PRP injections did not experience UTI or dysuria after treatment. However, only half of the study cohort had a GRA of $\geq$2 at the six-month follow-up, and the remaining patients sought additional bladder therapy to improve symptoms. Although the therapeutic efficacy for IC/BPS at 6 months was similar between PRP and BoNT-A, the patients who received the BoNT-A injection had a greater potential risk for UTI after treatment.

The pathophysiology of IC/BPS is complicated and not completely understood. The recent IC Data Base study noted that loss of epithelial integrity is a predominant histopathologic finding in patients with IC/BPS. The epithelial damage may precede other histopathologic findings, such as suburothelial inflammation and sensory nervous activation in the bladder wall, leading to increases in the sensation of bladder fullness and pain in response to bladder inflammation [9,15]. The inflammation of IC/BPS might increase the sensory neuropeptides release from the suburothelial nervous network and integrate the signal transmission from urothelium to the detrusor muscles. In animal models of chemical cystitis or human studies of IC/BPS, detrusor injection of BoNT-A has been shown facilitate an increase in bladder capacity and relief of bladder pain [16,17]. Inhibition of sensory fiber neuroplasticity and inflammation in the suburothelial space by BoNT-A injections provides good therapeutic efficacy in patients with IC/BPS [18]. However, a single BoNT-A injection might not be adequate to provide long-term durability for IC/BPS. Our previous study also demonstrated that four consecutive BoNT-A injections provide a longer therapeutic duration than that of treatment with fewer injections [19].

An intravesical injection of 100–200 U of BoNT-A followed by cystoscopic hydrodistention has been reported effective in decreasing bladder pain and nocturia in patients with IC/BPS [20]. A randomized, double-blind clinical trial demonstrated that 100 U of BoNT-A is safe and effective for treatment of IC/BPS [21]. Patients who received BoNT-A treatment had a significantly greater improvement in bladder pain reduction and bladder capacity increase than that of those in the placebo group. The therapeutic effects of BoNT-A on IC/BPS are result from inhibition of the noxious neurotransmitter releases [17]. Based on the above clinical and basic science evidence, BoNT-A injection was listed as the fourth-line therapeutic option in the treatment of IC/BPS in the AUA guidelines [22].

Although the BoNT-A injection seems promising for treating symptoms of IC/PBS, long-term results have not revealed a successful outcome [21]. The limited successful result is possibly due to inadequate control of chronic inflammation inside the urinary bladder [17]. Repeated intravesical BoNT-A injections were recently performed for patients with refractory IC/PBS, and the therapeutic effects appear promising. Approximately 70% of patients with non-ulcer type IC/PBS may benefit from repeated BoNT-A injections every six months [23]. A previous immunohistochemistry study also confirmed the reduction in inflammatory biomarkers and pro-apoptotic proteins, such as Bax and Bad expressions, after repeated BoNT-A injections. Furthermore, the adhesive protein E-cadherin and junction protein zonula occludens were increased after repeat BoNT-A injections. These immunohistochemistry changes correlated well with the improvement in clinical symptoms [24].

Autologous PRP is growing in the treatment to augment wound healing, fasten the recovery speed of muscle and joint injuries, and enhance surgical repair recovery [25]. PRP is extremely rich in several essential growth factors and cytokines, which regulate tissue reconstruction, and has been studied extensively among trauma patients and trauma experimental models [26]. Tissue regeneration can be improved by the local application of autologous bone marrow derived progenitor cells and PRP. In addition, PRP eliminates neuropathic pain primarily by platelet- and stem cell-released factors. These factors initiate the complex cascade of wound healing events, starting with the induction of enhanced inflammation and its complete resolution, including tissue remodeling, wound repair, and axon regeneration, resulting in neuropathic pain elimination; some of these same factors also act directly on neurons to promote axon regeneration, thereby eliminating neuropathic pain [27].

PRP injecting into the bladder wall could initiate the wound healing process, induce a new inflammation, complete the wound healing, resolve previous inflammation, and promote the relief of neuropathic pain. The cytokines and growth factors released from PRP could induce a new inflammation, which might override the residual inflammation, and increase tissue regeneration [25]. Our previous clinical trial demonstrated that multiple low-dose PRP injections were effective in patients with IC/BPS. The PRP injections could effectively decrease IC symptoms and VAS bladder pain scores from 3.38 ± 2.89 at baseline to 1.10 ± 1.85 at 3 months after PRP injections [28]. The elevated urinary cytokines and inflammatory proteins could also be reduced after repeated PRP injections [29]. Moreover, the ultrastructural deficits in IC/BPS urothelial could also recovered after intravesical PRP injections [30].

Although this was not a head-to-head randomized trial, the results of this comparative case series study reveal that PRP and BoNT-A are equally effective in reducing IC symptoms. Based on the therapeutic mechanism of PRP and BoNT-A on IC/BPS, either treatment can reduce chronic inflammation and improve urothelial regeneration [12]. Therefore, IC symptoms and urinary inflammatory cytokines can decrease after treatment [29]. However, BoNT-A has a more potent inhibitory effect on the release of noxious inflammatory neuropeptides and could better reduce bladder pain, compared to the effect of the PRP injection. On the other hand, BoNT-A reduces detrusor contractility by inhibiting acetylcholine from efferent nerves; thus, a larger PVR may develop after treatment [17]. Nevertheless, the inhibitory effect of BoNT-A on detrusor contractility in IC/BPS bladders was less than that observed in patients with overactive bladders [31]. Although the increased PVR is not clinically significant, this adverse event might lead to a higher rate of difficult urination and increase the risk of UTI after BoNT-A injections.

Both PRP and BoNT-A treatments are novel and currently off-labeled therapies for IC/BPS refractory to conventional therapy. The long-term efficacy has not been well investigated. Although fewer adverse events were reported following treatment with PRP than with BoNT-A, the therapeutic effect of PRP on chronic inflammation and for promoting recovery of defective urothelium was limited. As shown in this study, the GRA increased with the increasing number of PRP injections, suggesting the therapeutic efficacy needs an adequate PRP dose to achieve a therapeutic level. Therefore, repeated intravesical PRP injections every month are necessary to achieve a therapeutic efficacy similar to that of BoNT-A at six months. However, repeated monthly PRP injection treatment requires frequent anesthesia, which might place a tremendous burden on the patients. Four monthly injections might also increase the complications related with bladder injections, including hematuria and UTI. Although therapy with a single high-dose injection of PRP has been attempted, the efficacy on symptom improvement was inferior to that of four monthly low-dose PRP injections [14]. In addition, the economic burden of frequent admission, anesthesia, and the cost of preparing the PRP might be much higher than that of a single BoNT-A injection within a six-month treatment period. Therefore, although the BoNT-A injection bears a greater potential for detrusor underactivity and UTI, repeated BoNT-A injections every six months have the advantage of greater bladder pain improvement and less of an anesthesia burden, with the same efficacy as that of PRP treatment. Single BoNT-A injection only provides short-term therapeutic effect, whereas repeat injections provide a higher success rate in long-term follow-up. Before recommending either treatment to patients with refractory IC/BPS, patients should be thoroughly informed as to the efficacy and potential adverse events of both treatments to allow for shared decision-making.

Limitations of this study are small case numbers, the lack of a control arm, and the non-randomization of the study design. The treatment option was based on patients' choice after informing advantage and disadvantages of the treatment outcome and potential adverse events. Because all patients were chronic IC/BPS and had received many different conventional therapies, they might have had high expectations to BoNT-A or PRP injection. Further, all patients were not selected with a strict inclusion criterion as in the clinical trials but were diagnosed according to their present symptoms and past history. Therefore, the patients in this retrospective study are highly heterogeneous with varying severity of disease. Finally, although a GRA $\geq$2 was reported in around 50% of patients treated with BoNT-A or PRP and the ICSI and ICPI also showed improvement, the decrease in bladder pain VAS was limited. The higher VAS in the baseline of the BoNT-A group could have resulted in bias in the VAS reduction between PRP and BoNT-A group. Because this was a retrospective analysis, patients were informed of the advantages and disadvantages of treatment at baseline, and patients were allowed to choose treatment; therefore, more patients who had a higher bladder pain VAS might have chosen the BoNT-A injection. Although a significant reduction in bladder pain VAS was observed in the BoNT-A group, the difference of VAS changes with time between PRP and BoNT-A groups was not significant. Nevertheless, the results of this study may reflect the treatment outcome of BoNT-A and PRP injection in a real-life practice.

In clinical trials for functional urology such as in IC/BPS, OAB, or LUTS, the subjective primary endpoint and objective secondary endpoints are usually not equally improved. Although the primary endpoint can reach a significant result, a placebo effect of up to 30% can usually be found in clinical trial. In this study we found the treatment success was limited in GRA improvement and the other objective variables such as voiding diary parameters, bladder volume increment, and bladder pain reduction were very mild. These results bring a message that, in real-life practice, treatment with a single small dose of BoNT-A or PRP might not be as successful as that in clinical trials. Nevertheless, the safety endpoints also revealed that both treatments were safe and tolerable. With repeated injections of BoNT-A or PRP, the treatment success might be improved. In the future, randomized controlled trials with different doses might be necessary and a search for prognostic factors could help urologists select IC/BPS patients for a good response to PRP or BoNT-A injections.

4. Conclusions

The results of this comparative case series study revealed that intravesical injections of either PRP or BoNT-A were safe and effective for improving IC/BPS symptoms without significantly increasing the PVR, but the bladder pain reduction was limited. Only half of the study cohort had a GRA $\geq$2 at six months. Repeat treatment of PRP or BoNT-A would be necessary to achieve long-term success. The BoNT-A injection carries a potential risk of UTI after treatment compared with that of the PRP injection.

5. Materials and Methods

A total of 56 female patients with confirmed IC/BPS who had failed conventional treatments received either a single intravesical BoNT-A 100 U injection (n = 26) or four monthly PRP injections (n = 30) within the two previous years. The IC/BPS was diagnosed according to the characteristic symptoms and cystoscopic findings after hydrodistention under anesthesia [32]. All patients had previously received at least two types of treatment modalities, including oral medication and intravesical treatment in recent years, with persistent bothersome symptoms and bladder pain. All potential patients received detailed urological examinations and were excluded if the diagnosis failed to meet the criteria of the National Institute of Diabetes and Digestive and Kidney Diseases (NIDDK) [33]. The patients were not randomly allocated to the BoNT-A or PRP group but were treated based on their choice. This study was approved by the Research Committee of Hualien Tzu Chi Hospital (IRB: 111-257-B, dated 15 December 2022). The requirement for informed consent was waived because this study was a retrospective analysis of data.

Patients' preferred treatment was scheduled after a discussion regarding the advantages and potential adverse effects of each treatment type. They were treated with either (1) an intravesical injection of 10 mL PRP (which was extracted from 50 mL of patient's blood) at 20 sites every month for four months, or (2) one intravesical dose of BoNT-A 100 U at 20 injection sites. Both treatments were followed by cystoscopic hydrodistention in the operation room. The primary endpoint was the global response assessment (GRA) recorded at six months after the first treatment day. The GRA scale included 6 items: worsening of symptoms (less than 0%), no change (0%), mild improvement (less than 50%), moderate improvement (50–75%), marked improvement (more than 75%), and completely cured (100%) [34].

All patients were asked to maintain a three-day voiding diary at baseline for recording the functional bladder capacity (FBC), urinary frequency, and nocturia. The IC symptoms were assessed by the O'Leary-Sant symptom score (OSS), including IC symptom index (ICSI) and IC problem index (ICPI) [35]. The bladder painwas scored by a self-assessed 10-point visual analog scale (VAS) system [36]. A videourodynamic study (VUDS) and a potassium chloride sensitivity test were routinely performed to exclude patients with detrusor overactivity or bladder outlet obstruction. All patients were informed of potential complications related to anesthesia and bladder injections, such as gross hematuria, micturition pain, and increased bladder pain after PRP or BoNT-A injection. Patients were also informed that the BoNT-A injection could lead to a greater reduction in bladder pain, and both BoNT-A and PRP injection could reduce the frequency episodes after treatment. However, BoNT-A injection might have adverse events of difficulty in urination, increased PVR, and UTI after injection, which had not been observed in our previous clinical trials of PRP injection.

The VUDS was performed at baseline and time-points after intravesical injections. The VUDS was performed with an infusion rate of 20 mL/min, and the procedures and terminology were according to the International Continence Society recommendations [37]. After the VUDS study, a potassium chloride (KCl) test using 0.4 M KCl solution infused into the bladder was performed. A positive KCl test was considered when a patient perceived a painful (VAS score of ≥2) or urgency sensation (urgency severity score increased by ≥1) [38].

PRP was prepared according to previously reported standard procedures [17]. In brief, 50 mL of whole blood was withdrawn at the same day of treatment. The blood was sent to the central laboratory and the blood was centrifuged twice with a slow spin (190× *g*, 20 min, <20 °C) and fast spin (2000× *g*, 20 min, <20 °C) of the supernatant plasma containing platelets. The lower third of the tube comprised PRP, and the upper part was platelet poor plasma (PPP). The platelet pellets were added to the plasma to obtain the desired concentration of PRP. In this study, 6 mL of sterile PRP was obtained. We sent 1 mL of PRP for culture and platelet count. The remaining 5 mL of PRP was used for intravesical injection. A total of 20 suburothelial injections of the PRP solution were performed, with 0.25 mL of PRP at each site, using a 23-gauge needle and a rigid injection instrument (22 Fr, Richard Wolf, and Knittlingen, Germany). The injection was approximately 1 mm in depth into the suburothelium equally distributed at posterior and lateral bladder walls, Cystoscopic hydrodistention was performed immediately after PRP injection to activate the injected platelets and determine the maximal bladder capacity (MBC). The PRP injection procedure was repeated every month for four months. A total of 10 mL of sterile normal saline was used to dissolve the BoNT-A powder to a concentration of 5 U at each site. The BoNT-A solution was gently shaken and then slowly withdrawn and injected at 20 well-distributed sites at posterior and lateral bladder wall followed by cystoscopic hydrodistention as previously reported [17]. After the PRP or BoNT-A injections, a urethral catheter was indwelled overnight, and oral antibiotics were taken for three days.All patients were followed up at one, three, and six months after the first injection day. Urinalysis was routinely checked at each time point and UTI was considered if patients had bladder pain or micturition pain and a white blood cell count >10/high power field in urinalysis.

The three-day voiding diary data (including FBC, daily frequency and nocturia episodes), ICSI, ICPI symptom score, and bladder pain VAS were recorded at baseline (first PRP and BoNT-A injection), and at one, three (fourth PRP injection), and six (three months after fourth PRP, and six months after BoNT-A injection) months. At the one-, three-, and six-month (primary endpoint) follow-up, patients reported any improvement in IC symptoms and adverse events were recorded. An excellent treatment outcome was considered when patients reported a GRA of ≥2 or no bladder pain (VAS = 0). The outcome was considered improved if there was improvement in the GRA by = 1 or the pain VAS score reduced by two or more and there was at least a 25% decrease in urinary frequency and nocturia. Patients with excellent and improved results were considered as having a successful treatment. After the primary endpoint assessment, the patients were continuously followed up with medications, such as anti-inflammatory agents and pain killers only. If the patient's IC symptoms exacerbated and they requested bladder therapy, the duration from the first injection day to the consecutive bladder therapy was recorded as the effective duration.

The data of voiding diary, VUDS parameters, symptom score, and bladder pain VAS score at baseline, one, three, and six months after the first injection day were compared in each group. A successful result was assessed by a self-reported improvement in GRA and pain VAS score. The data were presented as the mean ± standard deviation. Comparisons between PRP and BoNT-A groups were analyzed by the Student's t-test to compare numerical data, and the Chi-square test for categorical data. Cumulative success rate was also calculated using Kaplan–Meier survival curves to compare the success rates from the initial treatment day to receiving additional treatment between groups. All statistical analyses were performed using the statistical package SPSS for Windows (Version 12, SPSS, Chicago, IL, USA). A *p*-value of less than 0.05 was considered statistically significant.

Author Contributions: Concept: H.-C.K.; investigation: J.-F.J. and W.-R.Y.; design: H.-C.K.; draft writing: J.-F.J.; manuscript writing and supervision: H.-C.K. All authors have read and agreed to the published version of the manuscript.

Funding: This research was funded by Buddhist Tzu Chi Medical Foundation grant TCMF-SP-108-01, and grant TCMF-MP-110-03-01.

Institutional Review Board Statement: This study was approved by the Research Committee of Hualien Tzu Chi Hospital (IRB: 111-257-B, dated 15 December 2022).

Informed Consent Statement: The informed consent form was waived because of the nature of retrospective analysis.

Data Availability Statement: Data can be obtained with permission of the corresponding author.

Conflicts of Interest: The author declares no conflict of interest.

References

1. Hanno, P.M.; Sant, G.R. Clinical highlights of the National Institute of Diabetes and Digestive and Kidney Diseases/Interstitial Cystitis Association scientific conference on interstitial cystitis. *Urology* **2001**, *57*, 2–6. [CrossRef] [PubMed]
2. Payne, C.K.; Mosbaugh, P.G.; Forrest, J.B.; Evans, R.J.; Whitmore, K.E.; Antoci, J.P.; Perez-Marrero, R.; Jacoby, K.; Diokno, A.C.; O'Reilly, K.J.; et al. Intravesical resiniferatoxin for the treatment of interstitial cystitis: A randomized, double-blind, placebo controlled trial. *J. Urol.* **2005**, *173*, 1590–1594. [CrossRef] [PubMed]
3. Nickel, J.C.; Barkin, J.; Forrest, J.; Mosbaugh, P.G.; Hernandez-Graulau, J.; Kaufman, D.; Lloyd, K.; Evans, R.J.; Parsons, C.L.; Atkinson, L.E. Randomized, double-blind, dose-ranging study of pentosan polysulfate sodium for interstitial cystitis. *Urology* **2005**, *65*, 654–658. [CrossRef] [PubMed]
4. Sant, G.; Propert, K.; Hanno, P.; Burks, D.; Culkin, D.; Diokno, A.; Hardy, C.; Landis, J.R.; Mayer, R.; Madigan, R.; et al. A pilot clinical trial of oral pentosan polysulfate and oral hydroxyzine in patients with interstitial cystitis. *J. Urol.* **2003**, *170*, 810–815. [CrossRef]
5. Hanno, P.M.; Buehler, J.; Wein, A.J. Use of amitriptyline in the treatment of interstitial cystitis. *J. Urol.* **1989**, *141*, 846–848. [CrossRef] [PubMed]
6. Sairanen, J.; Forsell, T.; Ruutu, M. Long-term outcome of patients with interstitial cystitis treated with low dose cyclosporine A. *J. Urol.* **2004**, *171*, 2138–2141. [CrossRef] [PubMed]
7. Keay, S.; Zhang, C.-O.; Kagen, D.; Hise, M.; Jacobs, S.; Hebel, J.; Gordon, D.; Whitmore, K.; Bodison, S.; Warren, J. Concentrations of specific epithelial growth factors in the urine of interstitial cystitis patients and controls. *J. Urol.* **1997**, *158*, 1983–1988. [CrossRef]
8. Tomaszewski, J.E.; Landis, J.; Russack, V.; Williams, T.M.; Wang, L.-P.; Hardy, C.; Brensinger, C.; Matthews, Y.L.; Abele, S.T.; Kusek, J.W.; et al. Biopsy features are associated with primary symptoms in interstitial cystitis: Results from the interstitial cystitis database study. *Urology* **2001**, *57*, 67–81. [CrossRef]
9. Brady, C.; Apostolidis, A.; Harper, M.; Yiangou, Y.; Beckett, A.; Jacques, T.; Freeman, A.; Scaravilli, F.; Fowler, C.; Anand, P. Parallel changes in bladder suburothelial vanilloid receptor TRPV1 and pan-neuronal marker PGP9.5 immunoreactivity in patients with neurogenic detrusor overactivity after intravesical resiniferatoxin treatment. *BJU Int.* **2004**, *93*, 770–776. [CrossRef]
10. Ikeda, Y.; Zabbarova, I.V.; Birder, L.A.; de Groat, W.C.; McCarthy, C.J.; Hanna-Mitchell, A.T.; Kanai, A.J. Botulinum neurotoxin serotype A suppresses neurotransmitter release from afferent as well as efferent nerves in the urinary bladder. *Eur. Urol.* **2012**, *62*, 1157–1164. [CrossRef]
11. Lin, C.C.; Huang, Y.C.; Lee, W.C.; Chuang, Y.C. New frontiers or the treatment of interstitial cystitis/bladder pain syndrome-Focused on stem cells, platelet-rich plasma, and low-energy shock wave. *Int. Neurourol. J.* **2020**, *24*, 211–221. [CrossRef]
12. Jhang, J.-F.; Jiang, Y.-H.; Hsu, Y.-H.; Ho, H.-C.; A Birder, L.; Lin, T.-Y.; Kuo, H.-C. Improved urothelial cell proliferation, cytoskeleton and barrier function protein expression in the patients with interstitial cystitis/bladder pain syndrome after intravesical platelet-rich plasma injection. *Int. Neurourol. J.* **2022**, *26*, S57–S67. [CrossRef] [PubMed]
13. Abrar, M.; Pindoria, N.; Malde, S.; Chancellor, M.; DeRidder, D.; Sahai, A. Predictors of poor response and adverse events following botulinum toxin A for refractory idiopathic overactive bladder: A systematic review. *Eur. Urol. Focus* **2021**, *7*, 1448–1467. [CrossRef] [PubMed]
14. Jiang, Y.-H.; Jhang, J.-F.; Lin, T.-Y.; Ho, H.-C.; Hsu, Y.-H.; Kuo, H.-C. Therapeutic efficacy of intravesical platelet-rich plasma injections for interstitial cystitis/bladder pain syndrome-A comparative study of different injection number, additives and concentrations. *Front. Pharmacol.* **2022**, *13*, 853776. [CrossRef] [PubMed]
15. Cockayne, D.A.; Hamilton, S.G.; Zhu, Q.-M.; Dunn, P.M.; Zhong, Y.; Novakovic, S.; Malmberg, A.B.; Cain, G.; Berson, A.; Kassotakis, L.; et al. Urinary bladder hyporeflexia and reduced pain-related behaviour in P2X3-deficient mice. *Nature* **2000**, *407*, 1011–1015. [CrossRef]
16. Çayan, S.; Coşkun, B.; Bozlu, M.; Acar, D.; Akbay, E.; Ulusoy, E. Botulinum toxin type A may improve bladder function in a rat chemical cystitis model. *Urol. Res.* **2003**, *30*, 399–404. [CrossRef] [PubMed]
17. Kuo, H.-C.; Jiang, Y.-H.; Tsai, Y.-C.; Kuo, Y.-C. Intravesical botulinum toxin-A injections reduce bladder pain of interstitial cystitis/bladder pain syndrome refractory to conventional treatment-A prospective, multicenter, randomized, double-blind, placebo-controlled clinical trial. *Neurourol. Urodyn.* **2016**, *35*, 609–614. [CrossRef]
18. Steers, W.D.; Tuttle, J.B. Mechanisms of disease: The role of nerve growth factor in the pathophysiology of bladder disorders. *Nat. Clin. Pract. Urol.* **2006**, *3*, 101–110. [CrossRef]

19. Kuo, H.C. Repeated onabotulinumtoxin-a injections provide better results than single injection in treatment of painful bladder syndrome. *Pain Phys.* **2013**, *16*, E15–E23. [CrossRef]
20. Smith, C.P.; Radziszewski, P.; Borkowski, A.; Somogyi, G.T.; Boone, T.B.; Chancellor, M.B. Botulinum toxin A has antinociceptive effects in treating interstitial cystitis. *Urology* **2004**, *64*, 871–875, discussion 875. [CrossRef]
21. Giannantoni, A.; Porena, M.; Costantini, E.; Zucchi, A.; Mearini, L.; Mearini, E. Botulinum A toxin intravesical injection in patients with painful bladder syndrome: 1-year followup. *J. Urol.* **2008**, *179*, 1031–1034. [CrossRef]
22. Hanno, P.M.; Erickson, D.; Moldwin, R.; Faraday, M.M. American Urological Association. Diagnosis and treatment of interstitial cystitis/bladder pain syndrome: AUA guideline amendment. *J. Urol.* **2015**, *193*, 1545–1553. [CrossRef]
23. Lee, C.L.; Kuo, H.C. Long-term efficacy and safety of repeated intravescial onabotulinumtoxinA injections plus hydrodistention in the treatment of interstitial cystitis/bladder pain syndrome. *Toxins* **2015**, *7*, 4283–4293. [CrossRef]
24. Shie, J.H.; Liu, H.T.; Wang, Y.S.; Kuo, H.C. Immunohistochemical evidence suggests repeated intravesical application of botulinum toxin A injections may improve treatment efficacy of interstitial cystitis/bladder pain syndrome. *BJU Int.* **2013**, *111*, 638–646. [CrossRef]
25. Mussano, F.; Genova, T.; Munaron, L.; Petrillo, S.; Erovigni, F.; Carossa, S. Cytokine, chemokine, and growth factor profile of platelet-rich plasma. *Platelets* **2016**, *27*, 467–471. [CrossRef]
26. Amable, P.R.; Carias, R.B.V.; Teixeira, M.V.T.; da Cruz Pacheco, Í.; Amaral, R.J.F.C.D.; Granjeiro, J.M.; Borojevic, R. Platelet-rich plasma preparation for regenerative medicine: Optimization and quantification of cytokines and growth factors. *Stem. Cell Res. Ther.* **2013**, *4*, 67. [CrossRef]
27. Wang, B.; Geng, Q.; Hu, J.; Shao, J.; Ruan, J.; Zheng, J. Platelet-rich plasma reduces skin flap inflammatory cells infiltration and improves survival rates through induction of angiogenesis: An experiment in rabbits. *J. Plast. Surg. Hand Surg.* **2016**, *50*, 239–245. [CrossRef]
28. Jhang, J.; Lin, T.; Kuo, H. Intravesical injections of platelet-rich plasma is effective and safe in treatment of interstitial cystitis refractory to conventional treatment–A prospective clinical trial. *Neurourol. Urodyn.* **2019**, *38*, 703–709. [CrossRef]
29. Jiang, Y.-H.; Kuo, Y.-C.; Jhang, J.-F.; Lee, C.-L.; Hsu, Y.-H.; Ho, H.-C.; Kuo, H.-C. Repeated intravesical injections of platelet-rich plasma improve symptoms and alter urinary functional proteins in patients with refractory interstitial cystitis. *Sci. Rep.* **2020**, *10*, 15218. [CrossRef]
30. Lee, Y.-K.; Jiang, Y.-H.; Jhang, J.-F.; Ho, H.-C.; Kuo, H.-C. Changes in the ultrastructure of the bladder urothelium in patients with interstitial cystitis after intravesical injections of platelet-rich plasma. *Biomedicines* **2022**, *10*, 1182. [CrossRef]
31. Kuo, Y.C.; Kuo, H.C. Adverse events of intravesical onabotulinumtoxinA injection between patients with overactive bladder and interstitial cystitis-Different mechanisms of action of Botox on bladder dysfunction? *Toxins* **2016**, *8*, 75. [CrossRef]
32. Homma, Y.; Akiyama, Y.; Tomoe, H.; Furuta, A.; Ueda, T.; Maeda, D.; Lin, A.T.; Kuo, H.-C.; Lee, M.-H.; Oh, S.-J.; et al. Clinical guidelines for interstitial cystitis/bladder pain syndrome. *Int. J. Urol.* **2020**, *27*, 578–589. [CrossRef]
33. Hanno, P.-M.; Landis, J.-R.; Matthews-Cook, Y.; Kusek, J.; Nyberg, L., Jr. The diagnosis of interstitial cystitis revisited: Lessons learned from the National Institute of Health Interstitial Cystitis Database study. *J. Urol.* **1999**, *161*, 553–557. [CrossRef]
34. Parsons, C.L.; Benson, G.; Childs, S.J.; Hanno, P.; Sant, G.R.; Webster, G. A quantitatively controlled method to study prospectively interstitial cystitis and demonstrate the efficacy of pentosanpolysulfate. *J. Urol.* **1993**, *150*, 845–848. [CrossRef]
35. Lubeck, D.P.; Whitmore, K.; Sant, G.R.; Alvarez-Horine, S.; Lai, C. Psychometric validation of the O'Leary-Sant interstitial cystitis symptom index in a clinical trial of pentosan polysulfate sodium. *Urology* **2001**, *57*, 62–66. [CrossRef]
36. Gülpınar, O.; Kayış, A.; Süer, E.; Gökçe, M.İ.; Güçlü, A.G.; Arıkan, N. Clinical comparision of intravesical hyaluronic acid and hyaluronic acid-chondroitin sulphate therapy for patients with bladder pain syndrome/interstitital cystitis. *Can. Urol. Assoc. J.* **2014**, *8*, E610–E614. [CrossRef]
37. Abrams, P.; Cardozo, L.; Fall, M.; Griffiths, D.; Rosier, P.; Ulmsten, U.; Van Kerrebroeck, P.; Victor, A.; Wein, A. The standardisation of terminology of lower urinary tract function: Report from the Standardisation Sub-Committee of the International Continence Society. *Neurourol. Urodyn.* **2002**, *21*, 167–178. [CrossRef]
38. Parsons, C.L.; Greenberger, M.; Gabal, L.; Bidair, M.; Barme, G. The role of urinary potassium in the pathogenesis and diagnosis of interstitial cystitis. *J. Urol.* **1998**, *159*, 1862–1866. [CrossRef]

Disclaimer/Publisher's Note: The statements, opinions and data contained in all publications are solely those of the individual author(s) and contributor(s) and not of MDPI and/or the editor(s). MDPI and/or the editor(s) disclaim responsibility for any injury to people or property resulting from any ideas, methods, instructions or products referred to in the content.

toxins

MDPI

Review

Liposome-Encapsulated Botulinum Toxin A in Treatment of Functional Bladder Disorders

Fan-Ching Hung [1] and Hann-Chorng Kuo [2,*]

1 Department of Urology, National Taiwan University Hospital Yunlin Branch, Douliu 64041, Taiwan
2 Department of Urology, Hualien Tzu Chi Hospital, Buddhist Tzu Chi Medical Foundation, Tzu Chi University, Hualien 97004, Taiwan
* Correspondence: hck@tzuchi.com.tw; Tel.: +886-3-8561825 (ext. 2113); Fax: +886-3-8560794

Abstract: Botulinum toxin A (BoNT-A) intravesical injections have been used to treat patients with refractory functional bladder disorders such as overactive bladder (OAB) and interstitial cystitis/bladder pain syndrome (IC/BPS), but the risk of adverse events and the need for repeated injections continue to prevent widespread application of this treatment. Liposomes are vesicles that comprise concentric phospholipid layers and an aqueous core; their flexible compositions enable them to adsorb and fuse with cell membranes and to deliver drugs or proteins into cells. Therefore, liposomes have been considered as promising vehicles for the less invasive delivery of BoNT-A. In previous placebo-controlled trials including patients with OAB refractory to medical treatment, it was shown that liposomal BoNT-A could significantly decrease the frequency and urgency of urination. In patients with IC/BPS, it was shown that liposomal BoNT-A could also improve bladder pain, but the therapeutic efficacy was not superior to that of the placebo. As the therapeutic mechanisms of BoNT-A include the decreased expression of nerve growth factors, P2X3 receptors, and vanilloid receptors on C-fibers, liposomal BoNT-A might play a more promising role in the treatment of bladder oversensitivity. This article features the contemporary literature regarding BoNT-A, liposomes, and liposomal BoNT-A treatment for functional bladder disorders and potential clinical applications in the future.

Keywords: botulinum toxin A; liposome; bladder oversensitivity; interstitial cystitis; detrusor overactivity

Key Contribution: Intravesical instillation of liposome-encapsulated botulinum toxin A can be a potential treatment option to treat functional bladder disorders such as OAB, IC/BPS, and bladder oversensitivity.

Citation: Hung, F.-C.; Kuo, H.-C. Liposome-Encapsulated Botulinum Toxin A in Treatment of Functional Bladder Disorders. *Toxins* **2022**, *14*, 838. https://doi.org/10.3390/toxins14120838

Received: 12 October 2022
Accepted: 29 November 2022
Published: 1 December 2022

Publisher's Note: MDPI stays neutral with regard to jurisdictional claims in published maps and institutional affiliations.

Copyright: © 2022 by the authors. Licensee MDPI, Basel, Switzerland. This article is an open access article distributed under the terms and conditions of the Creative Commons Attribution (CC BY) license (https://creativecommons.org/licenses/by/4.0/).

1. Introduction

Functional bladder disorders are a group of lower urinary tract disorders with unclarified structural etiologies, including overactive bladder (OAB) syndrome, bladder hypersensitivity, and interstitial cystitis/bladder pain syndrome (IC/BPS). These disorders are characterized by a relapsing–remitting course and require multiple treatments [1].

The prevalence rate of OAB ranges from 10.8% to 27.2% in men and 12.8% to 43.1% in women [2–6]. OAB is characterized by frequency, urgency, and nocturia, with or without urgency urinary incontinence (UUI). Behavioral therapies, oral antimuscarinics, and oral β3-adrenoceptor agonists are often offered as the first- and second-line treatments [7]. However, there are high withdrawal rates when using these OAB medications due to unsatisfactory symptom control or undesirable adverse effects [8].

Population-based studies conducted in the USA revealed that the prevalence of IC/BPS is 2% to 4.2% in men and 2.7% to 6.3% in women [9,10]. The definition of IC/BPS according to the Society for Urodynamics and Female Urology (SUFU) is the perception of pain, pressure, or discomfort in the urinary bladder caused by lower urinary tract symptoms lasting for over six weeks, without other identifiable causes [11]. American Urological Association (AUA) guidelines have suggested behavior modification; pain management; specialized manual physical therapy; oral agents such as amitriptyline, cimetidine, hydroxyzine, and pentosan polysulfate sodium; and intravesical therapy including dimethylsulfoxide (DMSO), heparin, and lidocaine as initial therapeutic approaches [12].

Intravesical botulinum toxin subtype A (BoNT-A) injections have been considered as an effective treatment option for patients with OAB and IC/BPS refractory to conventional medications or therapies. However, the risk of adverse events after BoNT-A injection and the need for repeated injections continue to prevent the widespread application of this treatment [13,14]. Clinicians have been searching for a less invasive treatment modality for the delivery of BoNT-A to achieve treatment efficacy without intravesical injection and adverse events [15].

Liposomes are vesicles that comprise concentric phospholipid layers and an aqueous core; their flexible compositions enable them to adsorb and fuse with cell membranes and deliver drugs or proteins into cells. Therefore, liposomes have been considered as promising vehicles for the less invasive delivery of BoNT-A to achieve a therapeutic effect without intravesical injection or the development of adverse events. In this article, we aim to review the current literature regarding the management of functional bladder disorders via liposomal BoNT-A instillation.

2. Botulinum Toxin A Mechanism and Clinical Applications

2.1. The Urinary Bladder and Botulinum Toxin A Mechanism

The bladder wall comprises urothelium, detrusor muscle, and adventitia, from the lumen to the outer surface. The bladder urothelium serves as an impermeable barrier preventing the penetration of urine and waste content into the submucosal layer [16]. From the apical to the detrusor side, the urothelium is constituted of umbrella cells, intermediate cells and basal cells [17]. Tight junctional proteins, uroplakins, and a glycosaminoglycan (GAG) mucin layer cover the umbrella cells, which help to establish the barrier function.

Botulinum toxin is a neurotoxic protein produced from Clostridium botulinum; the subtype A (BoNT-A) is the most popular clinically used form, with a 50 kDa light chain and a 100 kDa heavy chain bridged by a disulfide bond [18]. The heavy chain of BoNT-A binds to synaptic vesicle glycoprotein 2 (SV2) receptors on the surface of the parasympathetic nerve terminal and is then endocytosed into synaptic vesicles. The light chain is released from the vesicle to cleave synaptosomal-associated protein, 25 kDa (SNAP-25) and prevents the vesicles from fusion with the nerve terminal membrane, thereby inhibiting acetylcholine release and detrusor muscle contraction [19]. The accumulation of BoNT-A can decrease the bladder sensation by inhibiting ATP release into the suburothelium, indicating its mechanism of action may also involve inhibition of neurotransmitter release from afferent nerve terminals and the urothelium [20].

2.2. Botulinum Toxin A Injection for OAB

BoNT-A has been commonly utilized to treat bladder muscular hypercontractility and modulate sensory and inflammatory function [21]. In the last decade, the FDA approved the intradetrusor injection of 200 units of BoNT-A for the treatment of neurogenic detrusor overactivity (NDO) and the injection of 100 units of BoNT-A for the treatment of idiopathic OAB [22]. It was shown that BoNT-A 100 U intradetrusor injections significantly improved all OAB symptoms, including urgency, UUI, and health-related quality of life [23–25]. It was found that male gender, a baseline post-void residual (PVR) volume of more than 100 mL, and medical comorbidity are independent risk factors of acute urinary retention or large PVR after intravesical BoNT-A injections for the treatment of idiopathic OAB [26]. Subjectively successful treatment outcomes of intravesical BoNT-A injection for patients with OAB were associated with improvements in OAB symptoms but not with increases in bladder capacity, PVR volume, or voiding efficiency [27]. The balance of the therapeutic and adverse effects of BoNT-A injections can be modified by amending the dose and changing the injection site [28]. It was shown that BoNT-A injection at the bladder base and trigone could relieve the sensation of urgency but did not increase the PVR volume or the bladder capacity. After intravesical BoNT-A injections, the duration of their effect on OAB symptoms is about 6–9 months; therefore, repeated injections are necessary to maintain the efficacy of this treatment [29].

2.3. Botulinum Toxin A Injection for IC/BPS

The clinical symptoms of IC/BPS, such as frequency, urgency, and bladder pain, are considered to result from urothelial dysfunction and increased urothelial permeability [30]. There are higher levels of urothelial cell apoptosis, mast cell activation, abnormal E-cadherin expression, and less cell proliferation in patients with IC/BPS [31]. Increased urinary nerve growth factor levels were noted in patients with IC/BPS, and decreased levels in successful BoNT-A treatment responders, suggesting neurogenic inflammation might be involved in the pathogenesis of IC/BPS [32]. Intravesical injection of BoNT-A followed by cystoscopic hydrodistention significantly improved the clinically successful treatment response rate compared with cystoscopic hydrodistention alone [33]. Repeated intravesical BoNT-A injections in patients with IC/BPS resulted in significantly reduced numbers of apoptotic cells and the activation of mast cells [34]. The immunohistochemical findings were associated with the improvement of the maximal bladder capacity and glomerulation grade after cystoscopic hydrodistention. Patients who received repeated BoNT-A injections experienced an increase in functional bladder capacity and had longer-term pain relief than the relief that a single injection provided, without the increased prevalence of adverse events [35]. In patients with refractory IC/BPS, compared with the placebo-controlled group, suburothelial injections of 100 U of BoNT-A plus cystoscopic hydrodistention significantly reduced bladder pain symptoms [14]. In the AUA guidelines for IC/BPS, it is recommended to administer intradetrusor BoNT-A injections if other treatments provide an inadequate improvement of symptoms, while patients should be informed of the possibility of intermittent self-catheterization. In real-life practice, there is very little need for intermittent self-catheterization after BoNT-A injection for patients with IC/BPS [14,33,35]. Evidence showed that a reduced morbidity rate was reported with the dose of 100 U [12].

3. Liposome Mechanism and Applications to Functional Bladder Disorders

Urothelium serves as a barrier that prevents urine constituents and solutes from penetrating into the submucosal layer. Substances move across the urothelium via one pathway through cells and another through tight junctions and lateral intercellular spaces [17]. Alterations in either cellular or tight junction permeability change the urothelium barrier's characteristics [36]. Liposomes are microlevel vesicles that consist of concentric phospholipid layers and an aqueous core, with the ability to adsorb and merge with cells. Their flexible compositions make them suitable delivery vehicles for various molecules, including proteins, nucleotides, and small drug molecules [16]. Liposomes not prepared with drugs could form a molecular film on cell surfaces, and their wound-healing properties on skin were confirmed with animal models [37,38].

In a rat model of protamine-sulfate/potassium-chloride-induced bladder hyperactivity, it was shown that the intravesical instillation of liposomes could reverse the high micturition frequency [39]. Intravesical liposome infusion significantly reversed the decrease in the intercontractile interval in rats with chemically induced bladder hyperactivity, showing superior beneficial effects compared to DMSO and pentosan polysulfate sodium [40]. It was hypothesized that liposomes might reinforce the barrier function of a leaky urothelium and gain resistance against the penetration of irritants. In a comparative study, it was shown that the intravesical instillation of liposomes could achieve similar efficacy to oral pentosan polysulfate sodium for patients with IC/BPS. The instillation of 80 mg of liposomes in 40 mL of distilled water once weekly for 4 weeks was shown to improve the symptoms of pain and urgency for up to 8 weeks [41]. In a study comparing once-a-week or twice-a-week treatment within a 4-week period, 6 of 12 patients and 4 of 5 patients responded to liposome treatment, respectively. More frequent instillation was tolerable and had a potential benefit with regard to symptom flare-up, while the effects after 8 weeks of follow-up were not clear [42]. An open-label clinical evaluation also revealed symptom improvement without treatment-related adverse events [43].

4. Mechanism and Clinical Effects of Liposome Encapsulated Botulinum Toxin A

Although the therapeutic effects of intravesical BoNT-A injections on OAB and IC/PBS have been established, the need for a novel delivery method with lower risk became apparent due to certain adverse effects related to these injections, such as hematuria, injection pain, urinary tract infection, the uneven distribution of the drug, and drug leakage outside the bladder [44,45]. Thus, intravesical instillation was proposed with potential advantages, such as extending duration of drug contact with urothelium, decreasing systemic toxicity side effects while achieving higher drug concentrations, and modulating urothelium repair, neurotransmission, and sensory nerve function [46].

The instillation of BoNT-A delivery via liposomes was first reported in a rat model [47]. Rats pretreated with liposomes and BoNT-A displayed a considerable decrease in the inter-contractile interval after acetic acid (AA) infusion, whereas those pretreated with liposome-encapsulated BoNT-A (liposomal BoNT-A) showed a significantly diminished response to AA instillation. The study results demonstrated that liposomal BoNT-A pretreatment could suppress AA-induced bladder overactivity. Histologically, less inflammatory cell accumulation and edematous changes were also observed in the liposomal BoNT-A pretreated group. The calcitonin-gene-related peptide (CGRP) is one of the sensory mediators that is released in response to toxic stimuli, and BoNT-A can inhibit its release [48]. CGRP immunostaining in the bladder mucosal layer revealed that intravesical liposomal BoNT-A instillation inhibited CGRP release from afferent nerve terminals. The expression of SNAP-25 was also significantly decreased in the liposomal BoNT-A pretreated group compared to that in the liposome or BoNT-A pretreated groups, indicating that liposomal BoNT-A pretreatment could cleave SNAP-25. The concept of using liposomes as vehicles for BoNT-A delivery was supported by these results, while the actual mechanism of liposomal BoNT-A adsorption and transport in the urothelium remains to be discovered (Figure 1).

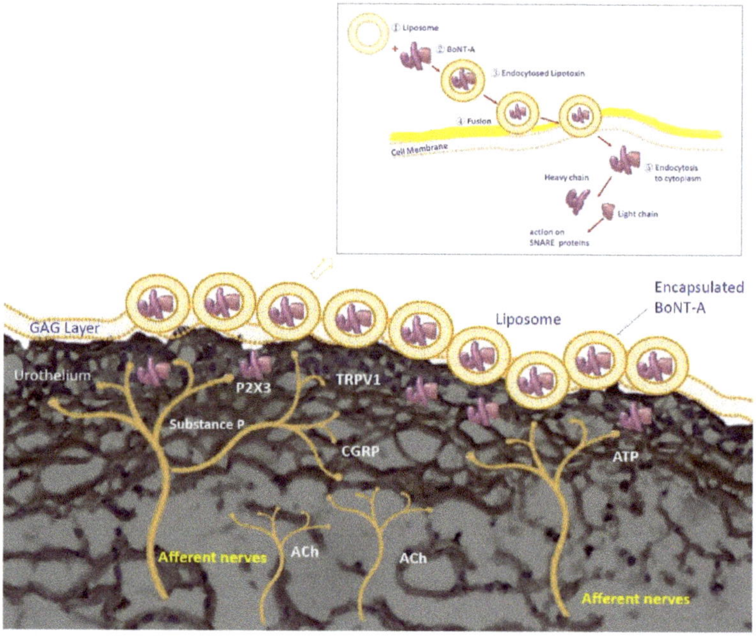

Figure 1. Empty liposomes mixed with botulinum toxin A (BoNT-A) solution yields encapsulated BoNT-A. After fusion with the phospholipid layer of the cell membrane of urothelial cells, the BoNT-A protein is endocytosed and transferred into the cytoplasm of the urothelial cells. The BoNT-A protein is cleaved into a heavy chain and a light chain; the latter acts on the SNARE protein complex, inhibits the releases of neurotransmitters, including acetylcholine (ACh), adenosine triphosphate (ATP), calcitonin-gene-related peptide (CGRP), and substance P, from the sensory nerve terminals, and suppresses the expression of transient receptor potential vanilloid receptor subfamily 1 (TRPV1) as well as purinergic receptor P2X3.

4.1. Liposome-Encapsulated Botulinum Toxin A for Treatment of OAB

The liposome encapsulated BoNT-A for clinical use was prepared with the following procedures. Sphingomyelin mixed with normal saline (N/S) creates a liposomal dispersion of sphingomyelin. Sphingomyelin liposomes are available for preparation at a concentration of 2 mg/mL (2.84 mM) in N/S containing 500 mM KCl (LP-08, Lipella Pharmaceuticals Inc., Pittsburgh, PA, USA). Lipotoxin was prepared before application by hydrating 80 mg freeze-dried LP-08 in 40 mL N/S and 200 U BoNT-A (Botox, Allergan, Irvine, CA, USA) in 10 mL N/S to make a total volume of 50 mL at room temperature [49].

In a double-blind, randomized, controlled trial, 24 patients with OAB received the intravesical instillation of liposomal BoNT-A (80 mg of liposomes and 200 U BoNT-A) or N/S (control group) [49]. The liposomal BoNT-A treatment was effective in reducing the number of frequency and urgency episodes 1 month after treatment, with an efficacy of 50% (6 out of 12 patients). No adverse events, such as urinary retention, large PVR volumes, or urinary tract infections (UTIs), were reported during the study period. In immunohistochemical staining and Western blotting, there were no significant differences in the synaptic vesicle protein 2A (SV2A) and SNAP-25 expressions at baseline and 3 months after liposomal BoNT-A treatment in the responders or non-responders. Another multicenter, double-blind, randomized, placebo-controlled study enrolled 62 patients with OAB inadequately treated with antimuscarinics to receive an intravesical instillation of liposomal BoNT-A or normal saline [50]. The results showed that treatment with liposomal BoNT-A reduced the number of episodes of voiding frequency, urgency, and overactive bladder symptom score (OABSS) but not urge incontinence 1 month after treatment. No urinary retention, increase in PVR, or any drug-related adverse events were noted. A study comparing the BoNT-A injection and liposomal BoNT-A instillation showed that there was decreased expression of ionotropic purinergic receptor P2X3 in the urothelia of responders, but no cleaved SNAP-25 was detected in the suburothelium 1 month after liposomal BoNT-A treatment [51]. To further enhance its clinical usability, the short therapeutic duration and depth of penetration require technical improvement in terms of instillation.

4.2. Liposome-Encapsulated Botulinum Toxin A for IC/BPS

A multicenter, double-blind, randomized, placebo-controlled study enrolled patients with refractory IC/BPS. In total, 96 eligible patients were assigned at a 1:1:1 ratio to three groups, including treatment with liposomal BoNT-A (BoNT-A 200 U with 80 mg liposome), BoNT-A 200 U in normal saline, or normal saline alone. Four weeks after treatment, liposomal BoNT-A instillation was associated with significant decreases in O'Leary–Sant symptom scores (including Interstitial Cystitis Problem Index [ICPI] and Interstitial Cystitis Symptom Index [ICSI]), and the visual analog scale for pain, as well as an increase in the global response assessment. However, no differences in the improvement rates among the three groups were found, suggesting a significant placebo effect might have existed in this study [52]. IC/BPS has multifactorial etiologies, including urinary, infection, organ-specific, neurological/systemic, tenderness, and psychosocial domains [53]. Multimodal treatment strategies and modified liposomal BoNT-A instillation concentrations may be necessary to provide more convincing outcomes in a future study.

4.3. Liposome-Encapsulated Botulinum Toxin A for Bladder Oversensitivity

Several sensory receptors have been found to be expressed in the bladder urothelial and suburothelial nerves, including substance P, P2X3, the transient receptor potential vanilloid receptor 1 (TRPV1), and the CGRP [54–56]. These receptors participate in the transmission of bladder sensation during the urine storage phase [57]. These sensory receptors are co-localized on the sensory fibers and urothelium. Capsaicin or its ultrapotent analog, resiniferatoxin, treatment targeting TRPV1 desensitization had been found to effectively decrease bladder oversensitivity and OAB symptoms [58–62]. Recent studies also revealed that acetylcholine (ACh) and ATP are involved in bladder filling and fullness transmission in response to the stretch of the bladder [63]. The release of ACh and ATP from urothelial cells increases with aging, which might be associated with the increased incidence of bladder oversensitivity and OAB in older people [64].

BoNT-A has both sensory and motor effects in treating patients with detrusor overactivity and OAB. Decreases in the expression of TRPV1 and P2X3 on the suburothelial sensory afferents were found after detrusor BoNT-A injections [27,65]. It was found that patients also experience reductions in the frequency and urgency of urination after BoNT-A injection [23]. Reduced TRPV1 and P2X3 receptor expressions on the suburothelial afferent nerves are likely to result in bladder oversensitivity alleviation. Bladder inflammation is also frequently found in patients with OAB, IC/BPS, and oversensitivity with symptoms of urgency and frequency [66]. Chronic neural plasticity due to unresolved bladder inflammation and sensory receptor activation may increase afferent activity by influencing antinociceptive activity and cause increases in nerve growth factor (NGF) levels and bladder oversensitivity [67,68].

As the pathophysiology of bladder oversensitivity involves chronic inflammation, neural hyperactivity, and sensory receptor overexpression, the intravesical instillation of liposomal BoNT-A might effectively inhibit the progress of these sensory receptors' expressions and subsequent neuroplasticity, further lowering the threshold of bladder sensation and hypersensitivity [69]. The weakness of liposomal BoNT-A in managing OAB and IC/BPS might become the strength of treatment for bladder oversensitivity, because the penetration of BoNT-A is limited to the urothelium without affecting detrusor contractility.

5. Future Perspectives for Liposome-Encapsulated Botulinum Toxin A for Functional Bladder Disorders

Liposomes can serve as vehicles to deliver BoNT-A across the cell membrane of the urothelium and may act on afferent nerves to reduce pain and inflammatory processing without directly impacting the detrusor. Based on previous studies, the intravesical instillation of liposomal BoNT-A could ameliorate lower urinary tract symptoms in patients with functional bladder disorders [70]. In addition to future studies, which are expected to reinforce the clinical efficacy in patients with OAB and IC/BPS, the potential expansion of liposomal BoNT-A can also be explored in further research.

Recent studies have explored the underlying pathophysiology of OAB and IC/BPS. Chronic inflammation and ischemic change in the urinary bladder might underlie these functional bladder disorders [71]. Due to the presence of chronic inflammation, urothelial cell proliferation, differentiation, and maturation are impaired, resulting in defective urothelia in IC/BPS bladders and the increased sensory expressions of the bladders of individuals with OAB [31,72]. As liposomal BoNT-A can only deliver the BoNT-A protein to the upper part of bladder urothelium, it is not likely this treatment will have an effect on the urotheliogenic OAB, but not on neurogenic, musculogenic, or central-nervous-system-related OAB. On the other hand, there are many different subtypes of IC/BPS that might result in different phenotypes with small or large maximal bladder capacities and different grades of glomerulations [73]. Treatment with liposomal BoNT-A can provide benefits to patients with IC/BPS who solely have urothelial dysfunction without bladder wall inflammation. For patients with IC/BPS who have small bladder capacities and Hunner's lesions, which are characterized by confined, crimson mucosal area with small vessels radiating toward a central scar [74], liposomal BoNT-A might not be an effective treatment. With this in mind, by carrying out patient selection using clinical presentation as well as urinary biomarkers to identify urotheliogenic OAB and pure urotheliogenic IC/BPS, we might effectively choose suitable patients with OAB or IC/BPS for this novel treatment [75].

Furthermore, although liposomes can encapsulate BoNT-A proteins and deliver the proteins across the cell membrane, their efficacy might be limited by the instillation time, the bladder volume during instillation, and the dose of BoNT-A. Preliminary data have shown that 200 U BoNT-A plus liposomes can have limited clinical efficacy in patients with OAB or IC/BPS, possibly due to this treatment's limited penetration depth into the urothelium [49,51]. If we increase the dose of BoNT-A and instillation duration to facilitate more liposomal BoNT-A to penetrate across the cell membrane, the therapeutic effect might be better than what has currently been shown. A recent study also revealed that applying low-energy shock waves on the bladder can increase the bladder urothelial permeability [76]. Pretreatment with low-energy shock waves might also enhance the penetration of liposomal BoNT-A into the urothelium and achieve a better treatment outcome. The classification of OAB and IC/BPS subtypes is important for the selection of suitable patients for the treatment [77].

BoNT-A has been utilized in the treatment of functional bladder disorders for over 20 years, although the limited number of licensed applications has prevented its clinical popularity. With various pharmacologic mechanisms, including inhibition of the release of neuropeptides, neuromodulation, and anti-inflammatory and anti-sense actions, BoNT-A can be an alternative treatment for lower urinary tract dysfunctions that are refractory to conventional medications or surgical procedures [78]. Detrusor BoNT-A injections could provide therapeutic effectiveness with regard to NDO due to spinal cord injury and multiple sclerosis [79], and they could modulate bladder afferent activity in patients with Parkinson's disease and spinal cord injury [80]. BoNT-A injections into the bladder neck and urethral sphincter have been reported to alleviate voiding symptoms and increase the maximal flow rate in patients with lower urinary tract symptoms and a small prostate [81]. The intravesical administration of liposomal BoNT-A can be a simpler and less invasive delivery method for these patients, with a potential decrease in the risk of urinary retention or UTIs. In the future, advancements in both basic science and clinical research will be required to expand the clinical application of liposomal BoNT-A in functional bladder disorders.

6. Conclusions

Intravesical instillation using liposomes to encapsulate BoNT-A proteins is a potential treatment option to treat functional bladder disorders such as OAB, IC/BPS, and bladder oversensitivity. Although current clinical data regarding liposomal BoNT-A instillation are still limited in terms of its clinical efficacy on OAB and IC/BPS, adverse events due to intravesical BoNT-A injection can be avoided. With the future adjustment of the dose of BoNT-A, an increase in the instillation duration, and pretreatment with low-energy shock waves, liposome plus BoNT-A might play an important role in the treatment of bladder oversensitivity, OAB, and IC/BPS refractory to conventional medication.

Author Contributions: F.-C.H.: literature search and manuscript writing, H.-C.K.: critical comments and manuscript rearrangement. All authors have read and agreed to the published version of the manuscript.

Funding: This study was supported by the grant from the Buddhist Tzu Chi Medical Foundation TCMF-MP-110-03-01.

Institutional Review Board Statement: Not applicable.

Informed Consent Statement: Not applicable.

Data Availability Statement: Not applicable.

Conflicts of Interest: The authors declare no conflict of interest.

Abbreviations

The following abbreviations are used in this manuscript: AA: acetic acid; ACh: acetylcholine; ATP: adenosine triphosphate; AUA: American Urological Association; BoNT-A: botulinum toxin subtype A; CGRP: calcitonin-gene-related peptide; DMSO: dimethylsulfoxide; IC/BPS: interstitial cystitis/bladder pain syndrome; ICPI: Interstitial Cystitis Symptoms Index; ICSI: Interstitial Cystitis Problem Index; Liposomal BoNT-A: liposome-encapsulated BoNT-A; NDO: neurogenic detrusor overactivity; NGF: nerve growth factor; N/S: normal saline; OAB: overactive bladder; OABSS: Overactive Bladder Symptom Score; PVR: post-void residual; SNAP-25: synaptosomal-associated protein, 25 kDa; SUFU: Society for Urodynamics and Female Urology; SV2: synaptic vesicle protein

2; SV2A: synaptic vesicle protein 2A; TRPV1: transient receptor potential vanilloid receptor 1; UTI: urinary tract infection; UUI: urgency urinary incontinence.

References

1. Leue, C.; Kruimel, J.; Vrijens, D.; Masclee, A.; van Os, J.; van Koeveringe, G. Functional urological disorders: A sensitized defence response in the bladder-gut-brain axis. *Nat. Rev. Urol.* **2017**, *14*, 153–163. [CrossRef] [PubMed]
2. Coyne, K.S.; Sexton, C.C.; Vats, V.; Thompson, C.; Kopp, Z.S.; Milsom, I. National community prevalence of overactive bladder in the United States stratified by sex and age. *Urology* **2011**, *77*, 1081–1087. [CrossRef] [PubMed]
3. Irwin, D.E.; Milsom, I.; Hunskaar, S.; Reilly, K.; Kopp, Z.; Herschorn, S.; Coyne, K.; Kelleher, C.; Hampel, C.; Artibani, W.; et al. Population-based survey of urinary incontinence, overactive bladder, and other lower urinary tract symptoms in five countries: Results of the EPIC study. *Eur. Urol.* **2006**, *50*, 1306–1314. [CrossRef]
4. Irwin, D.E.; Abrams, P.; Milsom, I.; Kopp, Z.; Reilly, K.; Group, E.S. Understanding the elements of overactive bladder: Questions raised by the EPIC study. *BJU Int.* **2008**, *101*, 1381–1387. [CrossRef] [PubMed]
5. Stewart, W.F.; Van Rooyen, J.B.; Cundiff, G.W.; Abrams, P.; Herzog, A.R.; Corey, R.; Hunt, T.L.; Wein, A.J. Prevalence and burden of overactive bladder in the United States. *World J. Urol.* **2003**, *20*, 327–336. [CrossRef]
6. Milsom, I.; Abrams, P.; Cardozo, L.; Roberts, R.G.; Thuroff, J.; Wein, A.J. How widespread are the symptoms of an overactive bladder and how are they managed? A population-based prevalence study. *BJU Int.* **2001**, *87*, 760–766. [CrossRef]
7. Lightner, D.J.; Gomelsky, A.; Souter, L.; Vasavada, S.P. Diagnosis and Treatment of Overactive Bladder (Non-Neurogenic) in Adults: AUA/SUFU Guideline Amendment 2019. *J. Urol.* **2019**, *202*, 558–563. [CrossRef]
8. Nambiar, A.K.; Bosch, R.; Cruz, F.; Lemack, G.E.; Thiruchelvam, N.; Tubaro, A.; Bedretdinova, D.A.; Ambuhl, D.; Farag, F.; Lombardo, R.; et al. EAU Guidelines on Assessment and Nonsurgical Management of Urinary Incontinence. *Eur. Urol.* **2018**, *73*, 596–609. [CrossRef]
9. Suskind, A.M.; Berry, S.H.; Ewing, B.A.; Elliott, M.N.; Suttorp, M.J.; Clemens, J.Q. The prevalence and overlap of interstitial cystitis/bladder pain syndrome and chronic prostatitis/chronic pelvic pain syndrome in men: Results of the RAND Interstitial Cystitis Epidemiology male study. *J. Urol.* **2013**, *189*, 141–145. [CrossRef]
10. Berry, S.H.; Elliott, M.N.; Suttorp, M.; Bogart, L.M.; Stoto, M.A.; Eggers, P.; Nyberg, L.; Clemens, J.Q. Prevalence of symptoms of bladder pain syndrome/interstitial cystitis among adult females in the United States. *J. Urol.* **2011**, *186*, 540–544. [CrossRef]
11. Hanno, P.; Dmochowski, R. Status of international consensus on interstitial cystitis/bladder pain syndrome/painful bladder syndrome: 2008 snapshot. *Neurourol. Urodyn.* **2009**, *28*, 274–286. [CrossRef] [PubMed]
12. Clemens, J.Q.; Erickson, D.R.; Varela, N.P.; Lai, H.H. Diagnosis and Treatment of Interstitial Cystitis/Bladder Pain Syndrome. *J. Urol.* **2022**, *208*, 34–42. [CrossRef] [PubMed]
13. Anger, J.T.; Weinberg, A.; Suttorp, M.J.; Litwin, M.S.; Shekelle, P.G. Outcomes of intravesical botulinum toxin for idiopathic overactive bladder symptoms: A systematic review of the literature. *J. Urol.* **2010**, *183*, 2258–2264. [CrossRef] [PubMed]
14. Kuo, H.C.; Jiang, Y.H.; Tsai, Y.C.; Kuo, Y.C. Intravesical botulinum toxin-A injections reduce bladder pain of interstitial cystitis/bladder pain syndrome refractory to conventional treatment—A prospective, multicenter, randomized, double-blind, placebo-controlled clinical trial. *Neurourol. Urodyn.* **2016**, *35*, 609–614. [CrossRef]
15. Kaufman, J.; Tyagi, V.; Anthony, M.; Chancellor, M.B.; Tyagi, P. State of the art in intravesical therapy for lower urinary tract symptoms. *Rev. Urol.* **2010**, *12*, e181–e189.
16. Tyagi, P.; Wu, P.C.; Chancellor, M.; Yoshimura, N.; Huang, L. Recent advances in intravesical drug/gene delivery. *Mol. Pharm.* **2006**, *3*, 369–379. [CrossRef]
17. Lewis, S.A. Everything you wanted to know about the bladder epithelium but were afraid to ask. *Am. J. Physiol. Renal. Physiol.* **2000**, *278*, F867–F874. [CrossRef]
18. Dolly, J.O.; O'Connell, M.A. Neurotherapeutics to inhibit exocytosis from sensory neurons for the control of chronic pain. *Curr. Opin. Pharmacol.* **2012**, *12*, 100–108. [CrossRef]
19. Dong, M.; Yeh, F.; Tepp, W.H.; Dean, C.; Johnson, E.A.; Janz, R.; Chapman, E.R. SV2 is the protein receptor for botulinum neurotoxin A. *Science* **2006**, *312*, 592–596. [CrossRef]
20. Cruz, F. Targets for botulinum toxin in the lower urinary tract. *Neurourol. Urodyn.* **2014**, *33*, 31–38. [CrossRef]
21. Apostolidis, A.; Dasgupta, P.; Fowler, C.J. Proposed mechanism for the efficacy of injected botulinum toxin in the treatment of human detrusor overactivity. *Eur. Urol.* **2006**, *49*, 644–650. [CrossRef] [PubMed]
22. Mangera, A.; Apostolidis, A.; Andersson, K.E.; Dasgupta, P.; Giannantoni, A.; Roehrborn, C.; Novara, G.; Chapple, C. An updated systematic review and statistical comparison of standardised mean outcomes for the use of botulinum toxin in the management of lower urinary tract disorders. *Eur. Urol.* **2014**, *65*, 981–990. [CrossRef] [PubMed]
23. Kuo, H.C. Clinical effects of suburothelial injection of botulinum A toxin on patients with nonneurogenic detrusor overactivity refractory to anticholinergics. *Urology* **2005**, *66*, 94–98. [CrossRef] [PubMed]
24. Nitti, V.W.; Dmochowski, R.; Herschorn, S.; Sand, P.; Thompson, C.; Nardo, C.; Yan, X.; Haag-Molkenteller, C.; Group, E.S. OnabotulinumtoxinA for the treatment of patients with overactive bladder and urinary incontinence: Results of a phase 3, randomized, placebo controlled trial. *J. Urol.* **2013**, *189*, 2186–2193. [CrossRef]

25. Chapple, C.; Sievert, K.D.; MacDiarmid, S.; Khullar, V.; Radziszewski, P.; Nardo, C.; Thompson, C.; Zhou, J.; Haag-Molkenteller, C. OnabotulinumtoxinA 100 U significantly improves all idiopathic overactive bladder symptoms and quality of life in patients with overactive bladder and urinary incontinence: A randomised, double-blind, placebo-controlled trial. *Eur. Urol.* **2013**, *64*, 249–256. [CrossRef]
26. Kuo, H.C.; Liao, C.H.; Chung, S.D. Adverse events of intravesical botulinum toxin a injections for idiopathic detrusor overactivity: Risk factors and influence on treatment outcome. *Eur. Urol.* **2010**, *58*, 919–926. [CrossRef]
27. Jiang, Y.H.; Kuo, H.C. Reduction of urgency severity is the most important factor in the subjective therapeutic outcome of intravesical onabotulinumtoxinA injection for overactive bladder. *Neurourol. Urodyn.* **2017**, *36*, 338–343. [CrossRef]
28. Kuo, H.C. Comparison of effectiveness of detrusor, suburothelial and bladder base injections of botulinum toxin a for idiopathic detrusor overactivity. *J. Urol.* **2007**, *178*, 1359–1363. [CrossRef]
29. Jiang, Y.H.; Liao, C.H.; Kuo, H.C. Current and potential urological applications of botulinum toxin A. *Nat. Rev. Urol.* **2015**, *12*, 519–533. [CrossRef]
30. Parsons, C.L. The role of a leaky epithelium and potassium in the generation of bladder symptoms in interstitial cystitis/overactive bladder, urethral syndrome, prostatitis and gynaecological chronic pelvic pain. *BJU Int.* **2011**, *107*, 370–375. [CrossRef]
31. Shie, J.H.; Kuo, H.C. Higher levels of cell apoptosis and abnormal E-cadherin expression in the urothelium are associated with inflammation in patients with interstitial cystitis/painful bladder syndrome. *BJU Int.* **2011**, *108*, E136–E141. [CrossRef] [PubMed]
32. Liu, H.T.; Tyagi, P.; Chancellor, M.B.; Kuo, H.C. Urinary nerve growth factor level is increased in patients with interstitial cystitis/bladder pain syndrome and decreased in responders to treatment. *BJU Int.* **2009**, *104*, 1476–1481. [CrossRef]
33. Kuo, H.C.; Chancellor, M.B. Comparison of intravesical botulinum toxin type A injections plus hydrodistention with hydrodistention alone for the treatment of refractory interstitial cystitis/painful bladder syndrome. *BJU Int.* **2009**, *104*, 657–661. [CrossRef] [PubMed]
34. Shie, J.H.; Liu, H.T.; Wang, Y.S.; Kuo, H.C. Immunohistochemical evidence suggests repeated intravesical application of botulinum toxin A injections may improve treatment efficacy of interstitial cystitis/bladder pain syndrome. *BJU Int.* **2013**, *111*, 638–646. [CrossRef] [PubMed]
35. Kuo, H.C. Repeated onabotulinumtoxin-a injections provide better results than single injection in treatment of painful bladder syndrome. *Pain Physician* **2013**, *16*, E15–E23. [CrossRef]
36. Giannantoni, A.; Di Stasi, S.M.; Chancellor, M.B.; Costantini, E.; Porena, M. New frontiers in intravesical therapies and drug delivery. *Eur. Urol.* **2006**, *50*, 1183–1193; discussion 1193. [CrossRef]
37. Lee, J.P.; Jalili, R.B.; Tredget, E.E.; Demare, J.R.; Ghahary, A. Antifibrogenic effects of liposome-encapsulated IFN-alpha2b cream on skin wounds in a fibrotic rabbit ear model. *J. Interferon Cytokine Res.* **2005**, *25*, 627–631. [CrossRef]
38. Jeschke, M.G.; Sandmann, G.; Finnerty, C.C.; Herndon, D.N.; Pereira, C.T.; Schubert, T.; Klein, D. The structure and composition of liposomes can affect skin regeneration, morphology and growth factor expression in acute wounds. *Gene Ther.* **2005**, *12*, 1718–1724. [CrossRef]
39. Fraser, M.O.; Chuang, Y.C.; Tyagi, P.; Yokoyama, T.; Yoshimura, N.; Huang, L.; De Groat, W.C.; Chancellor, M.B. Intravesical liposome administration–a novel treatment for hyperactive bladder in the rat. *Urology* **2003**, *61*, 656–663. [CrossRef]
40. Tyagi, P.; Hsieh, V.C.; Yoshimura, N.; Kaufman, J.; Chancellor, M.B. Instillation of liposomes vs dimethyl sulphoxide or pentosan polysulphate for reducing bladder hyperactivity. *BJU Int.* **2009**, *104*, 1689–1692. [CrossRef]
41. Chuang, Y.C.; Lee, W.C.; Lee, W.C.; Chiang, P.H. Intravesical liposome versus oral pentosan polysulfate for interstitial cystitis/painful bladder syndrome. *J. Urol.* **2009**, *182*, 1393–1400. [CrossRef] [PubMed]
42. Lee, W.C.; Chuang, Y.C.; Lee, W.C.; Chiang, P.H. Safety and dose flexibility clinical evaluation of intravesical liposome in patients with interstitial cystitis or painful bladder syndrome. *Kaohsiung J. Med. Sci.* **2011**, *27*, 437–440. [CrossRef]
43. Peters, K.M.; Hasenau, D.; Killinger, K.A.; Chancellor, M.B.; Anthony, M.; Kaufman, J. Liposomal bladder instillations for IC/BPS: An open-label clinical evaluation. *Int. Urol. Nephrol.* **2014**, *46*, 2291–2295. [CrossRef]
44. Kuo, H.C. Urodynamic evidence of effectiveness of botulinum A toxin injection in treatment of detrusor overactivity refractory to anticholinergic agents. *Urology* **2004**, *63*, 868–872. [CrossRef] [PubMed]
45. Mehnert, U.; Boy, S.; Schmid, M.; Reitz, A.; von Hessling, A.; Hodler, J.; Schurch, B. A morphological evaluation of botulinum neurotoxin A injections into the detrusor muscle using magnetic resonance imaging. *World J. Urol.* **2009**, *27*, 397–403. [CrossRef] [PubMed]
46. Janicki, J.J.; Chancellor, M.B.; Kaufman, J.; Gruber, M.A.; Chancellor, D.D. Potential Effect of Liposomes and Liposome-Encapsulated Botulinum Toxin and Tacrolimus in the Treatment of Bladder Dysfunction. *Toxins* **2016**, *8*, 81. [CrossRef]
47. Chuang, Y.C.; Tyagi, P.; Huang, C.C.; Yoshimura, N.; Wu, M.; Kaufman, J.; Chancellor, M.B. Urodynamic and immunohistochemical evaluation of intravesical botulinum toxin A delivery using liposomes. *J. Urol.* **2009**, *182*, 786–792. [CrossRef]
48. Chuang, Y.C.; Yoshimura, N.; Huang, C.C.; Chiang, P.H.; Chancellor, M.B. Intravesical botulinum toxin a administration produces analgesia against acetic acid induced bladder pain responses in rats. *J. Urol.* **2004**, *172*, 1529–1532. [CrossRef]
49. Kuo, H.C.; Liu, H.T.; Chuang, Y.C.; Birder, L.A.; Chancellor, M.B. Pilot study of liposome-encapsulated onabotulinumtoxina for patients with overactive bladder: A single-center study. *Eur. Urol.* **2014**, *65*, 1117–1124. [CrossRef]
50. Chuang, Y.C.; Kaufmann, J.H.; Chancellor, D.D.; Chancellor, M.B.; Kuo, H.C. Bladder instillation of liposome encapsulated onabotulinumtoxina improves overactive bladder symptoms: A prospective, multicenter, double-blind, randomized trial. *J. Urol.* **2014**, *192*, 1743–1749. [CrossRef]

51. Liu, H.T.; Chen, S.H.; Chancellor, M.B.; Kuo, H.C. Presence of Cleaved Synaptosomal-Associated Protein-25 and Decrease of Purinergic Receptors P2X3 in the Bladder Urothelium Influence Efficacy of Botulinum Toxin Treatment for Overactive Bladder Syndrome. *PLoS ONE* **2015**, *10*, e0134803. [CrossRef]
52. Chuang, Y.C.; Kuo, H.C. A Prospective, Multicenter, Double-Blind, Randomized Trial of Bladder Instillation of Liposome Formulation OnabotulinumtoxinA for Interstitial Cystitis/Bladder Pain Syndrome. *J. Urol.* **2017**, *198*, 376–382. [CrossRef] [PubMed]
53. Nickel, J.C.; Shoskes, D.; Irvine-Bird, K. Clinical phenotyping of women with interstitial cystitis/painful bladder syndrome: A key to classification and potentially improved management. *J. Urol.* **2009**, *182*, 155–160. [CrossRef] [PubMed]
54. Brady, C.M.; Apostolidis, A.N.; Harper, M.; Yiangou, Y.; Beckett, A.; Jacques, T.S.; Freeman, A.; Scaravilli, F.; Fowler, C.J.; Anand, P. Parallel changes in bladder suburothelial vanilloid receptor TRPV1 and pan-neuronal marker PGP9.5 immunoreactivity in patients with neurogenic detrusor overactivity after intravesical resiniferatoxin treatment. *BJU Int.* **2004**, *93*, 770–776. [CrossRef] [PubMed]
55. Brady, C.M.; Apostolidis, A.; Yiangou, Y.; Baecker, P.A.; Ford, A.P.; Freeman, A.; Jacques, T.S.; Fowler, C.J.; Anand, P. P2X3-immunoreactive nerve fibres in neurogenic detrusor overactivity and the effect of intravesical resiniferatoxin. *Eur. Urol.* **2004**, *46*, 247–253. [CrossRef] [PubMed]
56. Smet, P.J.; Moore, K.H.; Jonavicius, J. Distribution and colocalization of calcitonin gene-related peptide, tachykinins, and vasoactive intestinal peptide in normal and idiopathic unstable human urinary bladder. *Lab. Investig.* **1997**, *77*, 37–49.
57. Odle, T.G. Precision Medicine in Breast Cancer. *Radiol. Technol.* **2017**, *88*, 401M–421M.
58. Fowler, C.J.; Beck, R.O.; Gerrard, S.; Betts, C.D.; Fowler, C.G. Intravesical capsaicin for treatment of detrusor hyperreflexia. *J. Neurol. Neurosurg. Psychiatry* **1994**, *57*, 169–173. [CrossRef]
59. Kuo, H.C. Effectiveness of intravesical resiniferatoxin for anticholinergic treatment refractory detrusor overactivity due to nonspinal cord lesions. *J. Urol.* **2003**, *170*, 835–839. [CrossRef]
60. Avelino, A.; Cruz, C.; Nagy, I.; Cruz, F. Vanilloid receptor 1 expression in the rat urinary tract. *Neuroscience* **2002**, *109*, 787–798. [CrossRef]
61. Yiangou, Y.; Facer, P.; Ford, A.; Brady, C.; Wiseman, O.; Fowler, C.J.; Anand, P. Capsaicin receptor VR1 and ATP-gated ion channel P2X3 in human urinary bladder. *BJU Int.* **2001**, *87*, 774–779. [CrossRef]
62. Birder, L.A.; Kanai, A.J.; de Groat, W.C.; Kiss, S.; Nealen, M.L.; Burke, N.E.; Dineley, K.E.; Watkins, S.; Reynolds, I.J.; Caterina, M.J. Vanilloid receptor expression suggests a sensory role for urinary bladder epithelial cells. *Proc. Natl. Acad. Sci. USA* **2001**, *98*, 13396–13401. [CrossRef] [PubMed]
63. Gabella, G. The structural relations between nerve fibres and muscle cells in the urinary bladder of the rat. *J. Neurocytol.* **1995**, *24*, 159–187. [CrossRef] [PubMed]
64. Yoshida, M.; Miyamae, K.; Iwashita, H.; Otani, M.; Inadome, A. Management of detrusor dysfunction in the elderly: Changes in acetylcholine and adenosine triphosphate release during aging. *Urology* **2004**, *63*, 17–23. [CrossRef] [PubMed]
65. Apostolidis, A.; Popat, R.; Yiangou, Y.; Cockayne, D.; Ford, A.P.; Davis, J.B.; Dasgupta, P.; Fowler, C.J.; Anand, P. Decreased sensory receptors P2X3 and TRPV1 in suburothelial nerve fibers following intradetrusor injections of botulinum toxin for human detrusor overactivity. *J. Urol.* **2005**, *174*, 977–982. [CrossRef]
66. Fahad Ullah, M. Breast Cancer: Current Perspectives on the Disease Status. *Adv. Exp. Med. Biol.* **2019**, *1152*, 51–64. [CrossRef]
67. Liu, H.T.; Kuo, H.C. Urinary nerve growth factor levels are increased in patients with bladder outlet obstruction with overactive bladder symptoms and reduced after successful medical treatment. *Urology* **2008**, *72*, 104–108; discussion 108. [CrossRef]
68. Lowe, E.M.; Anand, P.; Terenghi, G.; Williams-Chestnut, R.E.; Sinicropi, D.V.; Osborne, J.L. Increased nerve growth factor levels in the urinary bladder of women with idiopathic sensory urgency and interstitial cystitis. *Br. J. Urol.* **1997**, *79*, 572–577. [CrossRef]
69. Katsura, C.; Ogunmwonyi, I.; Kankam, H.K.; Saha, S. Breast cancer: Presentation, investigation and management. *Br. J. Hosp. Med.* **2022**, *83*, 1–7. [CrossRef]
70. Jhang, J.F.; Kuo, H.C. Novel Applications of Non-Invasive Intravesical Botulinum Toxin a Delivery in the Treatment of Functional Bladder Disorders. *Toxins* **2021**, *13*, 359. [CrossRef]
71. Jiang, Y.H.; Jhang, J.F.; Hsu, Y.H.; Ho, H.C.; Wu, Y.H.; Kuo, H.C. Urine biomarkers in ESSIC type 2 interstitial cystitis/bladder pain syndrome and overactive bladder with developing a novel diagnostic algorithm. *Sci. Rep.* **2021**, *11*, 914. [CrossRef] [PubMed]
72. Liu, H.T.; Shie, J.H.; Chen, S.H.; Wang, Y.S.; Kuo, H.C. Differences in mast cell infiltration, E-cadherin, and zonula occludens-1 expression between patients with overactive bladder and interstitial cystitis/bladder pain syndrome. *Urology* **2012**, *80*, 225.e13–225.e18. [CrossRef]
73. Yu, W.R.; Jhang, J.F.; Ho, H.C.; Jiang, Y.H.; Lee, C.L.; Hsu, Y.H.; Kuo, H.C. Cystoscopic hydrodistention characteristics provide clinical and long-term prognostic features of interstitial cystitis after treatment. *Sci. Rep.* **2021**, *11*, 455. [CrossRef]
74. van de Merwe, J.P.; Nordling, J.; Bouchelouche, P.; Bouchelouche, K.; Cervigni, M.; Daha, L.K.; Elneil, S.; Fall, M.; Hohlbrugger, G.; Irwin, P.; et al. Diagnostic criteria, classification, and nomenclature for painful bladder syndrome/interstitial cystitis: An ESSIC proposal. *Eur. Urol.* **2008**, *53*, 60–67. [CrossRef]
75. Yu, W.R.; Jiang, Y.H.; Jhang, J.F.; Kuo, H.C. Use of Urinary Cytokine and Chemokine Levels for Identifying Bladder Conditions and Predicting Treatment Outcomes in Patients with Interstitial Cystitis/Bladder Pain Syndrome. *Biomedicines* **2022**, *10*, 1149. [CrossRef] [PubMed]

76. Wang, H.J.; Lee, W.C.; Tyagi, P.; Huang, C.C.; Chuang, Y.C. Effects of low energy shock wave therapy on inflammatory moleculars, bladder pain, and bladder function in a rat cystitis model. *Neurourol. Urodyn.* **2017**, *36*, 1440–1447. [CrossRef]
77. Veronesi, U.; Boyle, P.; Goldhirsch, A.; Orecchia, R.; Viale, G. Breast cancer. *Lancet* **2005**, *365*, 1727–1741. [CrossRef] [PubMed]
78. Kuo, H.C. Clinical Application of Botulinum Neurotoxin in Lower-Urinary-Tract Diseases and Dysfunctions: Where Are We Now and What More Can We Do? *Toxins* **2022**, *14*, 498. [CrossRef]
79. Kalsi, V.; Apostolidis, A.; Popat, R.; Gonzales, G.; Fowler, C.J.; Dasgupta, P. Quality of life changes in patients with neurogenic versus idiopathic detrusor overactivity after intradetrusor injections of botulinum neurotoxin type A and correlations with lower urinary tract symptoms and urodynamic changes. *Eur. Urol.* **2006**, *49*, 528–535. [CrossRef]
80. Conte, A.; Giannantoni, A.; Proietti, S.; Giovannozzi, S.; Fabbrini, G.; Rossi, A.; Porena, M.; Berardelli, A. Botulinum toxin A modulates afferent fibers in neurogenic detrusor overactivity. *Eur. J. Neurol.* **2012**, *19*, 725–732. [CrossRef]
81. Chen, J.L.; Chen, C.Y.; Kuo, H.C. Botulinum toxin A injection to the bladder neck and urethra for medically refractory lower urinary tract symptoms in men without prostatic obstruction. *J. Formos. Med. Assoc.* **2009**, *108*, 950–956. [CrossRef] [PubMed]

toxins

MDPI

Article

Preliminary Exploration of a New Therapy for Interstitial Cystitis/Bladder Pain Syndrome: Botulinum Toxin A Combined with Sapylin

Wenshuang Li [1,2,3,4,†], Zhenming Zheng [1,2,3,†], Kaiqun Ma [1,2,3,5,†], Caixia Zhang [1,2,3], Kuiqing Li [1,2,3], Paierhati Tayier [1,2,3] and Yousheng Yao [1,2,3,*]

1 Department of Urology, Sun Yat-Sen Memorial Hospital, Sun Yat-Sen University, Guangzhou 510120, China
2 Guangdong Provincial Key Laboratory of Malignant Tumor Epigenetics and Gene Regulation, Sun Yat-Sen Memorial Hospital, Sun Yat-Sen University, Guangzhou 510120, China
3 Guangdong Provincial Clinical Research Center for Urological Diseases, Guangzhou 510120, China
4 Department of Urology, The Eighth Affiliated Hospital of Sun Yat-Sen University, Shenzhen 518033, China
5 Department of Urology, Shantou Central Hospital, Shantou 515031, China
* Correspondence: yaoyoush@mail.sysu.edu.cn; Tel.: +86-1382-2213-262; Fax: +86-20-813-32505
† These authors contributed equally to this work.

Abstract: Interstitial cystitis/bladder pain syndrome (IC/BPS) is an intractable disease without long-term effective therapy. This study aims to evaluate the efficacy and safety of botulinum toxin A (BoNT/A) plus Sapylin, which might modulate the immune response of the bladder in the treatment of IC/BPS patients. We retrospectively investigated the clinical outcomes among 34 patients who accepted repeated Sapylin instillations after 200 U of BoNT/A submucosally injected into bladder walls (Mix group) and 28 patients who received BoNT/A alone (Control group). Each of the bladder walls (left, right, anterior and posterior) was injected six times with 8 U of BoNT/A per injection. The primary outcome measure was the global response assessment. The results showed that at 6 months post-injection, the response rate in the Mix group was remarkably higher than that in the Control group (58.8% vs. 28.6%, $p < 0.05$). The mean effective duration of the responders in the Mix group was apparently better than that in the Control group (27.5 (range 0–89) vs. 4.9 (range 0–11) months, $p < 0.05$). None of the patients experienced serious adverse events. In conclusion, repeated intravesical instillations of Sapylin after BoNT/A injection can produce significantly better clinical outcomes than BoNT/A alone in IC/PBS patients.

Keywords: bladder pain syndrome; botulinum toxin A; interstitial cystitis; Sapylin

Key Contribution: This is the first study to apply BoNT/A plus Sapylin to treat IC/BPS; this can produce significantly better clinical outcomes than BoNT/A alone.

Citation: Li, W.; Zheng, Z.; Ma, K.; Zhang, C.; Li, K.; Tayier, P.; Yao, Y. Preliminary Exploration of a New Therapy for Interstitial Cystitis/Bladder Pain Syndrome: Botulinum Toxin A Combined with Sapylin. *Toxins* **2022**, *14*, 832. https://doi.org/10.3390/toxins14120832

Received: 14 October 2022
Accepted: 28 November 2022
Published: 30 November 2022

Publisher's Note: MDPI stays neutral with regard to jurisdictional claims in published maps and institutional affiliations.

Copyright: © 2022 by the authors. Licensee MDPI, Basel, Switzerland. This article is an open access article distributed under the terms and conditions of the Creative Commons Attribution (CC BY) license (https://creativecommons.org/licenses/by/4.0/).

1. Introduction

Interstitial cystitis/bladder pain syndrome (IC/BPS) is a chronic disease with suprapubic pain or discomfort related to bladder filling, urinary frequency and urgency, resulting in a serious impairment of quality of life [1]. However, the current treatments for IC/BPS struggle to maintain long-term efficacy and the symptoms of IC/BPS are prone to recurrence because of its obscure etiology and pathogenesis [2].

It is proposed that an injured urothelium and neural hypersensitivity of the bladder might exacerbate chronic inflammation and immune responses in IC/BPS patients, causing persistent bladder pain and urinary frequency [3,4]. In fact, bladder pain or discomfort often drives urinary frequency and nocturia [5]. Botulinum toxin A (BoNT/A) might decrease the neural hypersensitivity of the bladder to relieve bladder pain and urination frequency and urgency [6]. However, the average effective duration of BoNT/A injection was only about 6 months, so repeated injection was required [7]. Therefore, a new therapy to extend the response duration is needed to reduce the burden on patients and health systems.

The immune and inflammatory responses might play a crucial role in the pathogenesis of IC/BPS [1]. Many researchers have shown that inflammatory factors, such as interleukin-6 and tumor necrosis factor-alpha (TNF-α), are significantly increased in the bladder tissue of IC/BPS patients [8–10]. In addition, Bosch's research demonstrated that subcutaneous certolizumab pegol, an anti-TNF-α agent, significantly improved patients' symptoms compared with placebo therapy [11]. Later, Mishra et al. pointed out that an intravesical instillation of tacrolimus had a significant effect on the treatment of IC/BPS by inhibiting the immune response [12]. These conditions show that immunotherapy for IC/BPS is a reasonable option.

Sapylin (OK-432) is a lyophilized preparation made from a low-virulence strain (Su) of Streptococcus pyogenes (group A) incubated with penicillin [13], which is successfully used as an immunotherapeutic agent in many malignant cancers [14,15]. In addition, many researchers found that Sapylin also had immunotherapeutic effects on bladder cancer, creating the possibility for it to treat bladder diseases [16–18]. In an animal study, researchers found that Sapylin might accelerate wound closure and promote angiogenesis, collagen synthesis and the remodeling process to improve wound healing and reduce seroma formation [19]. These promising results seemed to indicate a possibility that Sapylin might be used as an immunotherapeutic agent in IC/BPS by repairing injured urothelium.

At present, there are many therapeutic methods for relieving IC/BPS symptoms but these are symptomatic and their efficacy is not long lasting. As a consequence, most IC/BPS patients inevitably suffer again and continue to wait for an innovative formulation. Luckily, we found a new treatment scheme (repeated intravesical instillations of Sapylin after BoNT/A injection) that could more persistently improve the symptoms of IC/BPS patients. In this study, we would like to summarize and share the results of our preliminary exploration.

2. Results

2.1. Patient Characteristics

In Table 1, the baseline demographics and clinical characteristics of 62 patients with IC/BPS are compared between the Mix and Control groups, including 51 female and 11 male patients (female/male = 5:1), with a median age of 47 [26, 78] years. The median daytime frequency of urination and nocturia per 24 h were 25 [13, 40] and 5 [1, 13] times, respectively. Moreover, the participants' voided volume per micturition and functional bladder capacity were apparently decreased from normal individuals. Further, there were no significant differences in baseline characteristics between the Mix and Control groups.

Table 1. Baseline characteristics of the participants.

	Control (N = 28)	Mix (N = 34)	p-Value
Gender			
Male	5 (17.9%)	6 (17.6%)	1
Female	23 (82.1%)	28 (82.4%)	
Age (years)			
Mean (SD)	45.0 (12.5)	46.9 (14.2)	0.569
Median [Min, Max]	41.5 [26.0, 78.0]	48.5 [27.0, 72.0]	
BMI (kg/m^2)			
Mean (SD)	21.6 (3.5)	21.4 (3.4)	0.835
Median [Min, Max]	21.4 [16.0, 32.0]	20.8 [15.8, 28.2]	
Daytime frequency			
Mean (SD)	26.2 (6.8)	24.8 (7.1)	0.437
Median [Min, Max]	25.0 [13.0, 40.0]	23.0 [14.0, 40.0]	
Nocturia			

Table 1. *Cont.*

	Control (*N* = 28)	Mix (*N* = 34)	*p*-Value
Mean (SD)	5.6 (3.4)	5.5 (3.1)	0.909
Median [Min, Max]	5.0 [1.0, 13.0]	5.0 [1.0, 12.0]	
Mean voided volume per micturition (mL)			
Mean (SD)	56.2 (22.6)	57.1 (24.0)	0.883
Median [Min, Max]	54.0 [23.0, 125.0]	54.0 [22.0, 110.0]	
Maximal voided volume per micturition (mL)			
Mean (SD)	88.9 (26.6)	86.5 (25.2)	0.804
Median [Min, Max]	83.0 [57.0, 163.0]	83.5 [51.0, 152.0]	
Functional bladder capacity (mL)			
Mean (SD)	152.0 (49.3)	146.0 (48.8)	0.561
Median [Min, Max]	143.0 [90.0, 260.0]	138.0 [90.0, 255.0]	
QoL			
Mean (SD)	5.8 (0.5)	5.7 (0.4)	0.906
Median [Min, Max]	6.0 [4.0, 6.0]	6.0 [5.0, 6.0]	
VAS			
Mean (SD)	8.8 (1.3)	8.8 (1.3)	0.964
Median [Min, Max]	9.0 [6.0, 10.0]	9.0 [6.0, 10.0]	
PUF			
Mean (SD)	24.3 (4.4)	24.4 (4.6)	0.738
Median [Min, Max]	24.5 [15.0, 31.0]	25.0 [15.0, 31.0]	
ICSI			
Mean (SD)	16.1 (2.7)	16.1 (2.7)	0.971
Median [Min, Max]	16.0 [10.0, 20.0]	16.5 [10.0, 20.0]	
ICPI			
Mean (SD)	14.8 (1.5)	14.8 (1.6)	0.725
Median [Min, Max]	15.0 [9.0, 16.0]	15.5 [10.0, 16.0]	

BMI: body mass index; QoL: quality of life; VAS: visual analogue scale; PUF: pelvic pain and urgency/frequency patient symptom score; ICSI: O'Leary-Sant Interstitial Cystitis Symptom Index; ICPI: O'Leary-Sant Interstitial Cystitis Problem Index.

2.2. *Efficacy Assessment*

In Table 2, the overall GRA showed that at 3 months post-injection, 19 (67.9%) participants in the Control group and 23 (67.6%) participants in the Mix group had a significant response, without a statistical difference between the two groups. At 6 months, the response rate in the Mix group was remarkably higher than the rate in the Control group (58.8% vs. 28.6%, $\chi^2 = 5.7$, $p = 0.02 < 0.05$).

In Table 3, at 3 months post-injection, the clinical characteristics in each group had significantly improved from baseline and there was no statistical difference between the two groups. At 6 months, patients' QoL, VAS, ICSI and ICPI in the Control group had statistically improved from baseline, except for urinary frequency, bladder voided volume and PUF. In the Mix group, patients' urinary frequency, bladder voided volume, QoL, VAS, PUF, ICSI and ICPI had significantly improved from baseline, with a statistical difference from the Control group.

Table 2. Global response assessment at 3 and 6 months.

	Control (N = 28)	Mix (N = 34)	p-Value
3 Months			
7 = Markedly improved	2 (7.1%)	2 (5.9%)	
6 = Moderately improved	17 (60.7%)	21 (61.8%)	
5 = Slightly improved	4 (14.3%)	6 (17.6%)	
4 = No change	5 (17.9%)	5 (14.7%)	
3 = Slightly worse	0 (0.0%)	0 (0.0%)	
2 = Moderately worse	0 (0.0%)	0 (0.0%)	
1 = Markedly worse	0 (0.0%)	0 (0.0%)	
Non-responders (1 + 2 + 3 + 4 + 5)	9 (32.1%)	11 (32.4%)	1
Responders (6 + 7)	19 (67.9%)	23 (67.6%)	
6 Months			
7 = Markedly improved	2 (7.1%)	4 (11.8%)	
6 = Moderately improved	6 (21.4%)	16 (47.1%)	
5 = Slightly improved	6 (21.4%)	11 (32.4%)	
4 = No change	9 (32.1%)	3 (8.8%)	
3 = Slightly worse	5 (17.9%)	0 (0.0%)	
2 = Moderately worse	0 (0.0%)	0 (0.0%)	
1 = Markedly worse	0 (0.0%)	0 (0.0%)	
Non-responders (1 + 2 + 3 + 4 + 5)	20 (71.4%)	14 (41.2%)	<0.05
Responders (6 + 7)	8 (28.6%)	20 (58.8%)	

The mean effective duration of the responders in the Mix group was apparently better than that in the Control group (27.5 (range 0–89) vs. 4.9 (range 0–11) months, $p < 0.05$). The rates of the responders in the Mix therapy group were significantly higher than those in the Control group after 6 months of treatment (Figure 1A). In the Mix group, more than half of the participants could see a significant improvement within 6 months and a marked improvement at 12 months of treatment (Figure 1B). Furthermore, with repeated intravesical instillations of Sapylin, the great effect continues to maintain during the treatment. With a median follow-up of 32.5 [24.0, 92.0] months, the effective duration of the best responder in the Mix group was 89 months, which continues to last (symptom free).

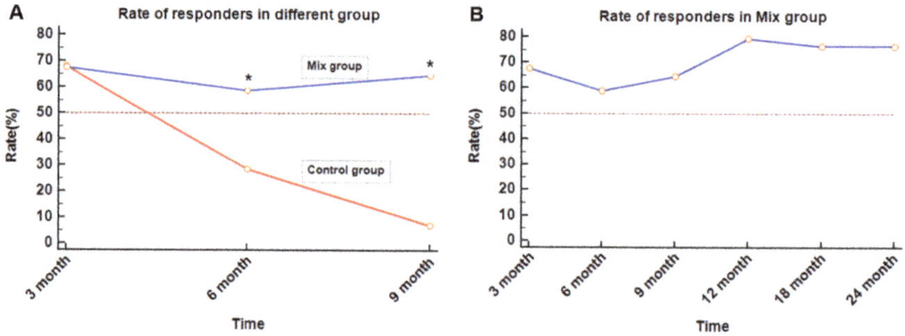

Figure 1. (**A**) * $p < 0.05$, the rates of the responders in the Mix therapy group are significantly higher than those in the Control group after 6 months of treatment. (**B**) In the Mix group, more than half of the participants see a significant improvement within 6 months and a marked improvement at 12 months of treatment. Furthermore, with repeated intravesical instillations of Sapylin, the effect is maintained during the treatment.

Table 3. Secondary outcome changes from baseline to 3 and 6 months after treatment.

	Baseline		3 Months		6 Months	
	Control (N = 28)	Mix (N = 34)	Control (N = 28)	Mix (N = 34)	Control (N = 28)	Mix (N = 34)
Daytime frequency						
Mean (SD)	26.2 (6.8)	24.8 (7.1)	13.5 (7.8) ^{b}	12.5 (6.7) ^{b}	21.5 (10.1)	11.7 (5.3) $^{a, b}$
Median [Min, Max]	25.0 [13.0, 40.0]	23.0 [14.0, 40.0]	10.0 [6.0, 35.0]	10.0 [5.0, 33.0]	24.0 [6.0, 35.0]	10.0 [4.0, 26.0]
Nocturia						
Mean (SD)	5.6 (3.4)	5.5 (3.1)	2.3 (2.1) ^{b}	2.3 (2.1) ^{b}	4.1 (3.2)	2.3 (1.7) ^{a,b}
Median [Min, Max]	5.0 [1.0, 13.0]	5.0 [1.0, 12.0]	2.0 [0.0, 9.0]	2.0 [0.0, 9.0]	3.5 [0.0, 11.0]	2.0 [0.0, 7.0]
Mean voided volume per micturition (mL)						
Mean (SD)	56.2 (22.6)	57.1 (24.0)	138.0 (69.9) ^{b}	144.0 (79.8) ^{b}	92.1 (73.5)	152.0 (91.7) ^{a,b}
Median [Min, Max]	54.0 [23.0, 125.0]	54.0 [22.0, 110.0]	143.0 [28.0, 301.0]	135.0 [34.0, 402.0]	59.0 [27.0, 289.0]	128.0 [39.0, 395.0]
Maximal voided volume per micturition (mL)						
Mean (SD)	88.9 (26.6)	86.5 (25.2)	171.0 (71.2) ^{b}	178.0 (79.7) ^{b}	120.0 (75.2)	188.0 (99.3) ^{a,b}
Median [Min, Max]	83.0 [57.0, 163.0]	83.5 [51.0, 152.0]	174.0 [63.0, 338.0]	170.0 [61.0, 438.0]	90.0 [56.0, 321.0]	174.0 [59.0, 432.0]
QoL						
Mean (SD)	5.8 (0.5)	5.7 (0.4)	2.7 (1.9) ^{b}	2.9 (2.0) ^{b}	4.4 (2.1) ^{b}	2.9 (1.9) ^{a,b}
Median [Min, Max]	6.0 [4.0, 6.0]	6.0 [5.0, 6.0]	2.0 [0.0, 6.0]	2.0 [0.0, 6.0]	5.0 [0.0, 6.0]	2.5 [0.0, 6.0]
VAS						
Mean (SD)	8.8 (1.3)	8.8 (1.3)	4.9 (2.2) ^{b}	5.1 (2.3) ^{b}	7.0 (3.1) ^{b}	4.9 (2.4) ^{a,b}
Median [Min, Max]	9.0 [6.0, 10.0]	9.0 [6.0, 10.0]	4.0 [1.0, 10.0]	4.5 [1.0, 10.0]	8.0 [1.0, 10.0]	5.0 [0.0, 9.0]
PUF						
Mean (SD)	24.3 (4.4)	24.4 (4.6)	13.8 (5.3) ^{b}	14.2 (5.6) ^{b}	20.1 (7.5)	14.0 (5.4) ^{a,b}
Median [Min, Max]	24.5 [15.0, 31.0]	25.0 [15.0, 31.0]	12.0 [6.0, 29.0]	12.0 [8.0, 28.0]	21.5 [8.0, 31.0]	12.5 [6.0, 26.0]
ICSI						
Mean (SD)	16.1 (2.7)	16.1 (2.7)	9.7 (3.5) ^{b}	9.7 (3.3) ^{b}	13.6 (4.5) ^{b}	9.5 (3.0) ^{a,b}
Median [Min, Max]	16.0 [10.0, 20.0]	16.5 [10.0, 20.0]	8.50 [3.0, 19.0]	8.0 [6.0, 19.0]	14.0 [6.0, 20.0]	9.5 [5.0, 16.0]
ICPI						
Mean (SD)	14.8 (1.5)	14.8 (1.6)	9.0 (3.0) ^{b}	9.2 (2.8) ^{b}	12.4 (3.8) ^{b}	8.9 (2.7) ^{a,b}
Median [Min, Max]	15.0 [9.0, 16.0]	15.5 [10.0, 16.0]	8.0 [4.0, 16.0]	9.0 [6.0, 15.0]	14.0 [5.0, 16.0]	9.0 [4.0, 14.0]

QoL: quality of life; VAS: visual analogue scale; PUF: pelvic pain and urgency/frequency patient symptom score; ICSI: O'Leary-Sant Interstitial Cystitis Symptom Index; ICPI: O'Leary-Sant Interstitial Cystitis Problem Index. ^{a} $p < 0.05$: Mix group compared to Control group. ^{b} $p < 0.05$: Mix or Control group compared to corresponding baseline.

2.3. Safety Assessment

None of the patients experienced serious adverse events. In the Mix group, mild or moderate adverse events related to the BoNT/A injection and Sapylin instillations occurred in 19 (19/34, 55.9%) cases, including 2 cases of acute urinary retention, 10 cases of dysuria, 3 cases of mild hematuria, 3 cases of urinary tract infection and 1 case of mild fever. In the Control group, mild or moderate adverse events related to BoNT/A injection occurred in 13 cases (13/28, 46.4%), including 1 case of acute urinary retention, 8 cases of dysuria, 2 cases of mild hematuria and 2 cases of urinary tract infection. The difference in the adverse events between the two groups had no statistical significance ($p > 0.05$) and they were cured spontaneously without any interventions, or with appropriate treatment, such as antibiotics.

3. Discussion

This long follow-up pilot study demonstrated that repeated intravesical instillations of Sapylin after BoNT/A injection could remarkably improve lower urinary tract symptoms and increase the bladder voided volume in IC/BPS patients with tolerable safety, for a long-term effective duration, which was apparently better than BoNT/A injection alone.

It is proposed that IC/BPS might be induced by the interaction among nervous, immune and endocrine factors [1]. The glycosaminoglycan layer protects the bladder mucosa as a chemical barrier against urine. When this layer is defective, it cannot protect the bladder mucosa from infiltrated urine that would induce submucosal inflammation, stimulate persistent sensory nerve hyperactivity and upregulate the urothelium permeability, contributing to urinary frequency and pain [3,4,20].

Previous studies demonstrated that BoNT/A was an effective therapy for IC/BPS; it was recommended by the American Urological Association [21] and the East Asian Urological Association [1]. BoNT/A can inhibit the release of neurotransmitters and neuropeptides (nerve growth factor, calcitonin gene-related peptide and substance P et al.) that regulate pain and inflammation from nerve fibers in the bladder wall and the urothelium to reduce neurogenic inflammation, alleviate neural hypersensitivity and inhibit bladder muscle contraction, which finally improves lower urinary tract symptoms [6]. In 2004, Smith et al. [22] studied 13 IC/BPS patients injected with BoNT/A into the trigone and bladder base, resulting in 69% of the patients seeing a significant improvement in pain. Later, Giannantoni et al. submucosally injected 200 U of BoNT/A into the trigone and bladder floor of 14 patients with IC/BPS. Among them, 12 patients (85.7%) reported subjective improvement at the 1- and 3-month follow-ups; however, the duration only lasted 3 months [23]. In the same group of patients, 13 were followed up with repeated BoNT/A injections for 2 years. A mean of 4.8 ± 0.8 injections were administered per patient, and the mean interval between two consecutive injections was 5.25 ± 0.75 months [24]. Another study reported that at the 5-month follow-up, the beneficial effects persisted in 26.6% of cases and at 12 months after treatment, pain recurred in all the patients [25]. These clinical studies show that the therapeutic duration of BoNT/A in IC/BPS patients is around 3–6 months. Similarly, our present study showed that the response rates of those participants who accepted only a BoNT/A submucosal injection at 3, 6, 9 and 12 months post-injection were 67.9%, 28.6%, 7.1% and 0%, respectively. Interestingly, a randomized comparative study enrolled 34 patients with refractory IC/BPS who were injected with 100 U BoNT/A, mainly into the suburothelial layer [26]. The response rate was 73.5% at 1 month, 58.8% at 3 months, 38.2% at 6 months and 20.6% at 12 months. However, in that study, patients who reported "slightly improved," "improved" or "remarkably improved," were considered as the responders to treatment. Further, the treated population might also differ between that study and ours.

Immunotherapy is a reasonable option for IC/BPS [27]. Many researchers found that Sapylin also had immunotherapeutic effects on bladder cancer by initiating marked lymphocytic infiltration around the tumor cells and inhibiting their growth [16,18]. These results suggested that Sapylin might regulate bladder immune and inflammatory responses.

In the present study, our results also demonstrated that the response duration of those who received BoNT/A with Sapylin was 27.5 months on average. This long-lasting effect might be attributable mainly to the repeated intravesical treatment of Sapylin. The mechanisms of Sapylin in the treatment of IC/BPS, however, were not investigated in this study. Interestingly, Kong et al. [28] demonstrated that Sapylin could stimulate the body to secrete a variety of cytokines to accelerate wound healing by promoting endothelial cell proliferation, migration and angiogenesis and increasing fibroblast migration and collagen deposition. These results are similar to an animal study [19]. These promising discoveries have encouraged us to explore whether Sapylin could induce immune responses in the bladder to stimulate the proliferation of bladder epithelial cells and inhibit the expression of those inflammatory factors initiated by infiltrated urine.

Our study has several limitations. This was a retrospective, preliminary and single-center pilot study. Although the present study has biases, it was designed as a pilot study to confirm a novel combined therapy for IC/BPS patients. Moreover, we did not directly compare BoNT/A plus Sapylin with other traditional treatments for IC/BPS. Moreover, post-void residual urine and other side effects need to be investigated comprehensively. Finally, we failed to compare the therapeutic effect between BoNT/A plus Sapylin and Sapylin alone. Further research comparing BoNT/A injection plus Sapylin instillation, BoNT/A alone, or Sapylin alone in the treatment of IC/BPS is warranted with a large, multicenter, randomized, placebo-controlled trial.

4. Conclusions

This long-follow-up pilot study shows that repeated intravesical instillations of Sapylin after BoNT/A injection can produce significantly better clinical outcomes than BoNT/A alone in IC/PBS patients. Further research comparing BoNT/A injection plus Sapylin instillation, BoNT/A alone, or Sapylin alone in the treatment of IC/BPS is warranted with a large, multicenter, randomized, placebo-controlled trial.

5. Materials and Methods

5.1. Participants and Ethics

From March 2015 to April 2020 in our hospital, 70 IC/BPS patients were selected according to the following: (1) diagnosed according to National Institute of Diabetes and Digestive and Kidney (NIDDK) guidelines [29]; (2) an O'Leary-Sant Interstitial Cystitis Symptom Index score (ICSI) of more than 9 and disease duration of more than 6 months; (3) previous adequate unsuccessful treatments in accordance with guidelines including oral anti-cholinergic agents, pain-killers, amitriptyline, intravesical hyaluronic acid, heparinoids and so on. Those patients with urinary cancers, bacterial genitourinary infections, bladder tuberculosis, radiation-induced or chemical cystitis, sexually transmitted diseases, pelvic inflammatory disease and endometriosis were excluded [30]. All patients were required to provide their informed consent to receive BoNT/A injection alone or BoNT/A plus Sapylin and they made their own decision about which treatment to receive. Furthermore, 8 cases were removed because of missing data. Finally, this study investigated 34 patients who received repeated intravesical instillations of Sapylin after BoNT/A injection (Mix group) and 28 patients who accepted a submucosal injection of BoNT/A alone (Control group).

After treatment, to evaluate its efficacy, we performed a questionnaire investigation of symptoms via telephone and outpatient interviews. The primary outcome was the global response assessment (GRA) at 3 and 6 months after treatment: "As compared to when you started the current study, how would you rate your overall pelvic symptoms now?", with seven response categories: 1 = Markedly worse, 2 = Moderately worse, 3 = Slightly worse, 4 = No change, 5 = Slightly improved, 6 = Moderately improved and 7 = Markedly improved. Participants who reported "moderately or markedly improved" were considered as the responders to the treatment. Others were defined as non-responders. The secondary outcomes were pelvic pain and urgency/frequency patient symptom score (PUF), visual analogue scale (VAS), O'Leary-Sant ICSI and Interstitial Cystitis Problem

Index (ICPI). Further, a 3-day urinary diary was used to evaluate the mean voided volume per micturition, maximal voided volume per micturition and mean urinary frequency per 24 h. Cystoscopy was performed under local anesthesia before treatment. Saline was delivered into the bladder until the patients' bladder pain or discomfort became intolerable. Then, the total saline delivery volume was calculated as the functional maximal bladder capacity.

5.2. Intervention

5.2.1. Submucosal Injection of BoNT/A

All the patients received a submucosal injection of BoNT/A (Lanzhou Biotechnology Development Co., Ltd., Lanzhou, China) under continuous epidural anesthesia. An amount of 200 U of BoNT/A was diluted in 20 mL of sterile saline in advance, resulting in 10 U of BoNT/A per 1.0 mL. The submucosal injection areas included the left, right, anterior and posterior bladder walls, sparing the trigone. Each of these four bladder walls was injected six times with 8 U of BoNT/A per injection. As dysuria was a common complication and urinary retention was a severe complication, catheterization was routinely applied and removed about 5 days after the operation. An oral antibiotic agent was prescribed for 7 days. Afterwards, the patients in the Mix group accepted intravesical instillation of Sapylin.

5.2.2. Intravesical Instillation of Sapylin

One week after the operation, all patients in the Mix group began to receive intravesical instillation of Sapylin (Sinopharm Group Luya (Shandong) Pharmaceutical Co., Ltd., Jining, China). Sapylin 5 KE (a unit of measure) was evenly dissolved in 40 mL of sterile saline. Mixed Sapylin was instilled into the bladder through a urinary catheter, which was removed after injection, and the Sapylin remained in the bladder until the occurrence of pelvic pain or discomfort but for no more than 2 h. It was instilled once a week within 6 weeks post-injection, then, once every 4 weeks for 2 years, totaling 29 intravesical doses.

5.3. Statistical Methods

The continuous variables are expressed as the mean value (standard deviation) and median [Min, Max] and the differences among groups were compared by Student's t-tests (normal distribution) or Mann–Whitney U test (non-normal distribution). In addition, categorical variables are represented as counts or percentages and the inter-block comparison was analyzed with a chi-squared test. A p value of <0.05 was considered statistically significant. SPSS version 26.0 (IBM, Armonk, NY) and MedCalc (MedCalc Software bvba) were used for the statistical analysis.

Author Contributions: Conceptualization, Y.Y.; Data curation, C.Z. and K.L.; Formal analysis, W.L., Z.Z. and K.M.; Funding acquisition, Y.Y.; Investigation, W.L., Z.Z. and K.M.; Methodology, Y.Y.; Resources, W.L., Z.Z., K.M. and P.T.; Software, C.Z. and K.L.; Supervision, Y.Y.; Validation, C.Z. and K.L.; Visualization, C.Z. and K.L.; Writing—original draft, W.L., Z.Z. and K.M.; Writing—review and editing, P.T. and Y.Y. All authors have read and agreed to the published version of the manuscript.

Funding: This study was funded by the Natural Science Foundation of Guangdong Province (2016A030313300) and Guangdong Provincial Clinical Research Center for Urological Diseases (2020B1111170006).

Institutional Review Board Statement: This retrospective study was approved by the Ethics Committee of the Sun Yat-sen Memorial Hospital of Sun Yat-sen University (Approval number: SYSEC-KY-KS-2022-156, Date: 11 May 2022) and performed following the 1975 Declaration of Helsinki, revised in 2013.

Informed Consent Statement: Informed consent was obtained from all subjects involved in the study.

Data Availability Statement: The data presented in this study are available on request from the corresponding author. The data are not publicly available.

Acknowledgments: We are grateful to the nurses and staff of Sun Yat-sen Memorial Hospital, as well as the patients involved in this study. Additionally, we are very grateful to the reviewers of our manuscript. We appreciate the providers of the grants; they were not involved in the writing of this manuscript.

Conflicts of Interest: The authors declare no conflict of interest.

References

1. Homma, Y.; Akiyama, Y.; Tomoe, H.; Furuta, A.; Ueda, T.; Maeda, D.; Lin, A.T.; Kuo, H.-C.; Lee, M.-H.; Oh, S.-J.; et al. Clinical guidelines for interstitial cystitis/bladder pain syndrome. *Int. J. Urol.* **2020**, *27*, 578–589. [CrossRef]
2. Patnaik, S.S.; Laganà, A.S.; Vitale, S.G.; Butticè, S.; Noventa, M.; Gizzo, S.; Valenti, G.; Rapisarda, A.M.C.; La Rosa, V.L.; Magno, C.; et al. Etiology, pathophysiology and biomarkers of interstitial cystitis/painful bladder syndrome. *Arch. Gynecol. Obstet.* **2017**, *295*, 1341–1359. [CrossRef]
3. Parsons, C.L.; Lilly, J.D.; Stein, P. Epithelial Dysfunction in Nonbacterial Cystitis (Interstitial Cystitis). *J. Urol.* **1991**, *145*, 732–735. [CrossRef]
4. Liu, H.T.; Tyagi, P.; Chancellor, M.B.; Kuo, H.C. Urinary nerve growth factor level is increased in patients with interstitial cystitis/bladder pain syndrome and decreased in responders to treatment. *BJU Int.* **2009**, *104*, 1476–1481. [CrossRef]
5. van de Merwe, J.P.; Nordling, J.; Bouchelouche, P.; Bouchelouche, K.; Cervigni, M.; Daha, L.K.; Elneil, S.; Fall, M.; Hohlbrugger, G.; Irwin, P.; et al. Diagnostic criteria, classification, and nomenclature for painful bladder syndrome/interstitial cystitis: An ESSIC proposal. *Eur. Urol.* **2008**, *53*, 60–67. [CrossRef]
6. Jhang, J.F. Using Botulinum Toxin A for Treatment of Interstitial Cystitis/Bladder Pain Syndrome-Possible Pathomechanisms and Practical Issues. *Toxins* **2019**, *11*, 641. [CrossRef]
7. Pinto, R.; Lopes, T.; Frias, B.; Silva, A.; Silva, J.A.; Silva, C.M.; Cruz, C.; Cruz, F.; Dinis, P. Trigonal injection of botulinum toxin A in patients with refractory bladder pain syndrome/interstitial cystitis. *Eur. Urol.* **2010**, *58*, 360–365. [CrossRef]
8. Schrepf, A.; O'Donnell, M.; Luo, Y.; Bradley, C.S.; Kreder, K.; Lutgendorf, S. Inflammation and inflammatory control in interstitial cystitis/bladder pain syndrome: Associations with painful symptoms. *Pain* **2014**, *155*, 1755–1761. [CrossRef]
9. Song, Y.; Cao, J.; Jin, Z.; Hu, W.; Wu, R.; Tian, L.; Yang, B.; Wang, J.; Xiao, Y.; Huang, C. Inhibition of microRNA-132 attenuates inflammatory response and detrusor fibrosis in rats with interstitial cystitis via the JAK-STAT signaling pathway. *J. Cell. Biochem.* **2019**, *120*, 9147–9158. [CrossRef]
10. Wu, K.; Wei, P.; Liu, M.; Liang, X.; Su, M. To reveal pharmacological targets and molecular mechanisms of curcumol against interstitial cystitis. *J. Adv. Res.* **2019**, *20*, 43–50. [CrossRef]
11. Bosch, P.C. A Randomized, Double-blind, Placebo-controlled Trial of Certolizumab Pegol in Women with Refractory Interstitial Cystitis/Bladder Pain Syndrome. *Eur. Urol.* **2018**, *74*, 623–630. [CrossRef]
12. Mishra, N.N.; Riedl, C.; Shah, S.; Pathak, N. Intravesical tacrolimus in treatment of intractable interstitial cystitis/bladder pain syndrome—A pilot study. *Int. J. Urol.* **2019**, *26*, 68–72. [CrossRef]
13. Okamoto, H.; Shoin, S.; Koshimura, S.; Shimizu, R. Studies on the anticancer and streptolysin S-forming abilities of hemolytic streptococci. *Jpn. J. Microbiol.* **1967**, *11*, 323–326. [CrossRef]
14. Kikkawa, F.; Hawai, M.; Oguchi, H.; Kojima, M.; Ishikawa, H.; Iwata, M.; Maeda, O.; Tomoda, Y.; Arii, Y.; Kuzuya, K.; et al. Randomised study of immunotherapy with OK-432 in uterine cervical carcinoma. *Eur. J. Cancer* **1993**, *29*, 1542–1546. [CrossRef]
15. Maehara, Y.; Okuyama, T.; Kakeji, Y.; Baba, H.; Furusawa, M.; Sugimachi, K. Postoperative immunochemotherapy including streptococcal lysate OK-432 is effective for patients with gastric cancer and serosal invasion. *Am. J. Surg.* **1994**, *168*, 36–40. [CrossRef]
16. Liu, Z.-H.; Zheng, F.-F.; Mao, Y.-L.; Ye, L.-F.; Bian, J.; Lai, D.-H.; Ye, Y.-L.; Dai, Y.-P. Effects of programmed death-ligand 1 expression on OK-432 immunotherapy following transurethral resection in non-muscle invasive bladder cancer. *Oncol. Lett.* **2017**, *13*, 4818–4824. [CrossRef]
17. Fujita, K. The role of adjunctive immunotherapy in superficial bladder cancer. *Cancer* **1987**, *59*, 2027–2030. [CrossRef]
18. Fujioka, T.; Aoki, H.; Yoshida, M.; Ohhori, T.; Kubo, T. Antigenic relationship between streptococcal preparation OK-432 and tumors and its effect on immunotherapy with OK-432 in patients with superficial bladder tumor. *Urol. Int.* **1989**, *44*, 198–204. [CrossRef]
19. Huijing, H.; Deguang, K.; Yu, L.; Qiuxia, C.; Kun, W.; Dan, Z.; Wang, J.; Zhai, M.; Yan, J.; Zhang, C.; et al. Sapylin promotes wound healing in mouse skin flaps. *Am. J. Transl. Res.* **2017**, *9*, 3017–3026.
20. Dupont, M.C.; Spitsbergen, J.M.; Kim, K.B.; Tuttle, J.B.; Steers, W.D. Histological and neurotrophic changes triggered by varying models of bladder inflammation. *J. Urol.* **2001**, *166*, 1111–1118. [CrossRef]
21. Hanno, P.M.; Erickson, D.; Moldwin, R.; Faraday, M.M.; American Urological, A. Diagnosis and treatment of interstitial cystitis/bladder pain syndrome: AUA guideline amendment. *J. Urol.* **2015**, *193*, 1545–1553. [CrossRef]
22. Smith, C.P.; Radziszewski, P.; Borkowski, A.; Somogyi, G.T.; Boone, T.B.; Chancellor, M.B. Botulinum toxin a has antinociceptive effects in treating interstitial cystitis. *Urology* **2004**, *64*, 871–875, discussion 5. [CrossRef]
23. Giannantoni, A.; Costantini, E.; Di Stasi, S.M.; Tascini, M.C.; Bini, V.; Porena, M. Botulinum A toxin intravesical injections in the treatment of painful bladder syndrome: A pilot study. *Eur. Urol.* **2006**, *49*, 704–709. [CrossRef]

24. Giannantoni, A.; Mearini, E.; Del Zingaro, M.; Proietti, S.; Porena, M. Two -Year Efficacy and Safety of Botulinum a Toxin Intravesical Injections in Patients Affected by Refractory Painful Bladder Syndrome. *Curr. Drug Deliv.* **2010**, *7*, 1–4. [CrossRef]
25. Giannantoni, A.; Porena, M.; Costantini, E.; Zucchi, A.; Mearini, L.; Mearini, E. Botulinum A toxin intravesical injection in patients with painful bladder syndrome: 1-year followup. *J. Urol.* **2008**, *179*, 1031–1034. [CrossRef]
26. Akiyama, Y.; Nomiya, A.; Niimi, A.; Yamada, Y.; Fujimura, T.; Nakagawa, T.; Fukuhara, H.; Kume, H.; Igawa, Y.; Homma, Y. Botulinum toxin type A injection for refractory interstitial cystitis: A randomized comparative study and predictors of treatment response. *Int. J. Urol.* **2015**, *22*, 835–841. [CrossRef]
27. Ogawa, T.; Ishizuka, O.; Ueda, T.; Tyagi, P.; Chancellor, M.B.; Yoshimura, N. Current and emerging drugs for interstitial cystitis/bladder pain syndrome (IC/BPS). *Expert Opin. Emerg. Drugs* **2015**, *20*, 555–570. [CrossRef]
28. Kong, D.; Zhang, D.; Cui, Q.; Wang, K.; Tang, J.; Liu, Z.; Wu, G. Sapylin (OK-432) alters inflammation and angiogenesis in vivo and vitro. *Biomed. Pharm.* **2019**, *113*, 108706. [CrossRef]
29. Gillenwater, J.Y.; Wein, A.J. Summary of the national institute of arthritis, diabetes, digestive and kidney diseases workshop on interstitial cystitis, National Institutes of Health, Bethesda, Maryland, 28–29 August 1987. *J. Urol.* **1988**, *140*, 203–206. [CrossRef]
30. Zhang, W.; Yao, Y.S.; Lin, M.E.; Xie, W.J.; Pan, W.W. Unexplained association between cystitis glandularis and interstitial cystitis in females: A retrospective study. *Int. Urogynecol. J.* **2015**, *26*, 1835–1841. [CrossRef]

MDPI
St. Alban-Anlage 66
4052 Basel
Switzerland
Tel. +41 61 683 77 34
Fax +41 61 302 89 18
www.mdpi.com

Toxins Editorial Office
E-mail: toxins@mdpi.com
www.mdpi.com/journal/toxins

www.ingramcontent.com/pod-product-compliance
Lightning Source LLC
LaVergne TN
LVHW070636100526
838202LV00012B/822
* 9 7 8 3 0 3 6 5 7 9 3 8 2 *